THE CASE MANAGER'S SURVIVAL GUIDE:

WINNING STRATEGIES FOR CLINICAL PRACTICE

 W9-BIB-206

DATE DUE

MAY - 6 1998			
MAY 2 8 1998			
GAYLORD			PRINTED IN U.S.A.

THE CASE MANAGER'S SURVIVAL GUIDE:

WINNING STRATEGIES FOR CLINICAL PRACTICE

TONI G. CESTA, PhD, RN
Director of Case Management
Saint Vincents Hospital and Medical Center
New York, New York

HUSSEIN A. TAHAN, MS, RN, CNA
Clinical Nurse Manager
Cardiac Care Center
Mount Sinai Medical Center
New York, New York

LOIS F. FINK, MA, RN, C
Director of Nursing
Mercy Medical Center
Rockville Center, New York

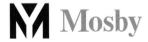

St. Louis   Baltimore   Boston   Carlsbad   Chicago   Minneapolis   New York   Philadelphia   Portland
London   Milan   Sydney   Tokyo   Toronto

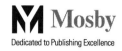
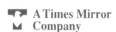

Vice President and Publisher: Nancy L. Coon
Editor-in-Chief: Darlene Como
Editor: Yvonne Alexopoulos
Developmental Editor: Dana Knighten
Associate Developmental Editor: Kimberly A. Netterville
Project Manager: John Rogers
Senior Production Editor: Lavon Wirch Peters
Designer: Yael Kats
Manufacturing Supervisor: Don Carlisle

Printed in the United States of America
Composition by Clarinda Company
Lithography/color film by Clarinda Company
Printing/binding by R.R. Donnelley & Sons

Mosby–Year Book, Inc.
11830 Westline Industrial Drive
St. Louis, Missouri 63146

ISBN 0-8151-1771-X

97 98 99 00 01 / 9 8 7 6 5 4 3 2 1

CONTRIBUTORS

TONIA DANDRY AIKEN, RN, BSN, JD
President
RN Development, Inc.
New Orleans, Louisiana

JULIA W. AUCOIN, DNS, RN, C
Faculty
North Carolina Central University
Durham, North Carolina

MARGUERITE WARD, MS, BSN, RN
Director of Nursing
Long Island College Hospital
Brooklyn, New York

The world is changing rapidly. Even the science and art of nursing are in the process of being transformed. One can see how rapid changes at times appear to overwhelm nurses as they care for people. Fortunately, out of the seeming chaos in society, nursing, and the health care system, the nurses of the future will emerge. And they will bring a new image of nursing that they can use to advance its science and practice. All of the changes we are experiencing can be seen as a hallmark in the renaissance of nursing. Ultimately, nurses will be recognized as the saviors of the health care system.

The rebirth of nursing will involve changes in education, in which nurses will obtain a broader knowledge that encompasses the arts and humanities. This knowledge is essential to the understanding of the human predicament. It will give depth to insights into the wholeness of people. Nurses who use this knowledge will be able to help people to be more aware of the many dimensions of their life, not just the health and curative ones. Nurses should be able to help people become more aware of the choices that enable them to participate in all aspects of their life process and actualize their potential.

The nurses of the future will realize that they can no longer confine themselves to aspects of medicine such as disease and illness. This realization will lead them to question some of the emerging roles of advanced practice nurses and to call for a close scrutiny of these roles. They will serve as guardians of the profession to ensure that its science and art are not eroded by obsolete views of nursing.

The nurses of the future will use their knowledge to create new theories and to design new strategies that enrich the art of nursing and its practice. There is no doubt that these nurses will be able to make clear distinctions between nursing and medicine and the differences in practice roles of each. These distinctions are already seen in the practice of some nurses, especially those who give primary care with a focus on the promotion of health rather than solely the prevention of disease. Physicians and nurses will work together in a harmonious way so that more needs of people will be met.

The nurses of the future will be recognized for the quality *nursing* care they give. The wisdom of nursing will be evident in their willingness to let go of "nursing" practices that have traditionally been delegated to them, mainly by physicians. They will have less anxiety about relinquishing more of the technical aspects of care already being assumed by new health care personnel, provided these staff members are properly educated and are not just an economic stopgap in the current budget crisis of the health care system. As these practices are performed expertly by other personnel, nurses will be able to regain the essence of nursing, which is giving *care* to people.

The nurses of the future will not fear the accelerating changes occurring in society, nursing, and the health care system but will recognize them as a phoenix, so that they can spread their wings and rise to become the protectors of the health care system and the angels of care. Nurses can soar to new heights as advocates of nursing, so its science and art can be used to care for all humanity.

John R. Phillips, RN, PhD
Associate Professor, New York University

Originally printed in *Visions,* Department of Nursing Newsletter, Long Island Jewish Medical Center, New Hyde Park, New York, October 1996. Reprinted with permission.

Today, nurses face challenges as never before. Managed care, such as HMOs and PPOs, continues to drive health care practices toward a more cost-effective care delivery system with emphasis on demonstrated quality. To meet these demands, health care providers have established networks and alliances with physicians and hospitals to create a continuum of care. In turn, these entities have implemented strategies such as patient-centered care to contain costs and case management to manage care across the continuum. These strategies raise critical issues in nursing practice, as well as personal views related to quality and caring.

As a practicing Community Nurse Case Manager and a Professional Development Specialist at Carondelet Health Network (CHN) in Tucson, Arizona, we have explored the opportunities available to enhance the network's systems. The excitement of this challenge has created a variety of diverse and eclectic programs and services that offer a multidisciplinary team approach with nursing as the hub.

One example of this community is the multiple sclerosis exercise program provided through CHN's Community Nurse Case Management Program, Community Volunteer Program, and the local National Multiple Sclerosis Society (NMSS). This program originated out of needs identified through a 1-year NMSS demonstration grant Carondelet received to provide case management for people with progressive MS. Although the study was completed over 5 years ago, the exercise program still receives private funding and has grown to a year-round, community-wide program accessible to anyone with MS. Several Carondelet nurse case managers lead an interdisciplinary team of community nurses, physical therapists, lifeguards, and volunteers in exercise and case management. The case managers also serve as consultants to a community-wide team of health professionals, provider networks, and community resources. Outcomes from the exercise programs have documented an improvement in functional status and community resource utilization. The successful approach is now being replicated for arthritis clients with a focus on preutilization and postutilization.

Case management has moved to the forefront as an innovative and dynamic method for providing a wide array of integrated services across the continuum. *The Case Manager's Survival Guide: Winning Strategies for Clinical Practice* is an essential tool every case manager will want to have to survive and succeed in these rapidly changing times. We all must learn to translate our successes into a language that businesses and health care providers mutually define and understand. This text offers an in-depth analysis on various nurse case management models and approaches. It also discusses practical skills such as communication, team building, and collaboration—all key components that lay the groundwork for continuous quality improvement. Finally, this text gives you a library of user-friendly guidelines, checklists, and report samples.

We encourage you to capitalize on your strengths. Reach out to demonstrate the essence of nursing—the art of caring. Nurse case management provides us with a multitude of experiences and opportunities. Take advantage of them.

Donna Zazworsky, RN, MS, CCM
Professional Nurse Case Manager
Carondelet Health Network

Carol Falk, RN, MS
Professional Development Specialist
Carondelet Health Network

In these changing and uncertain times, new and exciting opportunities abound for nurses in all settings across the continuum. The health care arena is changing its focus from one of disease and illness management to one of wellness and health promotion. This focus is not new to nurses. Registered nurses have always maintained a focus on education and helping people obtain their optimal level of wellness. The clinical case manager, advocating on behalf of the patient and family, can assist them to achieve their optimal levels of wellness within a cost-effective and reimbursable plan of care.

Nurse case managers are now found at all points along the continuum. Their roles ensure that patients receive the best quality of care at the lowest cost. This goal is important to the patient and the health care provider. Nursing is uniquely qualified to assess a person's needs, provide a plan of care, broker the resources and services required, and evaluate outcomes. This should not be a time of dismay for us, but a time of hope and opportunity unlike any we have seen in the history of our profession.

We, the authors, recognized the need to provide the hands-on clinical case manager with the tools necessary to answer the case management questions on the unit, in the clinic, in the home environment, or wherever the case manager is providing care to patients. We chose a format that is user friendly and a ready reference. Hiring case managers today includes the need to educate and mentor them in their role. Nationally, there are only a handful of colleges and universities providing formal education in case management. Most of today's case managers have learned their role through continuing education programs, home-grown orientation programs in their organizations, reading the literature, and trial and error. This text will help to add a substantial amount of usable information that will enhance the educational process.

Collectively, we have over 30 years of case management experience. Much of our knowledge has come through our own trial and error, research, and networking. We hope that this text will improve the skills and productivity of those who are currently functioning as case managers and ease the transition of the next generation of case managers who are just beginning to find their way in this exciting and worthwhile role.

We would like to thank our many colleagues who have helped mentor and guide us over the years, as well as our families and friends who have supported us.

Toni G. Cesta
Hussein A. Tahan
Lois F. Fink

CONTENTS

APPENDIXES, 167

GLOSSARY, 247

INDEX, 251

THE CASE MANAGER'S SURVIVAL GUIDE:

WINNING STRATEGIES FOR CLINICAL PRACTICE

CHAPTER 1

INTRODUCTION TO CASE MANAGEMENT

If you have purchased or borrowed this book, you must be a case manager, or you are thinking of becoming one. If you are *already working* in the field, you are probably beginning to experience many of the conflicts and confusions that come with this new role. If you are *thinking of becoming* a case manager, you are probably reading as much as you can about this delivery system and the role you will play in it.

Because case management is relatively new to many nurses, it may be difficult to find other nurses working with you or colleagues who have been case managers. Although there are thousands of case managers across the country, there may not be many in your organization or your part of the country. This book is written with you in mind. Although its overall objective is to provide comprehensive information on the role of the case manager and on case management, its format is designed so that it is a ready reference for on-the-job questions and issues you may face every day.

The case management process is often an intangible one—a behind-the-scenes process and outcomes role that is, at its worst, very stressful and, at its best, very rewarding. The role is complex and eclectic. It is not for the meek or mild. It requires confidence and comprehension of a vast array of topics, many of which will be reviewed in this book.

Although case management has become somewhat of a household word in health care, there is still a tremendous amount of confusion about what it is, how it applies to various settings, how its success can be measured, and what the role of the case manager is (Box 1-1). As a profession, we have yet to answer all these questions consistently. There are core components of the model and of the case manager role that can be taken and applied in a variety of ways. The objective is to find what works best for you and your organization without losing the essence of case management.

USING THIS GUIDE

The purpose of this book is to provide the hands-on information you will need to be an effective and success-

ful case manager. There is also a lot of information that can be used in the study of case management and in the implementation of case management models. To be a successful case manager you need to understand the role itself, but you also need to understand how case management fits into the bigger pictures of health care delivery and health care reform. Pick up this book whenever you have a general or specific question. Use it as a ready reference as you develop your expertise in case management.

Broad topics are addressed, and their specific implementation techniques and strategies follow. It is important to understand both the concepts and their application. We suggest you review both.

HEALTH CARE INDUSTRY IN CRISIS

The health care industry is in crisis—a chronic crisis of epic proportion, unprecedented in its history, and brought about by many factors (Box 1-2). The prospective payment system and managed care infiltration have both necessitated a reassessment of the industry's work, how it is organized, and how it is evaluated. The changing demographics of the patient population have also forced us to reexamine our values and our expectations or expected outcomes of the work we perform (e.g., patient care). These changes have come about as a result of an aging patient population, the HIV/AIDS epidemic, and a more educated patient as consumer of health care. Technology has driven up the cost of health care. Complex, high-tech surgery; expensive, life-prolonging treatments such as kidney dialysis; costly antibiotics; computerization; and the need for more and more durable medical equipment to support the care and recuperation of the elderly and the chronically ill have all contributed to escalating costs as we have never seen before.

The frenzy of activity going on in every health care setting across the country is an indicator of the need to bring massive and significant change to the industry. Many of the changes involve cost-cutting efforts that many criticize as compromising quality of care. **Man-**

---

box 1-1

Commonly Asked Questions About Case Management

1. What is it?
2. How does it apply to various health care settings?
3. How can its success be measured?
4. What is the role of the case manager?

---

box 1-2

Factors Affecting the Health Care Industry

1. Changes in health care reimbursement
2. An aging patient population
3. HIV/AIDS epidemic
4. Technology
5. Educated patients as consumers of health care

---

box 1-3

Evolutionary Process of Case Management Application

1. 1920—Psychiatry and social work; outpatient settings
2. 1930—Public health nursing
3. 1985—Acute care
4. 1990—All health care settings

---

aged care is one change that has been consistently criticized for its cost-cutting approach that has appeared to be less concerned with quality of care (Curtin, 1996). Other changes are intended to control both cost and quality. **Case management** is one such effort. It is designed to manage care, which results in a monitoring and control of resources and cost regarding management of the resources applied and the cost of the care. It is also an outcomes model, and it has as part of its methodology a close monitoring of the products of the care it manages and their effects on the patient and family. Case management is not equivalent to managed care. They are not interchangeable concepts or phrases. Whereas managed care is a system of cost-containment programs, case management is a process of care delivery sometimes used within the managed care system.

HISTORY OF CASE MANAGEMENT

Case management is not a new concept. It has been around for more than 50 years (Box 1-3). As a means of providing care, in the 1920s it originated out of the fields of psychiatry and social work and focused on long-term, chronic illnesses that were managed in the out-patient, community-based settings. Case management processes were also used by visiting nurses in the 1930s. The original public health nursing models used community-based case management approaches in their care of patients (Knollmueller, 1989). As a care delivery system, it is a relatively new concept to the acute care setting, having developed and flourished in the mid-1980s. Between the 1930s and the 1980s the model remained essentially in the community setting.

It wasn't until the introduction of the prospective payment system that the model shifted to the acute care, hospital-based setting.

Definition of Case Management

Whether case management is being applied in the acute care, community, or long-term care setting, its underlying principles and goals are consistent. As a system for providing patient care, case management is designed to ensure that quality care is provided in the most cost-effective manner possible. This is accomplished by improving the processes of care delivery, making them more efficient and effective. Other strategies involved include the management of product and personnel resources. By better administration and control over the ways in which care is provided and the resources used, outcomes can be achieved while ensuring that quality is maintained or improved.

There are a variety of definitions of case management, including the following:

A nursing care delivery system that supports cost-effective, patient outcome oriented care (Cohen and Cesta, 1997)

A clinical system utilized for selected individuals who are chosen based on a particular diagnostic category or targeted within a diagnostic category because they represent a higher risk than the rest of the population within that category. Ideally, case management should be employed across the continuum of care—over a variety of settings and over time—to coordinate the delivery of care (Kathleen Bowers, The Center for Case Management)

Case management is a system of health care delivery designed to facilitate achievement of expected patient outcomes within an appropriate length of stay. The goals of case management are the provision of quality health care along a continuum, decreased fragmentation of care across settings, enhancement of the client's quality of life, efficient utilization of patient care resources, and cost containment (American Nurses Association, 1988)

A multidisciplinary clinical system that uses registered nurse case managers to coordinate the care for select patients across the continuum of a health care episode (Frink and Strassner, 1996)

---

box 1-4

Goals of Case Management and the Case Manager's Role Functions

OVERALL GOALS

1. Manage cost and quality
2. Achieve positive patient outcomes

ROLE FUNCTIONS

1. Care coordination
2. Facilitation
3. Education
4. Advocacy
5. Discharge planning
6. Resource management
7. Outcomes management

A collaborative process which assesses, plans, implements, coordinates, monitors, and evaluates the options and services required to meet an individual's health needs, using communication and available resources to promote quality, cost-effective outcomes (Commission for Case Manager Certification, 1996)

Case Management and the Role of Case Manager

It is difficult to separate the model of case management from the role of the case manager. Case management, as a model, provides the system, but it is the **case manager** who implements the model and makes it come alive. In other words, the model provides the foundation and organizational structure within which the case manager role is implemented. This may be the reason for the added confusion related to what case management really is and how it works. It is difficult to understand the model without understanding the role, and vice versa. Once the various adaptations of the role and the model are mixed and matched, things really get complicated. The best way to understand the role and the model is to think of them in terms of what the goals of case management are (Box 1-4).

Regardless of the setting where case management is implemented, there are goals that can be identified that are consistent across the health care continuum (see Box 1-4). Whether it is a hospital, a nursing home, or a community care setting, the model attempts to address both cost and quality issues and to deliver the care in ways that result in the most positive patient outcomes.

The case manager accomplishes these goals by performing a number of complex role functions. These may include but are not limited to care coordination, facilitation, education, advocacy, discharge planning, resource management, and outcomes management.

---

box 1-5

Forces Driving the Move Toward Case Management

1. 1970s—Escalating health care costs
2. 1980s—Prospective payment system
3. 1990s—Managed care infiltration

These functions remain consistent across care settings along the continuum.

Case Management as an Outcomes Model

Case management is not only a process model but also an outcomes model in that it provides a prospective approach for planning the ways in which care will be provided, the steps in the care process, and the outcomes of care. In other words, for each step in the process, there is also an expected outcome that can be predetermined and managed. All steps in the process are designed to move the patient toward the desired outcome.

CHANGES IN REIMBURSEMENT: THE DRIVING FORCE BEHIND CASE MANAGEMENT

It wasn't until the 1980s that case management truly came into its own. Before 1983, health care costs were not of major concern to the health care provider. Because most health care reimbursement was based on **fee-for-service (FFS),** there were no financial incentives to reduce costs. In fact, because the use of resources was financially rewarded by the system, overuse abounded. This overuse and misuse of health care resources, particularly those in the acute care setting, resulted in spiraling costs for the consumers of care (Box 1-5). Concurrently, the costs of pharmaceuticals, radiology, and supplies continued to escalate with minimal management of those costs. In the 1990s, health care in the United States is a trillion-dollar business.

It is therefore no great surprise that the system eventually broke down. Consumers and **third-party payors** were no longer willing to pay these high costs when the quality of the services they were receiving was barely keeping pace. In fact, it appeared to most consumers of health care that the quality of the services they were receiving was diminishing and that the value of the care was reduced. The costs were rising while the value was subsiding.

The mid-1980s were witness to a flurry of activities all designed to figure out how to improve the quality of health care while reducing the cost. The expected result was an increase in value. On the payor side, we first saw the introduction of the prospective payment system with the **diagnosis-related groups (DRGs)** as the reimbursement scheme. Shortly after that, the western United States saw an increase in the use of managed care and **health maintenance organizations (HMOs).** DRGs and managed care are discussed in Chapter 2. Employers saw the use of HMOs as a way to reduce the cost of providing health care insurance to their employees. Several states, including Minnesota, California, Arizona, and Tennessee, have since adopted broad-based managed care programs. It is anticipated that managed care will be pervasive throughout the United States by the turn of the century.

Unfortunately, many of the efforts from changes in reimbursement and the introduction of managed care were perceived solely as cost-cutting. Although much lip service was given to the notion of quality, effective and consistent outcome measures, as well as measures of quality of care, were lacking. What did exist were financial parameters that guided outcomes evaluation, such as length of stay. Within 3 to 5 years, organizations began to recognize the need to incorporate quality into the agenda. Much of this came out of health care organizations themselves. Two major quality improvement models drove the quality initiatives. The first was total quality management and the use of continuous quality improvement methods. The second was case management. Ultimately, both of these concepts became the framework for redesign efforts and patient-focused care.

Continuous Quality Improvement and Case Management

Continuous quality improvement (CQI) and case management are linked in philosophy and practice. CQI methods are used to drive case management processes and to monitor outcomes (Cesta, 1993). Case management is now recognized as a system for delivering care that coordinates interdisciplinary care services, plans care, identifies expected outcomes, and helps facilitate the patient and family toward those expected outcomes. The case manager is responsible for ensuring that the patient's needs are being met and that care is being provided in the most cost-effective setting.

CQI can address both system and practice issues, looking for opportunities for improvement that will result in reduced cost and improved quality of care. Without addressing and improving these processes, case management as a delivery system will not be effective. When implemented, case management affects every part of the organization, every discipline, and every department. Therefore it is sometimes necessary to correct existing systems or interdisciplinary problems be-

fore the model can be successfully implemented. CQI can then be applied to measure and continuously monitor the progress of the model.

Nursing Case Management

Nursing case management evolved as a hospital-based care delivery system in 1985. Before that time there had been a number of other nursing care delivery systems, including functional, team, and primary nursing. It has been said that nursing case management incorporates elements of both team and primary nursing. In team nursing, a nurse team leader directs the care being provided by all the members of the nursing team, including registered nurses, licensed practical nurses, and nurse aides. The team leader generally does not provide direct patient care but directs the care being provided by the members of the team.

Move From Team to Primary Nursing

In the 1970s team nursing evolved to primary nursing. In primary nursing, the registered nurse (RN) is responsible for providing all aspects of care to an assigned group of patients. With the assistance of a nurse aide, the RN carries out all direct and indirect nursing functions for the patient. One of the goals of primary nursing is the reduction in fragmentation of nursing care. The primary nurse provides all facets of care to the patient but works independently. It was anticipated that primary nursing would enhance the professionalism of nursing by upgrading the level of autonomy and independent practice.

Breakdown of Primary Nursing

With the advent of the prospective payment system in 1983, primary nursing became increasingly difficult to implement. Although it provided a structure for the RN to function autonomously and independently, it did not address the cost/quality issues affecting the health care delivery system in the 1980s. As lengths of stay began to shorten, care activities had to be accelerated. At the same time the nursing profession began to experience a nursing shortage, and various strategies were put into place to recruit and retain nurses. One of these was flexible (flex) time, including 12-hour shifts. Twelve-hour shifts provided the RN with more flexibility in terms of the work schedule. This might mean more time to spend raising a family, or it might mean time to return to school. In any case, nurses working 3 days a week, combined with accelerated hospital stays, resulted in increasing difficulty in maintaining a primary nursing model. Continuity of patient care was all but destroyed as nurses worked only 3 days a week. With shortened lengths of stay, it was possible that the nurse who began caring for the patient on admission might not be the same nurse caring for the patient upon discharge. It was very expensive to staff nursing units to the extent necessary to maintain as much continuity as possible. In addition to the cost of personnel, primary nursing was not designed to manage care in shorter time frames or place an emphasis on the management of resources. Care was not outcome focused, and the health care providers were fragmented.

Early Hospital-Based Case Management

Two hospitals attempted to respond to the changing times by addressing the changes in health care reimbursement, shortened lengths of stay, and dwindling hospital resources. Carondelet St. Mary's Hospital in Tucson, Arizona, and New England Medical Center in Boston, Massachusetts, were the first to recognize the need to redesign their nursing departments. Each introduced nursing case management models that incorporated elements of both team and primary nursing within a context of controlled resources and shortened length of stay. The early case management models were structured on using hospital-based nurse case managers to monitor the patient's progress toward discharge.

Carondelet's model was initially designed as an acute care case management model. The job title *Professional Nurse Case Manager* described an RN with minimum educational preparation of a bachelor's degree. The case manager assumed responsibility for managing patients toward expected outcomes along a continuum of care. Carondelet collected data for the first 4 years after implementation of the model and found that quality and cost were both improved. Job satisfaction improved for nurses, and their job stress decreased. In addition, patient satisfaction increased (Ethridge, 1991).

Perhaps the most compelling finding was that some patients with chronic illnesses were not hospitalized at all (Ethridge and Lamb, 1989). Those who were admitted had lower acuity levels. They were immediately linked to the health care system so that the length of stay at the beginning of the hospitalization was decreased. This resulted in lower costs for the hospital (Ethridge, 1991).

These findings resulted in the development of the first nursing HMO. The initial program, begun in 1989, focused on case managing patients from a senior-care HMO. The nurse case manager screened all patients admitted under the Senior Plan contract. The assessment included determining the necessary nursing services before discharge, monitoring of any community services being provided, and a continuation of care in the community if necessary. Because the fees were **capitated,**

the case manager could match the patient's needs with the appropriate services.

New England Medical Center Hospitals (NEMCH) in Boston, Massachusetts, used RNs in positions of senior staff nurses to pilot the case manager role. The case managers carried a core group of patients for whom they provided direct patient care. They worked closely with physicians, social workers, utilization managers, and discharge planners. The core of the delivery system was that **outcomes** should drive the care process. Several versions of critical pathways were developed for planning, managing, documenting, and evaluating patient care. During those early years the "tools of the trade" moved more and more toward care management tools that structured the care process and outcomes and were more interdisciplinary (Zander, 1996).

Both models were deemed successes by their organizations. Across the country other hospitals began turning to these two role models for ideas, direction, and support. This was a watershed moment in health care delivery. Unprecedented numbers of health care organizations began to think about or implement case management. Its position in the health care arena was secured.

Although case management initially addressed the changes necessary for organizations to survive prospective payment, it was even more effective in its management of cases under a managed care system. In both reimbursement systems, patient care must be managed and controlled, with a tight rein on the use of resources, the length of stay, and continuing care needs.

The majority of the models of the 1980s did little in terms of changing the role functions of the other members of the health care team. Whereas nursing provided the driving force for the movement toward hospital-based case management, the other disciplines were slower in recognizing the value of such a system. Additionally, serious downsizing was only just beginning in the industry. Corporate America had already begun its massive layoffs and downsizing initiatives. Thousands of people lost their jobs. Health care had not yet begun to feel the economic pinch as it was being felt in other businesses. Therefore the incentives for merging and downsizing departments was not yet there.

Shortly after these early models, case management began to mature as more and more hospitals began to implement case management models. One could see a direct correlation between the degree of managed care infiltration and the use of case management. In nursing case management, the nurse essentially functions as the leader of the team, similar to the team nursing approach. The difference was that the team did not consist of nurses only. Now the team was an interdisciplinary one, and each health care provider had a say in terms of how a patient's care would be delivered and monitored.

History of Critical Paths

It has been more than a decade since the introduction of case management plans as a method of controlling cost and quality in health care. First known as critical pathways, these tools have grown in scope and sophistication over the years (Box 1-6). Critical pathways were originally designed and implemented by nursing departments as a paper-and-pencil system for outlining the course of events for treating a particular DRG for each day of hospitalization (Cohen and Cesta, 1997; Nelson, 1994; Zander, 1991).

In a broader fashion, critical pathways outlined the key or critical steps in the treatment of the DRG in a one-page summary. Because DRGs are broad groupings or classifications of similar types of patients, the critical pathway also had to be broad and nonspecific in nature (Edelstein and Cesta, 1993). The original critical pathways were mainly focused on nursing interventions and tasks. The daily interventions such as blood work or other diagnostics were outlined generically and were applicable to a host of different patient types. Because of the generic nature of the plans, they did little to control the use of resources, types of medications, route of administration, or other factors related to cost and quality. Although they did suggest the appropriate number of hospital days to allocate to the DRG, they did little beyond that to control the kinds of product resources applied to the particular broad grouping of patients.

Case Management Plans Today

Critical pathways were a good first attempt at providing a framework for controlling cost and quality within the prospective payment system. Subsequent adaptations of the critical pathway concept began to use more specific and direct clinical content in a multidisciplinary format. These more sophisticated case management plans

---

box 1-6
Elements of an Effective Case Management Plan

1. Interdisciplinary in nature
2. Outcomes based
3. Clinically specific
4. Care provider documentation included
5. Flexible enough to meet individual patient's care needs

---

are called multidisciplinary action plans (MAPs), clinical guidelines, practice guidelines, practice parameters, care maps, and so on. Today's case management plans are clinically specific, incorporate other disciplines, are outcome oriented, and may include care provider documentation. In addition to being more clinically specific, these plans are focused around specific clinical case types rather than DRGs. Thus the content applies to the clinical issue being planned out. This may be a medical problem, surgical procedure, or workup plan (Cohen and Cesta, 1997; Hampton, 1993; Tahan and Cesta, 1994). Chapter 7 contains more detailed information on the various adaptations of the current "tools of the trade" in case management. Appendixes A through G at the end of this book present examples of several different types of case management plans.

Benchmarking

Evolutionary changes involved much more specificity in terms of the content of the case management plan. Benchmarking is used as a strategy for understanding internal processes and performance levels; it provides a basis for understanding where the performance gaps are. It brings best ideas that identify opportunities and helps the organization to rally around a consensus of opinion. In addition, it results in the implementation of better-quality products and services (Czarnecki, 1994).

The clinical content for the case management plans should be based on benchmarks such as those established by the following:
- Professional societies
- Professional journals
- Health systems and hospital corporations
- Texts and manuals

One or more of these benchmarks can be used to develop any one plan. In this way much of the subjectivity is taken out of the plan of care, and instead the care is based on sound judgment, expert opinion, and research. With this step in the evolutionary process, the plans became much more clinically directive and began to provide a framework for controlling resource application for specific case types.

Multidisciplinary Care Planning

The next step in the evolutionary process was the introduction of plans that had a more multidisciplinary focus and that incorporated the plan of care for all disciplines represented (Adler et al, 1995; Goode and Blegan, 1993). The final step was the addition of expected outcomes of care that applied to the specific interventions on the plan. In other words, for each intervention there was an expected outcome for the patient to achieve before the patient could move on to the next phase of care (Sperry and Birdsall, 1994). Box 1-7 presents an example of expected outcomes.

CHOOSING A CASE MANAGEMENT TOOL

A variety of case management tools are available today. The tool chosen by any organization should be based on that organization's needs and goals. Some issues to be addressed during the design and implementation process are summarized in Case Manager's Tip 1-1 and described in more detail in the following paragraphs.

1. Format: critical path vs. MAP. A critical path is generally formatted as a one-page summary of the tasks to be accomplished for a specific DRG. It does not include outcomes and is usually not used as a documentation tool. In addition, it is customarily not a part of the patient's medical record. MAPs, however, are more comprehensive in nature, are usually a part of the patient's perma-

nent record, include outcomes, and are interdisciplinary.

2. Utility as a documentation system for nurses and other health care providers. The MAP is intended to be used as a documentation tool. This is most often accomplished by using the MAP in conjunction with a documentation-by-exception system, whereby the expected patient outcomes are prospectively identified and then charted against within the time frames established. To date, the majority of such documentation systems incorporate only nursing documentation. Some organizations have been successful in including other disciplines such as physical and occupational therapy. The format can be adjusted to include other disciplines such as physicians by including more narrative note space within the document.

3. Inclusion as a permanent part of the medical record. If the MAP is to be used as a documentation tool, then it clearly must be included as part of the permanent medical record. Some organizations, out of fear of legal liability, opt not to include the MAP as a part of the record. It is believed that this reduces their **liability**. In reality, if the plan is the standard of care for the organization, then the organization is responsible for producing the standard should a legal issue arise (Hirshfeld, 1993). If the MAP is used to guide the clinical care of a particular patient the hospital is being sued for, the court may demand that the MAP be made available. If the physician did indeed follow the MAP, then it will afford legal protection to the physician and the organization.

In any case, some organizations choose to test the MAP outside the medical record first before sanctioning it. In situations like this where the MAP has not been approved by the hospital, then patient consent may be necessary. Otherwise the use of two different standards of care cannot be justified.

Including the MAP as part of the medical record lends it more weight and credibility than not including it. Including it clearly gives the message that the organization stands behind it as the standard of care and believes that the MAP represents "state-of-the-art" care.

---

box 1-7

Expected Outcomes as They Might Appear on a Multidisciplinary Action Plan for Community-Acquired Pneumonia

INTERMEDIATE OUTCOMES (also known as milestones or trigger points)

Convert from intravenous to oral antibiotics when the patient:
1. Has two consecutive oral temperatures of less than 100.4° F obtained at least 8 hours apart in the absence of antipyretics
2. Shows a decrease in leukocytosis to less than 12,000
3. Exhibits improved pulmonary signs/symptoms
4. Is able to tolerate oral medications

DISCHARGE OUTCOMES

In less severe pneumonia, discharging the patient from the hospital may occur simultaneously or up to 24 hours of switch to oral antibiotics providing there is no deterioration or other reason for continued hospitalization.

---

case manager's tip 1-1 — Choosing a Case Management Tool

When choosing a case management tool, be sure to address the following issues during the design and implementation process:
1. Format: critical path vs. MAP
2. Utility as a documentation system
3. Inclusion as a permanent part of the medical record
4. Interdisciplinary nature
5. Legal issues related to care providers' use of the tool
6. Fulfillment of Joint Commission on Accreditation of Healthcare Organizations (JCAHO) requirements

4. Interdisciplinary nature, incorporating all disciplines in the care process and expected outcomes. Early case management plans did not include all disciplines but had a heavy nursing focus and emphasis. As case management has evolved and matured, case management plans have become more multidisciplinary. Although it may be more difficult to include all care provider documentation, it should be easier to include all disciplines in the actual plan itself. Expected outcomes for each discipline can be prospectively identified and incorporated. The biggest advantage to creating an interdisciplinary plan is that it reduces duplication and fragmentation. By being able to review the plan of each discipline in comparison to the others, opportunities to reduce redundancy become more obvious. This approach also enhances the use of existing personnel by ensuring that all are carrying out the care activities most appropriate to their disciplines. Areas in which this becomes obvious include patient education and **discharge planning,** in which there is greater likelihood that duplication of effort may take place.

Because quality and length of stay are affected by the efforts of each and every member of the health care team, it only makes sense to include all of them in the planning process.

5. Legal issues for physicians, nurses, and other providers. Many health care providers may feel anxiety related to the use of MAPs and other case management plans. This may be due to a lack of understanding related to the legal issues concerning these kinds of tools. Legal issues should be carefully discussed with the organization's risk management department after a thorough review of the literature is completed. Each organization must weigh the legal pros and cons and draw its own conclusions as to whether this is a concept that the physicians can adopt and embrace.

6. Fulfillment of JCAHO requirements for care planning, patient teaching, and discharge planning. The standards for the JCAHO focus on the incorporation of all disciplines into the plan of care for those tasks that are interdisciplinary in nature (JCAHO, 1996). The MAP, by nature of its format and philosophy, is deigned to ensure that all the disciplines are represented.

Physician Support

Physician support is a key component in the success or failure of any case management plan, no matter what format it takes. Although these plans were once feared as legally dangerous, physicians are beginning to realize some of their legal benefits. Conceptually, case management plans can meet physician, hospital, and patient needs in a number of ways.

Aid to shortening length of stay. To maintain financial viability, acute care settings must shorten the number of in-patient hospital days. Whether the reimbursement system is negotiated managed care or the prospective payment system, length of stay can translate to financial success or failure for any hospital in today's health care environment.

Selling tool for managed care/HMOs. An ability to demonstrate systems that control cost and quality is essential to any forward-thinking health care organization in the 1990s and beyond. Case management plans that are prospective and outcome oriented and outline both the appropriate length of stay and the appropriate use of resources for a particular case type provide a structure for controlling cost and quality. These plans can be shared with managed care organizations before admission to demonstrate how the hospital manages a particular case type, or they can be used as a concurrent review tool to justify the length of stay and resource allocation.

Means of legal protection. Practice guidelines and case management plans can protect physicians from a risk liability perspective in that they outline what is appropriate to do, as well as what is appropriate not to do. They provide for a plan of care that is supported by the organization in which they work (West, 1994).

Aid to regulatory agency compliance. Although not currently mandated by the JCAHO or other regulatory bodies, case management plans are recognized as an excellent vehicle for maintaining and improving quality. By outlining the expected clinical outcomes and documenting deviations form those outcomes, the organization can identify opportunities for clinical process improvements (JCAHO, 1996).

Means of providing a competitive edge. Clearly, the organizations that maintain market-share advantage will be the ones that will remain competitive in the managed care environment. If "covered lives" is the name of the game, a competitive edge will lie with those organizations that have captured the greatest market share. This means that they will have negotiated managed care contracts that provide for maximum reimbursement and that have large patient populations.

Source of practice parameters. A variety of respected organizations have developed practice guidelines (see section entitled "Benchmarking" earlier in this chapter). Physicians, nurses, and other providers can refer to their own specialty organizations regarding "state-of-the-art" guidelines (Holzer, 1990).

Benefits of Case Management

Internally, there are many reasons why **case management plans** spell success or failure (Case Manager's Tip 1-2).

1. Simplify care. Case management plans provide a systematic format for all disciplines to use in the treatment

Benefits of Case Management Plans

When soliciting support for case management plans, focus on the ways in which they can help to ensure the health care organization's success. Case management plans help to do the following:
1. Simplify care
2. Improve reimbursement
3. Objectify decision making
4. Contain cost
5. Prioritize resources

of specific case types. All disciplines involved in the care of the specific group of patients represented are included in one interdisciplinary plan of care. In some cases, documentation is also included so that the entire course of events is seen in one documentation tool (Adler et al, 1995) (see Appendixes).

2. Improve reimbursement. Because documentation is enhanced, there is greater opportunity for the medical record to be coded properly. Proper coding means maximization of reimbursement.

3. Objectify decision making. Although a tremendous amount of subjectivity and judgment goes into the art of practicing medicine, there still remains a core of safe and appropriate clinical practice that is based on research and "state-of-the-art" recommendations. Case management plans provide a vehicle for communicating these clinical recommendations in an objective manner.

4. Contain cost. Because case management plans provide a foundation for reducing variability in medical treatment, they serve as a tool for controlling cost. Care needs, both product and personnel, are prospectively determined, so that the organization can predict its resource needs and reduce the need for a variety of different brands and types of the same product. This ultimately has an effect on cost. The plans outline the expected length of stay, thereby controlling the number of hospital days, also resulting in cost savings to the hospital. Daily resource application is also outlined, which will translate to saved dollars for the organization (Edelstein and Cesta, 1993; Jijon and Jijon-Letort, 1995).

5. Prioritize resources. Resource use is closely tied to cost containment. By properly using resources, costs are reduced. Other issues involve the appropriate use of existing resources, both product and personnel. Case management plans can provide a framework for identifying which members of the health care team will provide which services. So much of the misutilization and/or overutilization of health care resources occurs because of lack of communication between departments and disciplines. Through case management, the work to be

done can be allocated to the most appropriate member of the team. Responsibilities are outlined prospectively rather than on a case-by-case basis. This reduces the opportunity for redundancy or for things to fall through the cracks and not be done at all. For example, discharge planning functions can be allocated to the most appropriate care provider, thereby using personnel most appropriately and as early in the process as possible (Tahan and Cesta, 1994).

INTERDISCIPLINARY TEAM

Case management has provided a structure for health care providers to develop teams that are truly interdisciplinary. In the past, various disciplines have either controlled the team, or the team was comprised of only one discipline. For example, "rounds" were generally physician dominated and focused on the medical plan. In team nursing, the team was composed of only nurses. The team leader was a nurse, members of the team were nurses, and so on. Discharge planning rounds were often interdisciplinary but were focused on the patient's discharge plan.

CHANGE PROCESS

Case management as a delivery model crosses all boundaries within the organization. Therefore it is critical that the members involved in the development of the team represent all those affected. The roles most closely affiliated with that of the case manager are utilization management, discharge planning, and home care. During the design process, an interdisciplinary team representing these departments should be brought together to examine current practice and look for opportunities to redefine role functions within the organization.

Logically, the membership should consist of those individuals who have the power and authority to make the necessary changes in the role functions of these departments. During the analysis phase, some disciplines may feel threatened or defensive about their current functions within the organization and may interpret the need to change as a criticism of their current job performance rather than as identifying opportunities to make the organization more productive and efficient. This period, while current processes are analyzed and critiqued, may cause some anxiety. How well this group works through the process will greatly depend on the members' interpersonal relationships, their vision, and their ability to collaborate.

Using the techniques of CQI will help to facilitate this process. CQI helps to place everyone on an equal playing field as processes are analyzed and changed (see Chapter 9). The team should first examine current practice by looking at what the various departments and disciplines are currently doing, where there may be overlap or redundancy, and where things may be falling through the cracks. Only then can opportunities for improvement be initiated. One useful tool for this technique is the flow diagram. The flow diagram provides the team with a visual representation of their current practice, where quality barriers may be, and where opportunities for improvement may lie (Figure 1-1).

The social worker and the case manager may be duplicating some discharge planning functions. There may be confusion between them in terms of who is doing what; specific tasks must then be negotiated as they arise. This results in confusion and delays as each episode requires an analysis, a discussion, and a resolution.

This executive-level team essentially designs the case management model after a thorough analysis has taken place. The role functions of each member of the team are clearly outlined and delineated prospectively before going further with the implementation process.

Once these role functions have been determined, then the members of the interdisciplinary case management team can be assembled to carry out a number of important functions. The team members are those clinicians and others who are directly involved in the care process. The team first prospectively develops the case management plan. The plan, as discussed in Chapter 7, is collaboratively developed by the team to manage the case as efficiently and cost effectively as possible. The team also individualizes the plan to the specific patient, and finally, the team implements the plan. The case manager serves as the thread that binds the interdisciplinary team together. The case manager does not lead the team but essentially guides the team and the patient/family toward the achievement of the expected outcomes as identified in the plan.

The members of the team are fluid and depend on the patient's location, clinical problem, and expected long-term needs. Core members of the team should al-

ways include the physician, nurse, case manager, social worker, discharge planner, and patient/family. Additional members depend on the picture presented. For example, orthopedic problems warrant the physical therapist's membership on the team; pulmonary problems necessitate the respiratory therapist. For the diabetic or other patient with metabolic problems, the nutritionist should be a member of the team. Clearly, members should be those health care providers who have some relevance to the case and who have something to contribute to the interdisciplinary plan of care.

In a time when containing costs has never been more important, a collaborative, interdisciplinary approach is critical to the success of any case management model. Without it, true case management can never take place.

MANAGED CARE

It has not been uncommon for the terms *case management* and *managed care* to sometimes be used interchangeably. There are specific differences between the terms. Although linked philosophically, managed care is a broader term that refers to an organized delivery of services by a select panel of providers (Rehberg, 1995). These services are managed under a prepayment arrangement between a provider of services and a managed care organization. Managed care is a system that provides the generalized structure and focus when managing the use, cost, quality, and effectiveness of health care services. HMOs and **preferred provider organizations (PPOs)** are the two most common types of managed care arrangements, which are essentially health insurance plans that link the patient to provider services. Their purpose is to improve the efficiency of the health care delivery system (Mullahy, 1995).

Because some physicians' only exposure to case managers has been through a managed care organization, they may see the two as synonymous. They may believe that case managers and case management means managed care. In reality, although case managers can be found in managed care organizations, they are also found in a wide variety of other practice settings (see Chapter 3).

Case management is a patient care delivery system. Perhaps the most profound difference between case management and managed care is the fact that managed care is a function of a health care reimbursement system, whereas case management is a structure for providing care within a managed care reimbursement system. Case management also applies to provider areas that are not reimbursed under managed care. *Managed care* is defined as a means of providing health care services within a defined network of providers. These

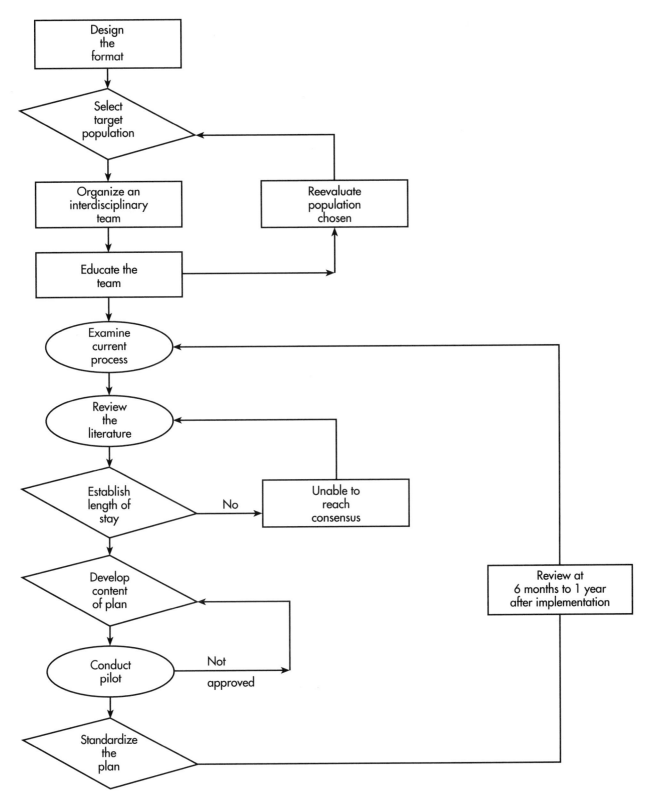

Key:
Box = Activities
Circle = Inputs to/outputs from
Diamond = Decision to be made (Yes/No)
Arrow = Direction of flow of activities

Fig. 1-1   Flow diagram: developing a case management plan.

providers are responsible for managing the care in a quality, cost-effective manner (Baldor, 1996).

The initial driving force for case management in the hospital setting was the prospective payment system because of the dwindling reimbursement associated with the DRGs. As managed care continues to proliferate, it has become an even greater force in the movement toward case management. Under full capitation, the incentive is greatest (see Chapter 2). In between full capitation and FFS we now find a wide variety of combinations of insurers, reimbursement systems, and service settings. It may be 5 years or more before the dust settles nationally, systems are in place and integrated, and the continuum of care has been defined.

KEY POINTS

1. Case management applications in the 1980s evolved out of changes in the health care reimbursement system.
2. Case management can be defined in a number of ways but is essentially a process and outcomes model designed to manage resources and maintain quality of care.
3. Case management tools such as pathways and guidelines can help faciliate the case manager role.
4. It is important for physicians to be part of the design, implementation, and evaluation processes related to case management.
5. Case management uses a team approach and incorporates elements of CQI.

References

Adler SL et al: Collaboration: the solution to multidisciplinary care planning, *J Orthop Nurs* 14(20):21-29, 1995.

American Nurses Association Task Force on Case Management, Kansas City, Mo, 1988, American Nurses Association.

Baldor RA: *Managed care made simple,* Cambridge, Mass, 1996, Blackwell Science.

Cesta TG: The link between continuous quality improvement and case management, *J Nurs Admin* 24(12):49-58, 1993.

Cohen EL, Cesta TG: *Nursing case management: from concept to evaluation,* ed 2, St Louis, 1997, Mosby.

Commission for Case Manager Certification: *CCM certification guide,* Rolling Meadows, Ill., 1996, Commission for Case Manager Certification.

Curtin L: The ethics of managed care—Part 1: proposing a new ethos? *Nurs Manage* 27(8):18-19, 1996.

Czarnecki MT: *Benchmarking strategies for health care management,* Gaithersburg, Md, 1994, Aspen.

Edelstein EL, Cesta TG: Nursing case management: an innovative model of care for hospitalized patients with diabetes, *Diabetes Educ* 19(6):517-521, 1993.

Ethridge P: A nursing HMO: Carondelet St Mary's experience, *Nurs Manage* 22(7):22-27, 1991.

Ethridge P, Lamb GS: Professional nursing case management improves quality, access and costs, *Nurs Manage* 20(3):30-35, 1989.

Frink BB, Strassner L: Variance analysis. In Flarey DL, Blancett SS, eds: *Handbook of nursing case management,* Gaithersburg, Md, 1996, Aspen.

Goode CJ, Blegan MA: Developing a CareMap for patients with a cesarean birth: a multidisciplinary approach, *J Perinat Neonat Nurs* 7(2):40-49, 1993.

Hampton DC: Implementing a managed care framework through care maps, *J Nurs Admin* 23(5):21-27, 1993.

Hirshfeld E: Use of practice parameters as standards of care and in health care reform: a view from the American Medical Association, *J Qual Improve* 19(8):322-329, 1993.

Holzer JF: The advent of clinical standards for professional liability, *Qual Rev Bull* 16(2):71-79, 1990.

Jijon CR, Jijon-Letort FX: Perinatal predictors of duration and cost of hospitalization for premature infants, *Clin Pediatr* 34(2):79-85, 1995.

Joint Commission on Accreditation of Healthcare Organizations: *The 1995 Joint Commission AMH Accreditation Manual for Hospitals,* Oakbridge Terrace, Ill, 1996, JCAHO.

Knollmueller RN: Case management: what's in a name? *Nurs Manage* 20(10):38-42, 1989.

Mullahy CM: *The case manager's handbook,* Gaithersburg, Md, 1995, Aspen.

Nelson MS: Critical pathways in the emergency department, *J Emerg Nurs* 19(2):110-114, 1994.

Rehberg CA: Managed care contracts: a guide for clinical case managers, *Nurs Case Manage* 1(1):11-17, 1996.

Sperry S, Birdsall C: Outcomes of a pneumonia critical path, *Nurs Econ* 12(6):332-345, 1994.

Tahan HA, Cesta TG: Developing case management plans using a quality improvement model, *J Nurs Admin* 24(12):49-58, 1994.

West JCC: The legal implications of medical practice guidelines, *J Health Hosp Law* 27(4):97-103, 1994.

Zander K: CareMaps: the core of cost and quality care, *New Definition* 6(3):3, 1991.

Zander K: The early years: the evolution of nursing case management. In Flarey DL, Blancett SS, eds: *Handbook of nursing case management,* Gaithersburg, Md, 1996, Aspen.

CHAPTER 2

FINANCIAL REIMBURSEMENT SYSTEMS

ORIGINS OF THE PROSPECTIVE PAYMENT SYSTEM: AN OVERVIEW

The prospective payment system and **diagnosis-related groups (DRGs)** were probably the strongest catalysts for the movement of case management from the community to the acute care setting. Under **fee-for-service (FFS)** plans there were no financial incentives for hospitals to reduce cost and length of stay. In the 1960s and 1970s public policy was focused on improving access to services. The **Medicare, Medicaid,** and other entitlement programs were designed to make services available to the poor, the disabled, and the elderly.

By the early 1980s cost containment had become the driving issue. Health care policy had begun to shift from the issues of access and entitlements to cost and fiscal monitoring. The prospective payment system was initiated to control hospital costs by providing a price-per-case reimbursement. The onus of responsibility was shifted to the provider to manage resource utilization as a set reimbursement would be allotted. The tool designed to determine the amount of reimbursement was the DRG. It was believed that the DRG would encourage physicians, nurses, ancillary departments, and administrators to work together to provide the most efficient care and to manage the patient through the system as efficiently as possible. It was also believed that the prospective payment system would help to standardize care and improve the efficiency of the care process. In reality, although the DRG controlled the payment rate the hospital was to receive, it did not control the cost of care. Despite these rather dramatic and strict reimbursement schemes, hospital costs continued to escalate.

USE OF DOCUMENTATION

Under the prospective payment system, it was believed that proper documentation could ensure that the DRG assignment would be timely and accurate and that the hospital would be reimbursed as quickly as possible. Therefore it became clear that much of the financial suc-

cess of the hospital would depend on accurate and appropriate documentation. Some hospitals introduced new positions known as *DRG manager* or *DRG coordinator.* The DRG coordinator/manager was responsible for disseminating information related to the DRGs, particularly data regarding how the hospital was doing in terms of **length of stay,** cost of care, and case mix. The coordinator, based on analytical findings, could make recommendations regarding areas for improvement in length of stay or cost, where the hospital might be able to maximize revenues, or where the hospital might work with the health care providers to help them enhance **coding** through improvements in their documentation.

In 1982 the Tax Equity and Fiscal Responsibility Act (TEFRA) enacted the DRGs (Richards, 1996). They were initially designed to set limits on Medicare reimbursement. The development of the methodology that would determine the reimbursement rates was intricate, complex, and laborious. The first generation of DRGs was based on the ICDA-8 (International Classification of Diseases, Adapted, Eighth Revision) and HICDA-2 (Hospital Adaptation of ICDA, Second Revision) diagnostic coding schemes. The second generation was based on the **ICD-9-CM** codes (International Classification of Diseases, Ninth Revision, Clinical Modification). The "I-8" was a four-digit scheme used to measure the incidence of disease, injury, or illness (Commission on Professional and Hospital Activities, 1975). The "I-9," introduced in 1979, is a five-digit scheme, and it added more specificity in terms of location and precision in the reporting of clinical conditions. For example, the I-8 described all fractures (e.g., fracture of the femur), whereas the I-9 added the actual location of the fracture (top or bottom). Tumors of the large intestine could be identified, as well as whether there was an associated obstruction.

DRGs

The DRGs are a patient classification scheme that provides a means of relating the type of patient a hospital treats (also known as its *case mix*) to the costs incurred by the hospital. The DRGs lump "like" patients together.

Patients are considered alike if they demonstrate similar resource utilization and length of stay. Resource utilization is defined by the product or personnel resources used to care for that type of patient. Product resources refer to things such as use of medications, laboratory tests, radiology, and so on. Personnel costs refer to the use of nursing hours per case or other personnel. Length of stay refers to the number of days that the patient remains in the hospital (also known as *bed days*).

Major Diagnostic Categories

The DRGs are categorized into major diagnostic categories (MDCs). The number of DRGs in each MDC varies from 1 to 20 or more. The MDCs are consistent with anatomical or pathophysiological groupings and/or the ways in which patients would be clinically managed. Examples include diseases of the central nervous system, diseases of bone and cartilage, and diseases and disorders of the kidney and urinary tract. The major diagnostic categories are broken down into either medical or surgical, meaning the presence or absence of a surgical procedure.

Relative Weights and Case Mix Index

Each DRG is assigned a **relative weight.** Weights are based on length of stay and cost. The assigned weight is relative to the number 1, meaning that the number 1 represents a DRG class using an average amount of resources. The assigned weight is intended to reflect the relative resource consumption associated with each DRG. The higher the relative weight, the greater the payment to the hospital. DRGs with relative weights above 1.00 represent those of greater **case mix complexity** and the use of greater amounts of resources. Those with a relative weight that falls below 1.00 represent lower resource use.

The weight assigned to the DRG for the hospital is based on the **case mix index (CMI).** The CMI is the sum of all DRG-relative weights divided by the number of cases. The higher the CMI, the higher the assumed case mix complexity of the hospital. Case mix is affected by the following:
- Severity of illness
- Prognosis
- Treatment difficulty
- Need for intervention
- Resource intensity

Measuring the Elements in Case Mix

Severity of illness and prognosis reflect the complexity of services or the types of services provided. **Severity of illness** is made up of objective, clinical indicators of the patient's illness that reflect the need for hospitaliza-

---

box 2-1
Severity of Illness Criteria

1. Clinical findings: chief complaints and working diagnosis identified on physical exam, direct observation, and patient interview
2. Vital signs: temperature, pulse, respiratory rate, and blood pressure
3. Imaging: diagnostic radiology, ultrasound, and nuclear medicine results
4. ECG
5. Hematology, chemistry, and microbiology results
6. Other (clinical parameters not identified in the above)

---

box 2-2
Intensity of Service Criteria

1. Physician evaluation
2. Monitoring (those clinical elements requiring direct observation and monitoring)
3. Treatments/medications
4. Scheduled procedures

---

tion (Box 2-1). Prognosis indicates the patient's likelihood of recovering and to what extent. Treatment difficulty, need for intervention, and resource intensity comprise the **intensity of service** or the number of services per patient day or hospital stay (Box 2-2). The case mix influences hospital costs. It is not the number of patients that affects the costs incurred by the hospital but rather the types of patients and their use of resources. Table 2-1 presents some examples of the components of a Medicare DRG.

Assigning the DRG

Assignment is made based on the documentation in the medical record. For the proper information to be obtained the record must be comprehensive and complete. The documentation must be timely, legible, and proper.

The DRG assignment is made after discharge. Once that assignment has been made, the hospital receives one lump-sum payment based on the relative weight (Case Manager's Tip 2-1). Some DRGs are given a higher relative weight based on existing complications or comorbidities. **Complications** are defined as conditions occurring during the hospitalization that prolong the length of stay at least 1 day in 75% of the cases. **Comorbidities** are preexisting conditions that increase the length of stay about 1 day in 75% of the cases.

case
manager's
tip   **2-1**   ## Elements of DRGs

1. The DRG is assigned after discharge
2. Payment to the hospital is made once the DRG has been assigned
3. One lump-sum payment is made for:
   • DRGs with complications or comorbidities
   • Cost and day outlier payments

TABLE 2-1
Examples of the Components of a Medicare DRG (HCFA, 1995)

DRG	Description	Relative weight	Mean LOS	Outlier
001	Craniotomy age > 17 except for trauma	3.1565	13.5	32
90	Simple pneumonia and pleurisy age > 17 without CC	0.6924	5.7	15

Outliers

Patients with atypically long or short lengths of stay are referred to as *outliers*. All other patients are considered inliers. The placement of a patient as an outlier depends on the trim points for the DRG. Each DRG has a high length-of-stay trim. Some DRGs also have a short length-of-stay trim. Trim points are based on medical and statistical criteria and represent the lowest and highest average lengths of stay for the DRG (see components of a DRG, above). Patients may also fall into a cost outlier category. These are patients who have fallen within the appropriate length of stay but who have used an exceptional amount of resources. This may be determined by a flat amount (such as $500) or by determining that the charges exceed the rate by at least 50%.

Managing the DRGs

In 1985 the prospective payment system was advanced to allow some states to designate reimbursement rates for Medicaid and all other **third-party payors.** Based on hospitals' experiences with the Medicare DRGs and the advent of the system at the state level, strong incentives appeared for the control of hospital resources. Regardless of the cost incurred for caring for a particular case type, the hospital would still be reimbursed a fixed amount of money based on the coded DRG.

It was recognized rather quickly that the registered nurse (RN) could play a vital role in managing these dwindling health care dollars. The RN's role became in-creasingly important in terms of the following:
   • Coordination of tests, treatments, and procedures
   • Confirmation of physician orders
   • Accurate documentation
   • Timely admissions
   • Timely discharges

In the past, much of the care process had a life of its own, running its course to completion. There were few financial incentives to control the health care process; in fact, there were disincentives. In an FFS environment, longer lengths of stay and greater use of product resources translated into greater revenue and financial success for the hospital. The prospective payment system changed all that. It became important to maximize the patient's hospital stay by coordinating the flow of patient care activities. This meant coordination of the patient's tests, treatments, and procedures so that delays could be avoided. Additional strategies included the confirmation of physician orders and/or questioning of their appropriateness when necessary. Getting the patient into the hospital on time and out of the hospital on time were other strategies for maximization.

Finally, documentation in the medical record, although always important, carried even greater weight under this system. Because reimbursement is contingent on the diagnoses and surgical procedures, charting must be complete and accurate. In some hospitals the utilization manager monitors the medical record documentation to ensure that it is accurate, timely, and reflective of what is currently happening in the case. Under case management this is often a role assigned to the case manager.

DRG Assignment

After discharge, the medical record coders review the patient's record. The DRG assignment requires a thorough accounting of the following:
- Principal diagnosis
- Secondary diagnosis
- Operating room procedures
- Complications
- Comorbidities
- Age
- Discharge status

The **principal diagnosis** (or primary diagnosis) is the condition determined to have been chiefly responsible for the admission to the hospital. The major diagnosis is that which consumed the most hospital resources. The principal diagnosis and the major diagnosis are not necessarily the same. The secondary diagnosis is the next priority in terms of resource consumption. **Principal procedures** are those performed to treat the chief complaint or complication rather than those performed for diagnostic purposes. If more than one procedure is performed, then the one most closely related to the principal diagnosis will become the principal procedure. Any other surgical procedures are considered as secondary. Operating room procedures other than those performed for diagnostic purposes are also considered as principal procedures. Complications and comorbidities, as defined above, are also considered. Age is a determining factor for about one fifth of the DRGs. Age 65 is a demarcation line for some. For a small number of DRGs, the patient's discharge status is considered. Discharge status refers to the final patient destination after discharge, such as nursing home, home, or home with services.

In some cases the DRG is used for **per diem** rate setting. States with these rate-setting programs use the DRGs to adjust per diem rates. In addition, there are some DRG-exempt categories in some states. These may include the following:
- HIV/AIDS
- Acute rehabilitation
- Psychiatry
- Pediatrics (if children's hospital)
- Other specialty hospitals (such as cancer hospitals)

Payments are calculated by multiplying the relative weight by the current reimbursement rate. The relative weight is determined by the final DRG coding. Short stays, or patients discharged below the short trim point, are paid at 150% of the daily rate. Outliers, those above the high trim point, are paid 60% of the daily rate for each day above (Box 2-3).

---

box 2-3

Calculating Payments*

EXAMPLE 1: AVERAGE RELATIVE WEIGHT

Payment = Relative weight × Current inlier rate
Payment = 1.0 × $1000.00
Payment = $1000.00

EXAMPLE 2: LIGHT RELATIVE WEIGHT

Payment = Relative weight × Current inlier rate
Payment = 0.5 × $1000.00
Payment = $500.00

EXAMPLE 3: HEAVY RELATIVE WEIGHT

Payment = Relative weight × Current inlier rate
Payment = 22 × $1000.00
Payment = $22,000.00

EXAMPLE 4: SHORT-STAY PAYMENTS BEFORE THE SHORT TRIM POINT

Short trim point = 2 Days
Average length of stay = 5 Days
Relative weight = 1.0
Current inlier payment = $1000.00
$$\text{Each day's payment} = \frac{1.0 \times 1000.00}{5 \text{ Days}}$$
Each day = $200.00
Patient stays in hospital 1 day
Payment = $200.00 × 150%
Payment = $300.00
Revenue loss = $700.00

EXAMPLE 5: OUTLIER PAYMENTS ABOVE THE HIGH TRIM POINT

Outlier point = Day 20
Average length of stay = 10 Days
Relative weight = 2.0
Current inlier payment = $1000.00
Payment = $2000.00
Each day = $200.00
Patient stays 2 days
Payment = DRG payment + $200.00 × 60%
Payment = $2000.00 + $120.00
Final payment = $2120.00

*Figures are for example only; they do not reflect actual hospital reimbursements. $1000.00 is used arbitrarily as the current inlier rate for the purpose of this illustration.

IMPACT OF THE DRGs ON THE HEALTH CARE INDUSTRY

In addition to the move toward case management after the institution of the DRG system, other changes have occurred in response to this reimbursement system.

Increased Number of Outpatient Procedures

For some low–relative-weight DRGs it is more financially lucrative for the hospital to treat patients on an outpatient basis. Generally the adjusted per diem rate will reimburse less than the DRG reimbursement but more than the short trim outlier payment. This finan-

Understanding Types of Health Insurance and Terminology

It is important for a case manager to understand the basic types of health insurance and the related terminology to better serve the patient and help provide the appropriate health care plan in accordance with a patient's insurance benefits.

cial incentive led many hospitals to open ambulatory or day surgery facilities, outpatient dialysis, and same-day surgery programs.

Reduced Length of Stay Via Preoperative Testing, Home Health Care, and Discharge Planning

The industry quickly realized that the management of the length of stay on the preadmission and postdischarge sides was extremely important. No longer could the focus be on the inpatient days only. Preoperative or preadmission testing departments were created to respond to these changes. The expense to the hospital and the reimbursement were greater if the hospital did as many tests before admission as possible. Conversely, the better the **discharge planning** process, as well as the availability of community-based programs, the sooner the patient could be discharged to a less-costly care setting.

Use of DRGs Today

Today we find a mixture of reimbursement systems and schemes. Although more and more patients are being reimbursed under managed care contracts, which is the subject of the next section, others remain under either state or federal reimbursement systems that use the DRG as a measuring stick for either flat rates of reimbursement for the hospital stay or in negotiating discounted rates.

Third-Party Payors/Managed Care Organizations

Like it or not, the health care system is taking on a brand new shape. Most health care institutions are scurrying to learn how to reduce their costs without reducing their quality.

Managed care has taken on many meanings over the past few years. It has grown to mean different things to different people. Business executives, financial controllers, and payors are viewing managed care as a means of reducing skyrocketing health care costs. Health care institutions may be viewing it as the mechanism for negotiating better discounted rates for the care of their patients but only if they can attract a larger volume of patients to their institution. To the physician base it prob-

ably seems like an external control over their previously unstandardized methods and treatment modalities. It is probably the patient who views managed care as a protective mechanism that helps keep health care costs down while maintaining quality services.

Before a discussion can take place about managed care, it is important to understand and be well versed in health insurance in general (Case Manager's Tip 2-2). Health insurance is the protection one seeks to provide **benefits** for an illness or injury. A person, group, or employer pays a price *(premium)* for protection from the potential expenses that could be incurred during an illness or injury. Lack of insurance coverage can mean going without needed health care, having to settle for lower-quality health care, or having to *pay out of pocket*—your own pocket—for health care. The insurance company gambles that it will take in much more in the way of premiums than it will pay out to the insured due to illnesses. The contract a person negotiates states the nature of the *benefits* or the *coverage* that is available. It also lists the conditions under which the insurer will cover expenses, either in part or less commonly in full. *Deductibles* and *co-payments* are those expenses the insured will be responsible for before and after the insurance carrier pays its portion of any medical bills.

The prominent types of health insurance are *group* and *individual* coverage. Group insurance is usually provided by an employer or professional organization to which one belongs. Employee group coverage is usually offered to spouses and dependents, as well as the employee. These policies vary from place to place and from one insurance company to another. Commercial or for-profit insurance companies dominate the group type of coverage. Individual health insurance is sometimes referred to as *personal* insurance. These policies also vary from provider to provider, and their premiums are often more expensive than group policies. Individuals may purchase individual insurance to supplement their group policy in areas that they identify as gaps in benefits (Enteen, 1992).

Currently the fastest-growing coverage option in the health care industry is the *prepaid health service plan*—commonly known as **health maintenance organizations (HMOs)** and **preferred provider organizations (PPOs).** In addition, government-paid coverage (i.e.,

Medicare, Medicaid, and veteran coverage) has recently undergone much scrutiny regarding its continued financial viability. These policies usually offer coverage for hospital expenses, surgical expenses, physician's expenses, and major medical (major illness or injury expenses). A person can also elect to pay larger premiums to supplement the basic plan for items not covered, such as home care benefits or durable medical equipment (Enteen, 1992).

It is important to discuss each type of insurance plan in more detail before moving on to an explanation of managed care. Each type of insurance plan has its advantages and disadvantages, and each is in such a state of flux right now that it is difficult to keep current and accurate on the various benefits. Definitions of each type of insurance as it is currently offered follow (Table 2-2), but it is important to remember that managed care reform can affect these definitions at any time.

HMOs vs. PPOs

Because HMOs and PPOs are the most commonly confused managed care organizations, it is helpful to detail them more fully. An HMO is an **indemnity** plan that delivers comprehensive, coordinated medical services to an enrolled membership in a defined geographic location on a prepaid basis. There are four models of HMOs: group model, **individual practice association (IPA)**, network plan (health plan), and staff model. A group-model HMO contracts with physicians organized in a partnership, corporation, or association. The plan compensates the medical group for services they have contracted at a negotiated rate, and the group is then responsible for compensating its physicians and for contracting with health care providers for their patients. The HMO and the group thus share in the risk. An HMO can also contract with an IPA to provide health care services for a negotiated fee. The IPA then contracts with physicians who practice in their individual or group practices. The IPA compensates the physicians on a **fee schedule** or an FFS basis. If the HMO contracts with more than one physician group, it is referred to as a *network health plan*. In this arrangement the physicians do not necessarily provide care exclusively to the HMO. The last HMO model is the staff model. In this type the physicians are employed by the HMO to provide health care services to its members. The physicians are paid a salary and are offered various incentive programs. The HMO is a good example of the **gatekeeper** model, in which a primary care provider is responsible for authorizing all specialist referrals. This serves to control costs and resource consumption.

Under a PPO agreement, a limited number of providers are contracted as part of a network. Members are

TABLE 2-2
Advantages and Disadvantages of Insurance Types

Insurance type	Advantages	Disadvantages
HMOs	Emphasis is on preventive care cost control	A referral is required for outside providers; the primary care is more limited
PPOs	Larger listing of providers since they are not exclusive to PPO providers	Cost is higher; not a prepaid plan
Medicare	Large numbers of providers; cost to patient is usually limited to co-payment and/or deductibles	Eligibility is usually dependent on age; costs are subject to customary charges
Medicaid	No out-of-pocket cost to patient	Eligibility requirements very specific: vary from state to state; may require spend down of personal assets or monies

Modified from Brucker MC, MacMullen NJ: Health insurance: a summary of basic types, *Home Health Care Nurs* 4(6):8-10, 1995.

encouraged to use the physicians and services of the PPO; however, they are permitted to go outside the network for their health care. Those members who do elect to use out-of-network services may be reimbursed at a lower rate than those who remain within the network. Therefore there is incentive for subscribers to remain in network, because those providers will be offering their services at a discounted rate as part of the PPO. Those cost savings are passed on to the consumer. There is a further incentive to employers to contract with a PPO as a means of reducing overall health care costs for their employees. PPOs have become more popular than HMOs, because their enrollees are less restricted regarding their choice of providers. Table 2-3 summarizes the two types of health care plans.

There has been an evolution of the health care market as it matures into the managed care environment. Managed care can be defined as a system of health care delivery aimed at managing the cost and quality of access to health care. Managed care is used by HMOs and PPOs to improve the delivery of services and contain costs (Mullahy, 1995). This so-called evolution has been mapped out and studied by the University Hospital Consortium and American Practice Management, Incorporated Management Consultants (1992). It has categorized the health care market and its evolution to managed care into four stages of development, with a pro-

---

TABLE 2-3
Summary of HMO and PPO Characteristics

Types	Flexibility	Premiums	Reimbursement	Rates	Provider risks
HMO	Must remain in network; less choice of providers	Prepaid; capitated	Not reimbursed out of network	Usually capitated; for profit or not for profit	High incentive to control costs; high risk sharing
PPO	Less restrictive; more choice of providers	Fee-for-service; not prepaid	Covers services out of network	Not usually capitated	Low incentive to control costs; less financial risk sharing

---

TABLE 2-4
Stages of Evolution of the Health Care Market

Stage I: Unstructured	Stage II: Loose framework	Stage III: Consolidation	Stage IV: Managed competition
Independent hospitals	HMO/PPO enrollment rise	A few large HMOs/PPOs emerge	Employer coalitions purchase health services
Independent physicians	Excess inpatient capacity	Provider margins erode	Integrated systems manage patient populations
Independent purchases, not price sensitive	Hospitals/physicians under pressure	Hospitals form systems	Continued consolidation of provider systems and health plans
	Provider networks form	Hospital systems align with physicians to form integrated systems	

Modified from University Hospital Consortium and American Practice Management, Incorporated Management Consultants: *Stages of market evolution,* 1992.

---

jection of a fifth stage on the horizon. Table 2-4 summarizes the various stages of evolution. *Stage I* of this market refers to the "now historical" perspective of health care when hospitals, physicians, employers, and HMOs were operating under a more *unstructured* FFS payment system. At this stage, more options were available to the client and more flexibility within this framework was permissible. The penetration of the HMO market was barely noticeable during Stage I. An example of an HMO at this point of development was the Health Insurance Plan (HIP), or the oldest HMO, Kaiser Permanente, in California.

Stage II of this market is referred to as the *loose framework*. Many areas of the country are currently in this stage and struggling with it. HMOs and PPOs are beginning to emerge in greater numbers, and enrollment has skyrocketed. They are no longer unnoticeable in the health care market of today. Due to their large enrollments, they now have the leverage to negotiate pricing and the ability to contract at lower reimbursement rates. During Stage II, the motivation is to lower the cost of providing health care so the value of the money received is not eroded. Several types of HMOs are developing. In the past, HMOs were organized to employ their own *staff* physicians and service provid-

ers and pay them a salary. Soon *groups* began to emerge, in which a number of physicians and other providers established partnerships and shared their profits. These groups usually practiced out of a common facility or location. Next came the independent practitioners who formed associations and contracted to be part of a group endeavor while still practicing out of their own offices. The last type of HMO to emerge is the *network,* in which large areas are covered, perhaps crossing various states or regions or even the entire United States. Networks are most popular among large conglomerates who want to obtain the benefits of HMOs for their employees with the same consistency at any of their sites.

At this stage of development the market moves into *Stage III, consolidation.* While HMOs are forming networks, hospitals are simultaneously forming systems and networks themselves. This now sets up the beginnings of a competitive market in which hospitals are aggressively recruiting physicians and practitioners. These groups of physicians and providers are more commonly becoming known as PPOs. The payment system is based on a per case, per diem **capitation** through the PPO. A contract is developed that outlines the cost per covered life in the plan. PPOs are now outgrowing the HMO market primarily due to their ability to offer greater savings for employers at a time when employers are extremely concerned about the cost of their employees' health benefits.

Many parts of the country, primarily the west coast, have lived through this phase and have now embarked onto *Stage IV, managed competition.* This is the phase where capitation prevails. In this market, purchasers contract with hospital/physician networks to provide a comprehensive health care package to their clients. These integrated systems contract with the purchasers to accept the financial risk for managing their **utilization** of services **(utilization management).** In other words, they bear the burden of controlling their costs to deliver health care. The next level of this system is capitation, where a set fee is given to provide comprehensive care to a given population. This puts an even greater burden on the ability to provide quality care while controlling cost. The managed organization is no longer taking the risk with its premiums; the risk has now shifted to the provider of the health care services within the network or physician care group. This phase of managed care is the most uncomfortable of them all, because this is where survival of the fittest comes into play. Competition is at its peak during this phase, because managed care organizations are searching for membership from the most frugal yet quality-driven establishments. Report cards are now the judgment mechanism of any managed care organization and can be the demise of any physician or hospital not meeting the standards of cost containment as set up by the managed care organizations. An example of capitation follows: 1000 HMO members sign up for a health care network as part of a full-risk contract. The network will reimburse approximately $400.00 per member per month to cover all of their health care needs regardless of how much or how little they access the health care system. It is the burden of the health care network to provide adequate resources to cover their health care needs at low cost.

Government provision of medical insurance is the final source when reviewing the options for our population at large. Both federal and state governments provide medical insurance benefits. The Medicare program under the federal government provides mandatory basic hospitalization benefits for most U.S. citizens over the age of 65 and some other special classes of individuals, such as the disabled. This coverage is referred to as *Medicare Part A,* and it can be supplemented by *Medicare Part B,* which provides for payment of doctor bills. These plans are not all inclusive enough for most senior citizens. Recently there have been growing cutbacks to Medicare, so it is prudent for any citizen over age 65 to supplement Medicare with another insurance

plan. Many HMOs/PPOs are now expanding their plans to offer a managed care Medicare component.

At the state level, insurance benefits are also offered. These are commonly referred to as the *Medicaid program of benefits for the indigent.* They are no longer associated with the stigma of the term *welfare,* because more and more citizens must apply for public assistance to cover their medical bills after they have exhausted their income and assets. Medicaid is a pool of funds used to provide insurance benefits for those who cannot afford health insurance. The amount of funds set aside for this purpose is most often a direct result of the economic status of a particular state. The amount of funding is undergoing a great deal of turmoil as many states are tightening their pocketbooks in anticipation of the full impact of managed care in a capitated environment.

A few examples of differing reimbursements for physician services are outlined in dollars in Figure 2-1. This is only a representative partial listing of potential physician fees and does not represent all practices or the many varieties of reimbursement schedules.

Other Health Benefit Plans

Worker's compensation. An additional type of government provision that can vary from state to state is the worker's compensation guidelines. Worker's compensation cases are different from group medical insurance in that the insurers and employers are mandated by legislature guidelines to reimburse for both medical costs and lost wages. It is imperative that a case manager working with worker's compensation claims be familiar with the state's laws, especially as they reflect the claimant's return to work.

Case manager's role in worker's compensation cases. The case manager must be aware that there is a two-pronged effort in worker's compensation cases. That is, the insurance carrier is not only interested in the timely results of medical care but also wants to minimize the outlay of lost wages. Therefore, getting the employee back to work as soon as possible becomes an additional motivational pressure on the case manager. At times the case manager may have difficulty balancing medical health and the timely return to the workforce. The case manager may be faced with the dilemma of a tight time frame to return someone to work if the salary losses are a greater expense to the insurer than the medical care expenses.

Case managers specializing in the field of worker's compensation must be well versed on orthopedic injuries, because these injuries dominate compensation cases. They must also be knowledgeable enough in rehabilitative medicine to recommend the resources nec-

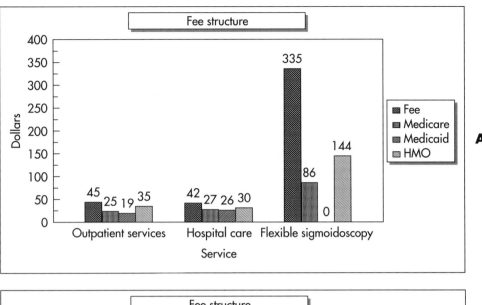

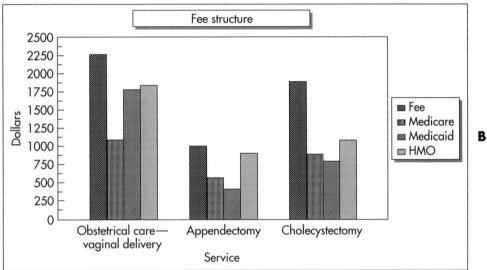

Fig. 2-1 Differing reimbursements for physician services.

essary to assist a patient in increasing functionality. It is the goal of the case manager to return an employee to the previous state of well-being or the optimum level of improvement obtainable. The case manager achieves this by ensuring that the appropriate treatment plan is in effect and progressing, along with verifying compliance by the employee. It is also important for the case manager to know the employee/claimant well enough to prevent the person from engaging in any untoward activities that would hinder or sabotage the progress or ultimate recovery.

Automobile insurance. As with worker's compensation guidelines, automobile policies and/or no-fault policies vary from state to state. Many rules depend on the location of the accident, where the person resides, or where the person's employment headquarters is located.

Case management usually becomes involved in mo-

tor vehicle accident cases when catastrophic injury has occurred. Case managers become very involved in the discharge planning and coordination, such as transfer from acute level of care to rehabilitative settings or decisions involving a chronic injury requiring adaptive equipment, home care, or home modifications.

Disability insurance. Disability plans are usually referred to as *short term, long term,* or *total disability.* Each type of plan varies in its amounts of salary replacement and length of time covered. Disability plans will require a case management review. Usually a case manager will become involved as the length of time for disability coverage is winding down. It will be the creativity of a case manager's skills that will determine if the financial plan and the medical plan will balance to the benefit of the insured and the employer.

Long-term care. This is a relatively new type of insurance offered. The policy holder has a variety of possibilities

case manager's tip 2-3

Case Management Caveat

Case management must not be the catchall for fixing all that ails a facility.

case manager's tip 2-4

Case Management's Focus

The focus must begin to go beyond illness to include wellness and preventive case management.

for nursing care coverage. Such care as skilled nursing, subacute care, custodial nursing care, extended home care, or nursing home provisions can be covered. The insurance company usually case manages a claim to confirm the need for services and approves benefit coverage accordingly.

Proactive Tactics to Counteract the Effects of Managed Care

Most strategies are incorporating a two-pronged approach to tackle all of the major areas that the managed care organizations seem to be concentrating on. One approach could fall under the overall heading of *operational management*. This is the area where efforts are initiated to control costs and to become more accountable for costs. Work redesigns and changes in the work delivery systems are becoming commonplace in organizations that are taking a more proactive approach. A more active performance and reward system is becoming evident and is attempting to integrate physician best practice with a functional integration system so that quality standards of care can be maintained at the least cost possible.

The second approach, and the area where case management will have the most direct impact on its overall success, is under the heading of *clinical management*. Nursing case management was the first tool used to oversee the patient's journey through the health care system. Without a clear system of managing the patient services and resources in the least costly way, particularly as we embark on capitation, funds will quickly be wiped out. Capitation clearly requires control over resources, utilization management, length-of-stay reduction, disease management, and clinical process improvement. All of these listed areas can be incorporated into the case management role (see Chapter 4).

The emergence of the case manager using the clini-

cal pathway was a major step toward a more cost-effective, efficient method of delivering care. By identifying variances to care, the case manager began to identify ways to continuously improve the delivery of care while not compromising quality. The use of clinical paths was the beginning initiative to control and reduce length of stay. An effective case management program can make a significant difference in managing and coordinating the clinical resources available for the patient (Case Manager's Tip 2-3) (Flarey and Blancett, 1996).

Integrating case management into managing a patient group or a specific disease entity is the next level of resource and clinical management. This strategy uses a multidisciplinary approach to care and requires input from the medical, clinical, ancillary, financial, and administrative teams. Many facilities have developed multidisciplinary teams to meet frequently on units and review the care of the patients to ensure that quality is being maintained while utilization of services is appropriate and cost efficient. Similarly, length-of-stay committees have been launched to discuss problem cases, high-cost patients or certain areas of overutilization, or more efficient methods of providing services at lower cost. Future strategies must expand efforts beyond the hospital walls to include community services and community-based initiatives of case management (Case Manager's Tip 2-4).

Differentiating between case management and managed care can be somewhat confusing at times, because the terms are used interchangeably in many arenas. In general terms, managed care is the umbrella for several initiatives of cost containment that include case management. Case management is a variation of the components that comprise managed care (i.e., managing cost, quality, and effectiveness of services) (Cohen and Cesta, 1997). Case management is a process that incorporates the components of managed care when attend-

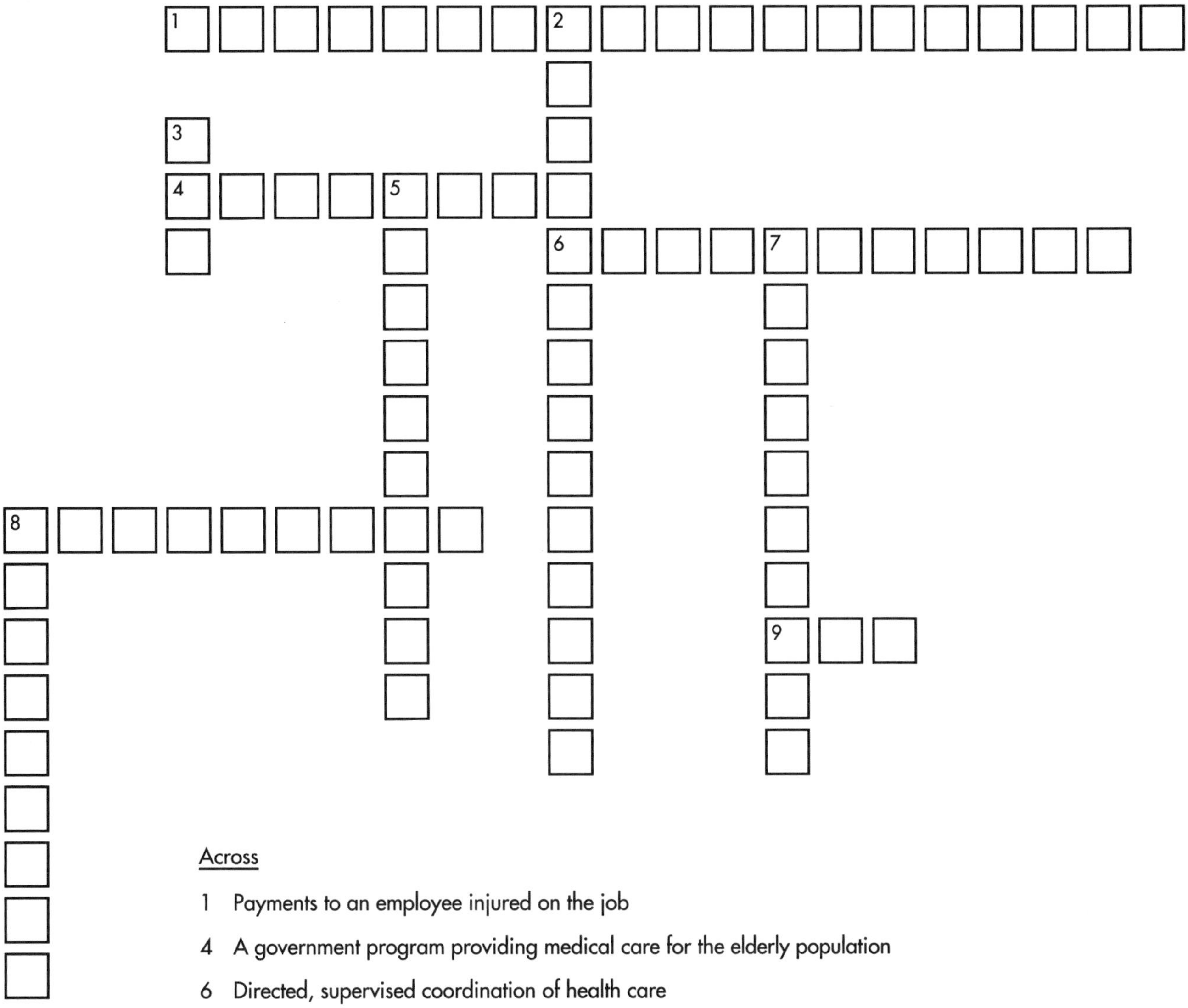

Across

1 Payments to an employee injured on the job

4 A government program providing medical care for the elderly population

6 Directed, supervised coordination of health care

8 Insurance against possible losses, damage, or injury

9 A plan that contracts with health care providers to offer services to a panel of patients

Down

2 A model to manage costs of health care and quality services that optimizes outcomes

3 Comprehensive medical services to enrolled membership on a prepaid basis

5 A set amount of money paid based on covered lives

7 A primary care physician who refers patients to specialists as needed

8 The protection one seeks to provide benefits for an illness or injury

Fig. 2-2 Crossword puzzle: a review of managed care terminology. (Answers appear in the footnote at the bottom of this page.)

Crossword puzzle (Figure 2-2) answer key. *Across:* 1, worker's compensation; 4, Medicare; 6, managed care; 8, indemnity; 9, PPO. *Down:* 2, case management; 3, HMO; 5, capitation; 7, gatekeeper; 8, insurance.

ing to the needs of patient care. It can be used in any form of patient delivery systems such as team, functional, primary, or alternative nursing care. Continuous monitoring of care rendered to a patient is maintained through interdisciplinary team meetings and analysis of variances from the outlined plan. Case management is effective because it coordinates, integrates, and evaluates the outcomes of the processes of care (Cohen and Cesta, 1997).

Summary

To have an effect on managed care, the case management model must take an active role in watching for quality outcomes. Benchmarking research used by managed care companies will be an important tool that a case manager must incorporate into the role as it will become clear that adequacy of care will be measured by outcomes. Case managers must demonstrate that they have the flexibility to ensure that care is delivered in a high-quality and cost-effective manner. They will undoubtedly play a vital role in the future of our health care industry and the survival of quality health care provided to its people.

Key Points

1. The prospective payment system was one of the forces leading acute care settings toward the adoption of case management models.
2. Case mix helps hospitals to determine their costs, as well as their types of patients and use of resources.
3. Regardless of the reimbursement system under which the patient is eligible, the length of stay will continue to need to remain short, and the use of resources will need to be monitored and controlled.
4. Health insurance is the protection one seeks to provide benefits for an illness or injury.

5. The insurance contract states the nature of the benefits or the coverage available to the insured.
6. An HMO delivers comprehensive medical services to an enrolled membership on a prepaid basis.
7. The PPO offers a more limited number of providers and encourages the use of physicians and services within the network, but patients are permitted to go outside the network for decreased reimbursement.
8. The evolution of the health care market has four stages of development in the managed care environment.
9. Work redesigns are becoming commonplace in organizations taking a proactive approach to managed care.
10. Managing patient services and resources in the least costly way while maintaining quality will be the primary goal of case management as it relates to managed care.
11. Managed care is the umbrella for several cost-containment initiatives that include but are not limited to case management.

The crossword puzzle shown in Figure 2-2 will help you review some of the key terms related to financial reimbursement systems. The answers appear in the footnote at the bottom of the page.

References

Blancett SS, Flarey DL: *Case studies in nursing case management: health care delivery in a world of managed care,* Gaithersburg, Md, 1996, Aspen.

Brucker MC, MacMullen NJ: Health insurance: a summary of basic types, *Home Health Care Nurs* 4(6):8-10, 1995.

Cohen EL, Cesta TG: *Nursing case management: from concept to evaluation,* ed 2, St Louis, 1997, Mosby.

Commission on Professional and Hospital Activities: *The international classification of diseases,* rev 8, 2 vols, Ann Arbor, Mich, 1975, CPHA (adapted for use in the United States).

Enteen R: *Health insurance: how to get it, keep it, or improve what you've got,* New York, 1992, Paragon House.

Flarey DL, Blancett SS: *Handbook of nursing case management,* Gaithersburg, Md, 1996, Aspen.

Mullahy CM: *The case management handbook,* Gaithersburg, Md, 1995, Aspen.

Richards S: A closer look at case management, *J Health Qual* 18(4):8-11, 1996.

University Hospital Consortium and American Practice Management, Incorporated Management Consultants: *Stages of market evolution,* 1992.

CHAPTER 3

CASE MANAGEMENT MODELS

ase management is a malleable and easily adapted model that applies to a variety of care delivery locations and systems. It is because of this flexibility that the model has been designed and implemented in various ways that respond to and meet the needs of the organization applying them. Although case management has been used in the community setting for the longest period of time, it is now commonly seen as an integrated care delivery model in the acute care setting. More and more hospitals are recognizing the model's ability to manage resources while maintaining or improving quality.

Clearly the most effective models are those that provide a mechanism for managing cases across the continuum of care, thereby providing a seamless, integrated care process. In a managed care environment, this is most easily done because of the integrated services inherent in a managed care system. The notion of managing cases in a variety of care settings is more difficult in other payor systems where there are no incentives for various settings to communicate and/or share resources. Managed care is traditionally viewed as a system that provides the generalized structure and focus when managing the use, cost, quality, and effectiveness of health care services. **Managed care** is the umbrella for cost-containment efforts such as case management. **Case management** is a process model. It is based on and contains elements of the managed care theme.

This is why many hospitals have opted to first implement case management in the acute care setting. This accomplishes a number of things. First, it allows the organization to design, implement, and perfect its case management system in a more easily controlled environment, the hospital. Although it provides greater challenges in terms of the clinical management of patients in the acute care setting, it is still a place where team members are part of a team that is "within the walls." In fact, the term *within the walls* has been used to aggregate those case management models that manage patients' care during the acute care portion of the ill-

ness. Among the many applications of the within-the-walls models are a host of types using the members of the team in various role functions. In most cases the registered nurse (RN) is used as **case manager.** It is the placement of the RN in the organizational structure and the associated role functions that differentiates the various models.

Case management is difficult to encapsulate because it describes many different approaches, including a patient care delivery system, a professional practice model, a defined group of activities performed by health care providers in a particular setting, and services provided by private practitioners (Goodwin, 1994).

TYPES OF CASE MANAGEMENT

Case management services can be provided in a variety of ways and care sites. There are basically four types: primary, medical/social, private, and **nurse case management.** Box 3-1 summarizes the types and the sites in which they typically occur.

Primary Care Case Management

In primary care case management the physician functions as the case manager. As case manager the physician is responsible for coordinating and managing patient care services. Some managed care organizations are using nurse practitioners as primary care case managers. Nurse practitioners are able to take on this role because of their ability to function independently under the supervision of a physician. The primary care case manager is the **gatekeeper** who plans, approves, and negotiates care for the patient.

In managed care organizations the case manager triages patients and determines their future needs and resource allocation. For example, the primary care case manager evaluating a newly diagnosed asthmatic patient will determine whether the patient needs to be seen by a specialist. This particular managed care function serves to control expenses by limiting the use of more expensive interventions.

box 3-1

Case Management Models and Sites in Which They are Used

PRIMARY CARE CASE MANAGEMENT

1. Health maintenance organizations (HMOs)
2. Preferred provider organizations (PPOs)
3. Physician hospital organizations (PHOs)
4. Private practice

MEDICAL/SOCIAL CASE MANAGEMENT

1. Acute care
2. Outpatient settings (including clinics and community health programs)

PRIVATE CASE MANAGEMENT

1. Direct referral for a variety of services and sites

NURSE CASE MANAGEMENT

1. Ambulatory care
2. Acute care
3. Home care
4. Long-term care
5. Rehabilitation
6. Managed care

Medical/Social Case Management

This type of case management focuses on the long-term care of patient populations at risk for hospitalization. The needs may be either medical or social in nature, and the case manager may be a physician, social worker, or RN. In some instances the case manager will follow the patient regardless of the setting in which services are being rendered.

Private Case Management

Private case management is used by patients who fall outside the traditional patient care programs. In this type of case management an RN will either be self-employed, an independent practitioner, or work on a case-by-case basis for a managed care organization or other **third-party payor.** The private case manager is contracted for services as needed. The case manager coordinates and manages the care for the patient regardless of the setting.

Because the case manager is independent of the organization, some believe that private case managers can provide the greatest level of completely unbiased services to the patient and family. The case manager functioning under this model is not advocating for anyone but the patient. This area is perhaps the newest addition to the case management arena. Many of the private case managers hired in the 1980s were master's prepared RNs or social workers (Knollmueller, 1989). In the 1990s

we find this trend continuing with case managers who are usually clinical nurse specialists (CNSs) or social workers. Often they are paid privately by the client or subcontracted by a third-party payor. The private case manager may coordinate services for the client, advocate on behalf of the client, and/or provide counseling (Clark, 1996).

Nurse Case Management

This approach to case management uses the RN as the case manager. The RN functions as the facilitator, coordinator, and manager of patient care services and expected outcomes.

HOSPITAL-BASED/ACUTE CARE MODELS
Primary Nurse Case Management

This model uses the staff nurse or primary nurse in the position of case manager. In addition to being responsible for hands-on, direct nursing care, the primary nurse case manager is also responsible for the indirect nursing functions that have often been the responsibility of other members of the health care team. Direct nursing functions include tasks such as physical assessments, medication administration, vital sign monitoring, intravenous administration, and patient/family education. Indirect functions include facilitation and coordination of services, discharge planning, monitoring of utilization of resources, **outcomes management, variance** analysis, and others. In this model many of the functions that would have been traditionally handed off to other departments or disciplines are collapsed under the staff nurse case manager role.

Traditionally the staff nurse's role has been focused on the acute care, clinical, hands-on component of the patient's illness. Some **discharge planning** may have been included in the job responsibilities, such as referrals to visiting nurse services. Other functions, such as **utilization,** continuing care placement, or patient/family education, might have been shared by others on the team. For example, **utilization management** would have been the responsibility of the utilization nurse. Discharge planning and placement issues might have been managed by the social worker or the dedicated discharge planner. Patient/family education might have been shared with CNSs such as the enterostomal CNS, the pain management specialist, or the medical-surgical CNS. These professionals were often called on to provide specific clinical expertise to augment that being provided by the staff nurse.

Functions such as **outcomes monitoring** and variance analysis were not core components of the traditional primary nursing models. Both outcomes manage-

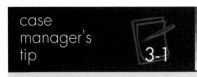

3-1   # Primary Nurse Case Management

In the primary nurse case management model, *all* patients must be case managed because of the reduction of other services and personnel.

ment and variance identification have evolved as by-products yet important elements of case management. Traditional nursing care plans did not include expected outcomes or identification of variations from the expected outcomes. In this model the staff nurse is expected to take responsibility for these role functions.

In some versions of the staff nurse model, the staff nurse may be given the responsibility for some of these additional role functions. In some cases, role functions such as utilization management are retained by the core department. The underlying principle of the staff nurse case manager model is that the staff nurse takes ultimate responsibility and accountability for the patient's hospital course and continuing stay needs.

The early primary nurse models were intended to place the RN in the position of being ultimately accountable for all aspects of the patient's care. The primary nursing models of the 1970s developed in response to nursing's evolution toward greater autonomy and professionalism. These responsibilities included those mentioned above as related to the direct, hands-on care. In addition, responsibilities may have included discharge planning. Utilization management responsibilities have not been traditional elements of the primary nurse role. Unfortunately, these models were unable to manage the cost and quality issues of the 1990s (Lynn-McHale, Fitzpatrick, and Shaffer, 1993).

In the primary nurse or staff nurse case management models, different levels of responsibility are placed on the staff nurse depending on the level of integration of other departments. For example, in a fully integrated hospital the staff nurse may be responsible for direct care and all related indirect nursing functions, including discharge planning, utilization management, variance analysis, and outcomes/quality improvement. In other cases, levels of responsibility may vary. Utilization management is the most common exception to this list, with some basic utilization functions often retained by a central department. Some of the functions may include telephone communication with managed care organizations or other insurers, continued stay revenues, or denials.

Despite the degree of responsibility delegated to the staff nurse, a tremendous amount of education must take place to prepare the staff nurse or primary nurse to assume these added responsibilities. The staff nurse may be responsible not only for providing care to a caseload of patients on the unit but also for managing the care of patients in other parts of the hospital, regardless of location (Davis, 1996).

The staff/primary nurse case manager model may also serve as a framework for a clinical ladder, which may be composed of several positions of increasing responsibility with the case manager as the top level. This may mean that the case manager oversees more comprehensive or complicated patients. *In this model, all patients must be case managed.* This is because of the reduction of other services and personnel, which means that these job responsibilities must be absorbed by the staff nurse (Case Manager's Tip 3-1).

Advanced Practice Case Management

The advanced practice case manager is an RN with an advanced practice degree; either a CNS or a nurse practitioner. The advanced practice nurse brings additional dimensions to the case manager role and a level of educational preparation not held by the majority of staff nurses. The master's prepared nurse's educational preparation has a wellness or health focus that is clinically specialized and care continuum based (Koerner, 1991). These nurses are also educated to bring their advanced educational skills and focus on patient/family education to the daily care of their patients (American Nurses Association, 1988).

This case management model removes the case manager from direct patient care. The case manager becomes concerned with the continuum of care and moves the patient from one phase of care to the next regardless of who is providing the specific care along the way. This facilitation/coordination role may also include discharge planning and/or utilization management responsibilities, depending on how the organization has been redesigned. Members of the team continually consult with each other, and the CNS case manager provides the coordination and facilitation role to the process. It is this cadre of additional and advanced skills that makes the advanced practice nurse a prime candidate for case management (Hamric, 1992).

To use existing personnel more efficiently, the organization may convert already existing CNS positions to case managers. In this case the current role functions of the CNS must be reevaluated. For example, mandatory Joint Commission continuing education functions may need to be redeployed to other staff developers. By doing so, the CNS case manager is truly freed up to perform advanced practice role functions, which may have been impossible when other job responsibilities were added onto the role.

CNS case managers can be either unit based or diagnosis (hospital) based. In either case they should be assigned based on their clinical specialty. If the clinical care units are specialty oriented, with cohorted, like-type patients, then a unit-based approach may work. If not, the case manager may need to be diagnosis based to remain within the clinical specialty, regardless of the patient's physical location.

The removal of case managers from direct patient care means that they have more time to dedicate to advanced case management functions such as outcomes management and research. They are also educated to perform these role functions. Their clinical expertise, advanced preparation including research, and a continuum of care focus are benefits that they bring to the role of case manager (Gaedeke Norris and Hill, 1991). The CNS case manager position allows the CNS to function in a way that is more purely a clinical specialist role than when a host of staff-development responsibilities are collapsed onto the role (Wells, Erickson, and Spinella, 1996). Because of their advanced clinical expertise, it is sometimes easier for the CNS to develop relationships with physicians that extend beyond the acute care setting. The advanced practice case manager, as part of the interdisciplinary team, may work with the team in the ambulatory setting, seeing patients after discharge from the hospital. The opportunity for the patient/family to develop a long-standing relationship with the case manager may mean greater compliance with their care regimen and more positive clinical outcomes over a longer period of time.

Nurse practitioners bring even more skills to the case manager role. With their ability to prescribe and discharge the patient from the hospital, the care process can be facilitated and less fragmented. The ambulatory care setting may be the most valuable place to use the nurse practitioner, particularly for those patients with chronic illnesses who are frequently accessing the health care system (Case Manager's Tip 3-2). The nurse practitioner's holistic approach with a focus on education and wellness may translate to reduced hospital admissions and a better quality of life for the patient in the community.

There are some commonalities and some differences between the two advanced practice roles of CNS and nurse practitioner. Case management models have been suggested that integrate the two roles (Schroer, 1991).

Commonalties between the roles include patient education, graduate-level preparation, practice, care coordination, referral, specialty practice, and autonomy. In contrast, the nurse practitioner has more of a focus on primary care, including the physical examination, history, and prescribing of medications. The title is protected by state regulations, and there can be reimbursement to primary care. The CNS is more inpatient focused and uses health promotion as a secondary consideration (Schroer, 1991).

Currently nurse practitioners work in primary care, outpatient clinics, **health maintenance organizations (HMOs),** and other specialty areas. CNSs work in inpatient settings (Diers, 1993). The differences and similarities described may suggest the use of the CNS case manager in the acute care setting and the use of the nurse practitioner case manager in the ambulatory setting.

Utilization Review Nurse Case Management

In this version of case management, some institutions have eliminated the traditional utilization review nurse and converted these positions to case managers. The first step in this process is the transition from utilization review to utilization management. This step is both philosophical and operational. Utilization review has been a retrospective process that attempted to correct problems after they occurred. The utilization review nurse would read and review medical records to determine appropriateness for hospitalization based on the physician's and other health care provider's documentation. In some cases the utilization review nurse would intervene when delay occurred in the care process. For

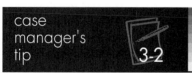
case manager's tip 3-2

Advanced Practice Case Management

The ambulatory care setting may be the most valuable place to use the advanced practice case manager, particularly for chronically ill patients who access the health care system frequently.

example, a delay in completion of a computerized axial tomography (CAT) scan might result in the utilization review nurse making a call to radiology to determine the cause of the delay. In these cases the nurse identified a delay once it had occurred and then tried to remedy the situation. In any case, the delay had already happened. Other functions included review of services for medical necessity and assurance that services were being provided in the most appropriate setting and at an acceptable quality standard level.

Implementation of utilization case management means that the utilization management/review functions must be picked up by the case manager. One method of implementing this model has come as a result of the hospital simply taking existing personnel and redeploying them as case managers. Responsibilities remain essentially the same without a reengineering of other departments/disciplines. In other cases the clinical case manager is given added responsibilities that include utilization management, after which the original positions are eliminated. Another approach may be to blend the discharge planning and utilization management functions together. All versions have the goal of eliminating redundant, currently existing positions and making the care process more efficient by streamlining the process and reducing the number of steps in the completion of tasks.

If financially feasible, maintaining a small utilization management core department is beneficial. The blending of all the utilization functions onto the case manager role may mean that the case manager gets completely absorbed in these functions and has less time to devote to the clinical dimensions of the role. Issues such as denial of **benefits** may remain within the purview of the utilization management core department. Retrospective insurance reviews may also be the responsibility of this department, to reduce fragmentation and delays in the care process. The case manager should take over those functions that are most closely related to the patient's current hospitalization, including admission and continued stay reviews. As many cases as possible should be concurrently reviewed. These **concurrent reviews** are performed by the case

manager every 3 days—or more frequently in the case of critical care areas. Among the functions performed during the concurrent review process are evaluations for severity of illness and intensity of service. Evaluation of severity of illness includes an evaluation of the patient's significant symptoms, any deviations from normal levels, or unstable or abnormal vital signs or laboratory values. Intensity of service includes evaluation of the plan of treatment, interventions, and expected outcomes. **Retrospective reviews** can be handled by the utilization management core department.

Including concurrent reviews as part of the case management process can help expedite the plan more quickly. The case manager has the most comprehensive knowledge and understanding of the case and is observing it in its totality rather than in a fragmented approach. Payor interactions can also be facilitated through such an integrated approach. Benefits identification and eligibility are becoming more cumbersome processes as the number of managed care organizations continues to rise. Each organization brings with it a host of different benefits. Even within one managed care organization, similar patients will be entitled to different benefits. Negotiating these benefits for the patient while in the hospital and after discharge can mean a smoother transition for the patient from the acute care to the community setting. This comes as a result of fewer "hand-offs" of the work from one provider to another.

Caution must be taken in the implementation of such a model so as not to overload the case manager. It is highly recommended that the tasks identified above as part of a centralized core utilization management department remain so, or the true case management focus will be lost in performing insurance reviews, dealing with denials, and so on (Case Manager's Tip 3-3).

Social Work Case Management

Social workers have used the title *case manager* for many years. In fact, after the RN, social workers are the other professionals most often seen in the role of case manager (Rantz and Bopp, 1996). The social worker, if functioning as the case manager, can focus on the patient's social, financial, and discharge planning needs.

---

case manager's tip	3-3	**Utilization Review Nurse Case Management**

In the utilization review nurse case management model it is easy for the case manager to become overloaded. Keeping the case manager's tasks part of a centralized core utilization management department can help prevent the true case management focus from being lost.

The social worker as case manager is effective in the outpatient setting, where many of the patient's needs are related more to financial or social issues and less to clinical ones. In the hospital setting, a dyad of RN and case manager can be an effective way to manage cases based on needs. If the prevailing issues are clinical or educational in nature, the RN may be more appropriate for case management. If the patient's needs are more social or financial, the social worker may be more appropriate to provide the necessary services.

In the dyad model the RN and social worker case managers assess the patient on admission to the hospital; based on that assessment it is determined which practitioner may be more appropriate to manage the case. In some cases it may be necessary for both disciplines to case manage the patient.

The case manager's initial assessment would be a clinical or biological review of systems, reason for hospitalization, relevant previous medical history, clinical issues that may affect discharge, and educational needs. The social worker would be focused on the social and psychological segments of the patient's overall clinical picture. A social assessment includes an evaluation of the patient's life-style, activities, and interests. Family support, living environment, and the patient's ability to return to the preadmission environment would be assessed by the social worker. The psychological assessment would consist of an evaluation of the patient's mental status; use of alcohol, tobacco, and drugs; and previous history of mental disorders.

When implementing this model, it is extremely valuable for both disciplines to sit down together and outline what their case management inclusion or selection criteria will be (Box 3-2). Through techniques such as case conferencing, an ongoing evaluation can be made as to the patient's progress toward the expected outcomes and an ongoing determination can be made as to whether additional providers may need to be added to the case.

This type of model, although extremely patient focused and beneficial to the patient and family, may be too costly for the organization to support. If so, the RN case manager can call the social worker on a referral basis for cases needing more comprehensive social-work–type interventions (Case Manager's Tip 3-4).

OUTPATIENT CASE MANAGEMENT MODELS
Home Care Case Management

Case management in the home is designed with the same goals in mind as case management in the acute care setting. The case manager in the home environment directs the members of the interdisciplinary

---

| box 3-2 |

Neonatal Case Management Team Role Responsibilities

SOCIAL WORK

1. Psychosocial assessment, including evaluation of family situation/home/financial support, other high-risk social factors. Clarify medical coverage. Advocate, refer for such coverage. Refer for appropriate entitlements. Advocate for patients with various systems.
2. Evaluation of coping with illness/hospitalization; evaluation of family support systems; provision of emotional support.
3. Referral to community support agencies/mental health services as indicated.
4. Coordinate child abuse/neglect cases, including substance abuse cases.
5. Act as part of NICU team in providing coordinated services to families with children in the NICU.

SHAREABLE SKILLS/TASKS FOR TEAM

1. Attend regular interdisciplinary NICU rounds to share information.
2. Decision making with family.
3. Identify system barriers and solutions.
4. Patient/team continuity.
5. Collaboration with utilization management.
6. Optimize patient's adjustment to NICU.

CASE MANAGER

1. Case management plan of care; length of stay.
2. Track data.
3. Follow clinical status.
4. Coordinate/facilitate plan of care.
5. Consultation for clinical issues.
6. Monitoring outcomes.
7. Track clinical resource utilization with team.
8. Discharge teaching (e.g., CPR, medications).
9. Discharge planning, including equipment, home care referrals.
10. Posthospital follow-up.
11. Transportation arrangements.

---

health care team toward the achievement of the best-quality care at the lowest possible cost. The home care case manager also makes visits to patients in their homes to ensure that they are receiving the appropriate services and that the expected outcomes are being met. During the home visit the case manager may decide to refer the patient to the physician or other health care providers as deemed necessary.

The home care case manager receives referrals from the hospital-based case manager. The home care case manager can obtain important information on the patient's condition and related care by visiting the patient in the hospital and/or attending the hospital patient planning or discharge planning rounds. If a face-to-face

case
manager's
tip **3-4** Social Work Case Management

Social work case management is beneficial to patients and families yet may be too costly for the organization to support. One solution is for the nurse case manager to call the social worker on a referral basis for cases that need more comprehensive interventions.

case
manager's
tip **3-5** Home Care Case Management

Home care case managers can help ensure that patients achieve expected outcomes without duplication or redundant use of resources by coordinating services and monitoring the patient's progress closely.

exchange of information is not practical or possible, then the home care and hospital case managers must develop good systems for sharing and exchanging information. Information to be shared should include the patient's medical history, physical symptoms and findings, financial information including entitlements, and relevant psychosocial issues including family support mechanisms (Brueckner and Glover, 1993).

Patients receiving home care are not acute enough for hospitalization and are not ambulatory enough for daily visits to a clinic setting or physician office. In most cases the cost of home care is a fraction of what a hospital stay would cost. In addition to monitoring the patient's progress during this phase of illness, the case manager will also ensure that the necessary services are being delivered in the home setting and that the patient's optimal level of wellness is being met. Under **fee-for-service (FFS)** reimbursement, there was no financial incentive for the home care agency to control the number of home visits. Just as hospital visits were relatively unlimited before the prospective payment system, the home care agencies are only now beginning to face reductions in resources and reimbursement for visits. Under **capitated** managed care the number of home visits are the most strictly controlled.

Research has shown that a variety of factors may influence home care nurses' decisions regarding management of their clients, including the appropriate number of visits or the necessity for referrals to social service or other agencies (Feldman et al, 1993). Home care agencies are beginning to develop home care protocols similar to those previously developed for hospital care (e.g., pathways and multidisciplinary action plans [MAPs]). These prospectively developed tools become the case manager's frame of reference as they outline

the appropriate number of visits for a particular disease entity or surgical procedure. Expected outcomes for each discipline are predetermined so that the number of patient care visits correlates with the expected outcomes. As a result, allotted visits are not arbitrary but can be validated, and the patient's progress toward these expected outcomes can be benchmarked. The termination point for the case is also clearly defined, and the expectations of the staff in terms of when to close the case are delineated. Cases kept open beyond the appropriate length of time become very costly to the home care agency. By prospectively identifying the criteria for case closure based on **outcomes,** the care provider no longer has to make a subjective decision regarding when to close the case. Closing cases in a timely fashion allows resources to be appropriated to those cases that truly need extended services beyond the norm.

Home care case managers can be assigned by disease entity or broader clinical specialty. Chronic illnesses such as diabetes, asthma, or congestive heart failure may require case management services in the home after an episode of acute exacerbation of the disease. Rehabilitation after joint replacement is another clinical grouping for which case management may work well. These patients will require the services of more than one discipline, such as nursing and physical therapy. The case manager, by coordinating these services and monitoring the patient's progress closely, can ensure that the patient is moving toward those outcomes as efficiently as possible without duplication or redundant utilization of resources (Case Manager's Tip 3-5).

Community-Based Case Management

Community case management models are focused on primary care and primary prevention. They are therefore predominantly focused on well individuals in the community who are at risk or who have the potential for needing health care services. These models can provide integrated services found nowhere else. Comprehensive, coordinated, community-based programs can interrelate the client's health, social, educational, employment, and recreational needs.

Community nursing centers are defined as those where the key management positions are filled by RNs. These centers can range in size from a staff of 1 to 115 RNs, with an average of 8 per agency (Barger and Rosenfeld, 1993). Some centers use a case management model and philosophy to guide the care delivery process. In nurse case management models, the practice may be an autonomous nursing one. Two thirds of the RNs employed in nursing centers are certified for advanced nursing practice (Barger and Rosenfeld, 1993). Nurse practitioners are able to provide primary care as the client's first contact with a health care provider (Aydelotte et al, 1987). The remaining practitioners are generally master's prepared social workers. Referrals are made to on-site and off-site physicians and other off-site health care providers. Other resource referrals may be on or off site.

The goal of community-based case management is to support and empower individuals to maximize their optimal level of wellness through the use of community resources (Case Manager's Tip 3-6). Health promotion may be incorporated into activities such as day care classes, youth and adult recreation programs, support groups, meals for elders, community development activities, or adult education programs.

Both formal and informal mechanisms can be used to provide case management services. These might include nonscheduled walk-in clinics, scheduled appointments, home visits, or telephone consults. All are focused on "continuous" rather than "episodic" care (Trella, 1996).

The community-based case manager can provide other important services to the patient, such as continuing the educational program initiated in the hospital setting. Patients in the hospital may not retain the information they learned due to anxiety or pain and may

therefore benefit greatly from reinforcement on returning to the community. The community-based case manager discusses topics the patient has been taught in the hospital and continues the educational process through repetition, reinforcement, or continuation of teaching related to the specific topic.

The ongoing education and support provided by the community-based case manager may mean that exacerbations of the patient's disease and/or readmissions can be reduced. Many programs are focused around specific disease entities such as diabetes, chemical dependency, or HIV. These programs are geared to already diagnosed individuals whose goal is to maintain their optimal level of wellness in the community for as long as possible.

SYSTEM MODELS

The system models are designed to provide case management services along the continuum. A continuum of care is defined as an integrated, client-oriented system of care composed of both services and integrating mechanisms that guides and tracks clients over time through a comprehensive array of health, mental health, and social services spanning all levels of intensity of care (Evashwick, 1987). The continuum contains seven access points to health care, as described in Box 3-3.

The case manager is assigned to the case at one of the seven access points, depending on where the patient entered the health care system. In most cases the case manager is responsible for the patient no matter where the patient is along the health care continuum. This may mean that the primary case manager communicates with the case manager in the setting where the patient currently is. For example, if a community-based case manager is following the patient, the responsibility for the case may be relinquished to the hospital-based case manager should the patient be admitted. The community-based case manager would share relevant information with the hospital-based case manager and might visit the patient. The ultimate responsibility for the management of the case while the patient was in the hospital would be the hospital-based case manager's.

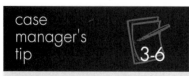

case manager's tip 3-6

Community-Based Case Management

By providing ongoing education and support to patients, the case manager can help ensure that the goal of community-based case management is met: to support and empower individuals to reach their optimal level of wellness through the use of community resources.

In organizations where the service line crosses the continuum and where there are multiple service programs, patient referrals and continuity of care are not necessarily automatic. In fact, the more complex the organization, the greater the need for client referral and

```
┌─────────────────────────────────────────┐
│              box 3-3                      │
│                                           │
│   Health Care Access Points and Types     │
│          of Care Offered                  │
│                                           │
│ PRIMARY CARE                              │
│                                           │
│  1. Clinics                               │
│  2. Health fairs                          │
│  3. Screening programs                    │
│  4. Health education programs             │
│                                           │
│ AMBULATORY CARE                           │
│                                           │
│  1. Physician offices                     │
│  2. Clinics                               │
│  3. Diagnostic centers                    │
│  4. Day surgery                           │
│                                           │
│ ACUTE CARE                                │
│                                           │
│  1. Hospitals                             │
│  2. Medical centers                       │
│  3. Emergency departments                 │
│                                           │
│ TERTIARY CARE                             │
│                                           │
│  1. Teaching hospitals                    │
│  2. Acute rehabilitation                  │
│  3. Specialty physicians                  │
│                                           │
│ HOME CARE                                 │
│                                           │
│  1. Visiting nursing services             │
│  2. Home medical equipment, including     │
│     intravenous therapy                   │
│  3. Community care programs               │
│                                           │
│ LONG-TERM CARE                            │
│                                           │
│  1. Nursing homes                         │
│  2. Subacute care facilities              │
│  3. Long-term rehabilitation centers      │
│  4. Adult homes                           │
│  5. Skilled nursing facilities            │
│                                           │
│ HOSPICE CARE                              │
│                                           │
│  1. Home hospice programs                 │
│  2. Hospital-based programs               │
│  3. End-stage group homes                 │
└─────────────────────────────────────────┘
```

tracking mechanisms (Evashwick, 1987). Continuity can be maintained by the case manager for clients at any point along the continuum (Case Manager's Tip 3-7).

CHRONIC CARE CASE MANAGEMENT

Chronic conditions are those the patient is expected to have for years or possibly for the rest of his or her life. These individuals may access and use a variety of health care services in a multitude of settings during the course of their illness. It is the use of these various services and settings for the chronically ill that places them at risk for receiving less-than-adequate, duplicative, or delayed health care services. Typical target populations for chronic care case management include the frail elderly, survivors of strokes, accident victims, mentally ill, and children and infants with congenital abnormalities (Evashwick, 1987).

Patients with chronic illnesses may access a wide range of services from acute care to social services, mental health, home care, or subacute care. It is during these transitions that the greatest opportunity for problems may arise. Case management integrates these wide-ranging services so that care, financing, and information are integrated. It provides a foundation for planning and managing care across settings (Case Manager's Tip 3-8). The focus is more than just providing the patient with access to the various services; it is also geared toward integrating these systems to provide a coordinated, continuing care approach.

The patient population at greatest risk for chronic care needs are the elderly, particularly the frail elderly. This group is at high risk for complex health needs, potential for physical or social complications, and continued use of health care resources. A multidisciplinary approach such as that provided by a case management model has been documented to reduce cost and improve outcomes for this population (Trella, 1993). The application of case management to this population may mean providing adult day care programs with transportation. The children of aging parents may be able to maintain their parents in the community if they have access to an adult day care program that provides a flexible structure so that they can drop parents off on their way to work and pick them up in the evening. Other

Chronic Care Case Management

The case manager can coordinate the wide range of services needed by chronically ill patients so that care, financing, and information are integrated. This provides a foundation for planning and managing care across settings.

---

box 3-4

Conditions Typically Considered Subacute

Emphasis on subacute care as a cost-saving mechanism is increasing. The conditions that typically are included in this category include the following:
1. Short-term complex medical problems
2. Short-term rehabilitative conditions
3. Long-term (chronic) conditions

---

necessary services may be meal preparation, delivery services, housekeeping, or shopping services (Mullahy, 1995).

LONG-TERM CARE CASE MANAGEMENT

Long-term care settings such as the nursing home, rehabilitation facility, or skilled nursing facility are settings in which case management can serve the purpose of slowing the deterioration process and functional status of the resident. In long-term care settings care has been task oriented (Smith, 1991), with different practitioners providing different services to the resident. Today's typical nursing home patient is sicker, requires more complex medical and nursing care, and will live longer.

Increasing focus is also being placed on other subacute care settings as managed care drives the need for less-expensive care settings appropriate to the needs of the patient (Stahl, 1996). Conditions that usually are considered subacute are listed in Box 3-4.

Short-term complex medical problems would include problems such as wound care, respiratory management, total parenteral nutrition, dialysis, intravenous therapies, and postsurgical recovery. The goal in case managing this group of patients is recuperative in nature. The expected outcome is to bring the patient to the optimal level of wellness.

Short-term rehabilitative subacute care focuses on clinical issues such as stroke, amputation, total hip/knee replacement, and brain injury. The case management goal for this clinical group is restorative, to bring the patient as close to the preinjury condition as possible.

Long-term (chronic) case management is preventive maintenance, assisting the patient to maintain the level of functioning without deterioration for as long as possible. Long-term chronic conditions include coma, ventilator dependence, and head injury.

In response to these changes, nursing homes are adapting and undergoing modifications to the way they provided care in the past. Case management has been used as a mechanism for not only improving patient outcomes in long-term care settings but also for improving the job satisfaction of the care providers in these settings (Deckard, Hicks, and Rountree, 1986). With the introduction of a case management model, a health care provider can coordinate the services being provided by nursing assistants, RNs, physical and occupational therapists, and nutritionists. Integrating these services and identifying interdisciplinary expected outcomes allows the resident's functional status to be closely monitored and managed. Care is managed using an interdisciplinary approach, and therefore goals can be more specific, realistic, and measurable. Furthermore, the move away from a task-oriented approach means that goals are patient focused instead of staff focused (Smith, 1991).

The case manager in the long-term care setting may not be an RN if there is a lack of RN staff in the facility. In some cases it may be necessary to use the licensed practical or licensed vocational nurse in the role of case manager. The case manager provides for ongoing monitoring and evaluation of the resident's progress. Progress is measured against an assessment of the patient's medical problems, functional capabilities, social supports, and psychosocial well-being (Zawadski and Eng, 1988).

Case management plans can be used to manage the care and expected outcomes. Plans should focus on such things as nursing needs, therapies, activities of daily living, and personal care (Case Manager's Tip 3-9). The chronicity of the residents may mean that the case management plans are reviewed at a maximum of every 3 months or whenever the resident's condition or change in progress warrants a review. The case manager provides an on-going evaluation process and liaisons between the resident, the physician, the family, and other members of the health care team.

case
manager's
tip
3-9 | **Long-Term Care Case Management**

To manage the care and expected outcomes of long-term care clients, focus the case management plan on nursing needs, therapies, activities of daily living, and personal care.

case
manager's
tip
3-10 | **Managed Care Case Management**

Managed care case managers usually function either as financial case managers (utilization managers), who may have a caseload of hundreds or even thousands, or as more clinically focused case managers, who have fewer cases but of higher intensity.

MANAGED CARE MODELS

Managed care is a broad, expansive term covering a wide variety of services. Its main objective is to contain costs by controlling utilization and coordinating care. It is used as the generic term for insurance plans offering managed health care services to an enrolled population on a prepaid basis. Access, cost, and quality are controlled by care "gatekeepers." The gatekeeper is usually a physician in primary care. This physician after assessing the patient will determine whether the patient needs additional services such as a specialty physician or other service controlled by the managed care organization. There are many types of managed care organizations, but the most common is the HMO. The four basic models are the group model, staff model, **individual practice association (IPA)** model, and network model (see Chapter 2).

In the various managed care models case managers are employed to carry out a variety of functions. Broadly speaking, the case management functions can be classified as either financial case management or clinical case management. The financial case manager functions in what might traditionally be classified as utilization management. This case manager is in communication with the hospital case manager or utilization manager determining the patient's admission eligibility, continued stay, or discharge disposition including eligibility of services. The case manager in this role advocates on behalf of the managed care organization and may have a caseload of hundreds or thousands of patients. This role is of a lower intensity–higher volume approach (Sampson, 1994).

Some managed care organizations supplement the patients being followed by a financial case manager with a more clinically focused case manager. These case managers tend to have a somewhat smaller caseload (Sampson, 1994). Their focus is more high intensity–low volume in nature. They may be assigned by high-risk patient populations as identified by the managed care organization. These may include such things as catastrophic illness or injury, high-user or high-volume members, chronic or disabling conditions, or cases with high annual cost projections ($25,000 to $50,000) (Hicks, Stallmeyer, and Coleman, 1993). Assisting in the management of these patients will hopefully prevent unnecessary admissions to the hospital and minimize misutilization of health care resources (Case Manager's Tip 3-10).

Some managed care organizations are focusing on the management of their older members. The elderly are at greater risk in terms of cost and care needs. It is hoped that case managing this population will enhance the health status of older adults while containing their use of health care resources (Pacala et al, 1995).

Whether introduced in the inpatient or outpatient setting, case management models can be adapted to meet the goals of quality patient care in a fiscally responsible environment. Selection of the most appropriate model will depend on the needs of the organization, the available resources, and the expected goals.

KEY POINTS

1. There are four basic types of case management, using RNs, physicians, or social workers as case managers.
2. Hospital-based models generally use the RN as case manager, but the RN can be a primary nurse, CNS or nurse practitioner, or utilization review nurse. In some cases the case manager may be a social worker.
3. Outpatient case management models can be applied in home care, the community, or along the continuum.

4. Some models focus on management of the chronically ill.
5. Long-term case management can take place in the sub-acute setting, rehabilitation facility, or chronic nursing home setting.
6. Managed care models use the case manager as either a utilization manager or clinical manager acting on behalf of the managed care organization.

References

American Nurses Association: *Nursing case management*, Kansas City, Mo, 1988, ANA.

Aydelotte MK et al: *The nursing center: concept and design*, Kansas City, Mo, 1987, American Nurses Association.

Barger S, Rosenfeld P: Models in community health care: findings from a national study of community nursing centers, *Nurs Health Care* 14(8):426-431, 1993.

Brueckner G, Glover T: Case management and the continuum of care. In Donovan MR, Matson TA, eds: *Outpatient case management*, Chicago, 1993, American Hospital Association.

Clark KA: Alternate case management models. In Flarey DL, Blancett SS, eds: *Handbook of nursing case management*, Gaithersburg, Md, 1996, Aspen.

Davis V: Staff development for nurse case management. In Cohen E, ed: *Nurse case management in the 21st century*, St Louis, 1996, Mosby.

Deckard GJ, Hicks LL, Rountree BH: Long-term care nursing: how satisfying is it? *Nurs Econ* 4(4):194-200, 1986.

Diers D: Advanced practice, *Health Manage Q* second quarter, 16-20, 1993.

Evashwick J: Definition of the continuum of care. In Evashwick J, Weiss L, eds: *Managing the continuum of care*, Rockville, Md, 1987, Aspen.

Feldman C et al: Decision making in case management of home healthcare clients, *J Nurs Admin* 23(1):33-38, 1993.

Gaedeke Norris MK, Hill C: The clinical nurse specialist: developing the case manager role, *Dimensions Crit Care Nurs* 10(6):346-353, 1991.

Goodwin DR: Nursing case management activities: how they differ between employment settings, *J Nurs Admin* 24(2):29-34, 1994.

Hamric A: Creating our future: challenges and opportunities for the clinical nurse specialist, *Oncol Nurs Forum* 19(suppl 1):11-15, 1992.

Hicks LL, Stallmeyer JM, Coleman JR: *Role of the nurse in managed care*, Washington, DC, 1993, American Nurses Publishing.

Knollmueller RN: Case management: what's in a name? *Nurs Manage* 20(10):38-42, 1989.

Koerner J: Building on shared governance: the Sioux Valley Hospital experience. In Goertzen IE, ed: *Differentiating nursing practice into the twenty-first century* Kansas City, Mo, 1991, American Academy of Nursing.

Lynn-McHale DJ, Fitzpatrick ER, Shaffer RB: Case management: development of a model, *Clin Nurs Spec* 7(6):299-307, 1993.

Mullahy CM: *The case manager's handbook*, Gaithersburg, Md, 1995, Aspen.

Pacala JT et al: Case management of older adults in health maintenance organizations, *J Am Geriatr Soc* 43(5):538-542, 1995.

Rantz MJ, Bopp KD: Issues of design and implementation from acute care, long-term, and community-based settings. In Cohen E, ed: *Nurse case management in the 21st century*, St Louis, 1996, Mosby.

Sampson EM: The emergence of case management models. In Donovan MR, Matson TA, eds: *Outpatient case management*, Chicago, 1994, American Hospital Association.

Schroer K: Case management: clinical nurse specialist and nurse practitioner, converging roles, *Clin Nurs Spec* 5(4):189-194, 1991.

Smith J: Changing traditional nursing home roles to nursing case management, *J Gerontol Nurs* 17(5):32-39, 1991.

Stahl DA: Case management in subacute care, *Nurs Manage* 27(8):20-22, 1996.

Trella B: Integrating services across the continuum: the challenge of chronic care. In Cohen E, ed: *Nurse case management in the 21st century*, St Louis, 1996, Mosby.

Trella RS: A multidisciplinary approach to case management of frail, hospitalized older adults, *J Nurs Admin* 23(2):20-26, 1993.

Wells N, Erickson S, Spinella J: Role transition: from clinical nurse specialist to clinical nurse specialist/case manager, *J Nurs Admin* 26(11):23-28, 1996.

Zawadski RT, Eng C: Case management in capitated long-term care, *Health Care Financ Rev* annual supplement, 1988.

CHAPTER 4

ROLE OF THE NURSE CASE MANAGER

The advent of the nurse case manager's role has improved health care delivery. It changed the provision of care from a multidisciplinary to an interdisciplinary one. The old days of *"parallel play"* in providing health care, where the different disciplines involved in patient care worked in isolation, are outdated. Today's customers demand high-quality care that can be best achieved through *"interactive play,"* where ongoing interaction and cooperation among members of the various disciplines is a key. With the creation of the nurse case manager's role as the focal point of the interdisciplinary approach to care, the age of isolation, territoriality, fragmentation, redundancy, duplication, lack of communication, and unnecessary tests/procedures is gone. The new age of patient care is characterized by collaboration, integration, coordination, continuity, consistency, interaction, and open communication. Today's health care customer is happier and more satisfied with the care received. Nurse case managers play an integral role in this accomplishment.

The role of the nurse case manager is designed to maximize these efforts. The role has been implemented in almost all care settings in the majority of health care organizations. Currently, nurse case managers can be found working in insurance companies and managed care organizations; acute, intensive, and ambulatory care settings (including emergency departments, nursing centers, and outpatient clinics); nursing and group homes; hospices; senior citizen centers; and home care. Their job descriptions may vary from one setting to another, but the roles, functions, responsibilities, and required skills for success in the role are very similar. This chapter presents a thorough description of the case management process through which the various roles and responsibilities assumed by nurse case managers are discussed.

The extent of responsibilities provided for **case managers** is dictated by the job description defined by each health care organization. Description of the role is affected by the operations of the organization, placement of the nurse case manager in the table of organization,

power embedded in the role, cost incurred, goals of the case management model implemented, and organizational and specific nursing goals. In addition, the focus of the role of the nurse case manager is determined by the area of practice or the care setting. Although the common theme is patient care management, there still exist some differences that are reflected by the type of services needed in relation to the care setting.

CASE MANAGEMENT PROCESS

The case management process is a set of steps and activities applied by nurse case managers in their approach to patient care management. It delineates the roles and responsibilities of case managers toward patient care from the time of admission until discharge and in some instances after discharge. The case management process is a modified version of the nursing process (Table 4-1). Both the case management and nursing processes are similar in that they identify the plan of care of patients by assessing needs, diagnosing the problem(s), planning and implementing the care, and evaluating **outcomes.** The nursing process is applied to the care of every patient by all nurses in any care setting regardless of the patient care delivery model followed by the organization. However, the case management process is used by nurse case managers in an environment where case management is the patient care delivery model, and it is applied only to a select group of patients who meet specific predetermined criteria.

The case management process is a systematic approach to patient care delivery and management (Figure 4-1). It identifies what should be done by the nurse case manager at which time of the patient's hospitalization or course of care. The process provides the framework for the role of the case managers. It also helps organize and simplify their work. Each step in the process requires the nurse case manager to be astute and to exhibit specific skills. The combination of these skills is the token for success in the role.

TABLE 4-1
Comparison of the Nursing and the Case Management Processes

Nursing process	Case management process
Assessment	Case finding/screening and intake Assessment of needs
Diagnosis	Identification of actual/potential problems
Planning	Interdisciplinary case conferencing Establishing the goals of treatment and expected outcomes of care Developing/individualizing the case management plan
Implementation	Implementing the case management plan/interdisciplinary plan of care Facilitation/coordination of patient care activities
Evaluation	Monitoring of the delivery of patient care services Evaluation of outcomes of care/patient responses to treatment Discharge/disposition Repeating the case management process

Nurse case managers are active members of interdisciplinary teams of various health care providers working toward a common goal (i.e., provision and management of cost-effective, efficient, and high-quality patient care). Membership of the interdisciplinary team varies based on the patient's problems and the plan of care. Some members are always represented, such as the nurse case manager, physician, house staff or physician extenders (nurse practitioners and physician assistants), registered nurses (RNs), and patients and their families. Other members are called upon in consultation, such as the social worker, physical therapist, occupational therapist, respiratory technician, and nutritionist.

Case Finding/Screening and Intake

The initial step in case management is case finding (i.e., identifying the patients who require case management services). The purposes of case finding/screening are to identify the patient problems and determine the needs for case management services and the patient's eligibility for these services (Bower, 1992). Nurse case managers may identify such patients in four different ways. They may (1) screen all admissions to select those who are in need for case management services; (2) screen only those patients who are referred for services by other health care providers; (3) not screen any patients but consider them all in need of some sort of case management services; or (4) respond to a referral made by the patients or families themselves.

It is important, however, for each organization to de-

fine the method of patient referrals/identification for such services. Guidelines or policies must be established at the same time case management systems are implemented and case manager roles are defined and established. The clearer the system for case finding is, the easier the role of the nurse case manager becomes and the faster the patients are referred or identified for case management services. The efficiency of the system impacts on the cost and increases the effectiveness of the case management model. To expedite case finding, interdisciplinary health care team members are encouraged to make referrals to nurse case managers within 24 hours of patients' admission to a hospital, subacute care facility, or long-term care facility. In other care settings such as clinics or emergency departments, patients should be referred as soon as their needs for case management services are identified. In home care settings, patients are referred for case management services in the home while still on the premises of a health care facility.

Patients can be referred by private physicians, house staff, primary nurses, social workers, utilization managers/reviewers, discharge planners, nurse practitioners, physician assistants, physical therapists, and nutritionists. Generally each nurse case manager is made responsible for identifying patients in his or her service or area of responsibility. Patient selection criteria can be predefined to make this responsibility easier. It is important to establish patient referral criteria, especially if the case management model followed identifies patient referrals as the major source for selection of patients for case management services rather than waiting for nurse case managers to screen every admission to the hospital. These criteria eliminate any confusion that may arise when a member of the interdisciplinary team evaluates whether a patient needs to be referred to the nurse case manager.

Box 4-1 presents a list of examples of patient selection criteria for case management services. Some of these criteria are generic, can be applied to any care setting, and are based on issues that may affect the patient in terms of quality of care and/or length of stay. Other criteria are service/setting based and are only appropriate to that specific service/setting. The list serves as a guide nurse case managers can use to establish the criteria specific to their area of responsibility.

Whatever the case finding method is, nurse case managers still have to evaluate the appropriateness of patients for case management services and determine the necessity for "intake." The decision of whether a patient requires case management services (i.e., intake) is made based on screening (initial assessment) of the patient's needs, review of the medical record, and a dis-

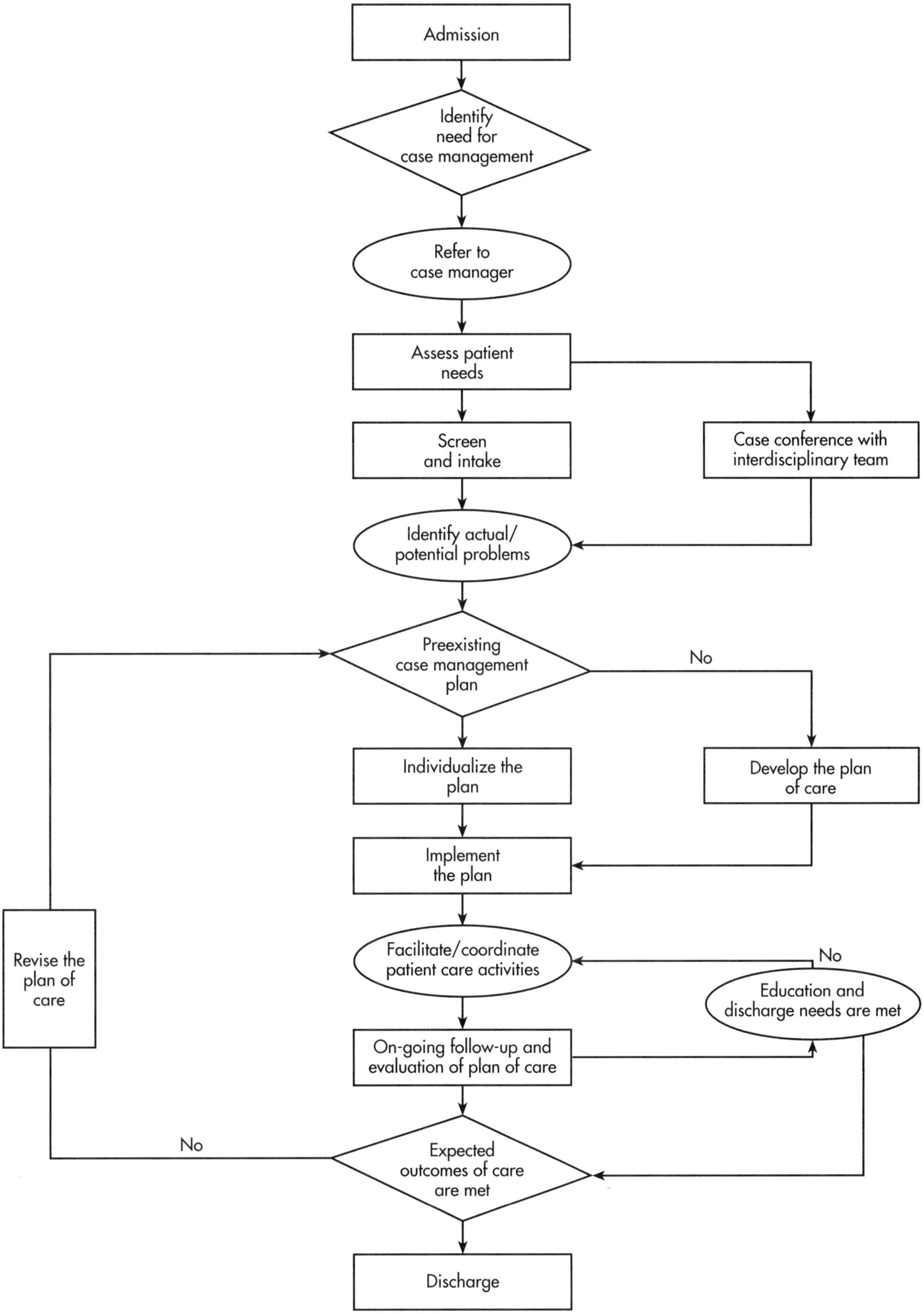

Fig. 4-1 Flow diagram: the case management process.

---

box 4-1

Criteria for Case Management Services

This is a list of examples of criteria for referral and/or acceptance of patients for case management services. It is not an exhaustive list. However, hospitals may adopt some of these criteria into their guidelines.

GENERIC CRITERIA

1. Physiological instability
2. Inability to assume self-care due to physical dependencies and/or neurological status
3. Mobility impairment/disability
4. Lack of support from significant other
5. History of noncompliance with medical/surgical regimen (e.g., medications, follow-up)
6. Pain management problems
7. Complexity of diagnosis
8. Fluctuating emotional status
9. Problem/complications prone
10. Involvement of several disciplines in the care
11. Multiple readmissions in a short period of time
12. Complex discharge, need for placement in a particular facility
13. Need for intensive health care education of patient/family
14. Death and dying, hospice care
15. Belong to managed care insurance companies
16. Medicare and Medicaid carrier
17. Financial risk to the hospital (i.e., inadequate health care coverage/financial support)
18. At risk for prolonged length of stay
19. Required treatment in various care settings in one hospitalization (e.g., intensive care unit, telemetry, regular unit)
20. Preexisting problems accessing health care
21. Noncompliance with medical/surgical regimen

SERVICE/UNIT-SPECIFIC CRITERIA
Emergency Department/Clinic

1. Homelessness
2. Lack of primary care physician

3. Inconsistency in medical follow-up
4. Requiring admission into the hospital
5. Multiple visits in a short period of time

Neonate/Pediatric

1. Age
2. Chronic illness (e.g., asthma, croup, HIV/AIDS)
3. Prematurity
4. Vaccination
5. Child abuse

Obstetric/Gynecology

1. First pregnancy
2. First baby, multiple newborns
3. High risk/complicated pregnancy (e.g., gestational diabetes, preeclampsia)
4. No prenatal follow-up

Geriatric

1. Requiring placement in a nursing home
2. Dementia/Alzheimer's disease
3. Frail elderly
4. No social support system
5. Elderly abuse

Intensive Care Unit(s)

1. Ventilator dependency/weaning
2. Organ transplant
3. Multisystem failure

Regular Unit

1. Diagnosis specific (e.g., stroke, heart failure)
2. First-time diagnosis

---

cussion with the referring personnel. It is then determined whether the patient meets any of the selection criteria for case management. When the intake decision is made, the nurse case manager flags the medical record identifying that the patient is accepted for case management services and writes an intake note in the patient's record.

Assessment of Needs of the Patient and Family

Once the nurse case manager has identified patients who meet the predetermined selection criteria, a case management assessment must take place. This assessment is comprehensive and covers a wide range of areas, including the following:

- The chief complaint that required the patient to seek medical attention

- The physical, mental, spiritual, and psychosocial status of the patient
- The health care insurance coverage and, when needed, whether the patient's admission has been approved (i.e., **precertification**) by the managed care organization
- The patient's social support systems and coping mechanisms
- Adjustment to illness and hospitalization
- The health education needs of the patient and family
- The projected discharge planning needs
- The resources required for caring for the patient and family

The assessment data that nurse case managers collect and analyze fall into two important categories, *sub-*

Effective Interviewing of Patients and Families

1. Introduce yourself, indicating your full name, your title and responsibility, and what you prefer to be called.
2. Inform the patient and family of the reasons of your visit.
3. Make them aware of what you can do to help them survive and cope well with the current episode of illness.
4. Review the medical record before you approach the patient.
5. Discuss the reasons for case management services with the person referring the patient before you conduct the interview.
6. Obtain as much information as possible about the patient and family before you interview them.
7. During the interview, ask open-ended questions to obtain an appropriate history of the problem/chief complaint. Also, ask direct questions based on the needs you may have identified during the chart review and the discussion with the person who referred the patient.
8. Maintain privacy and confidentiality during the interview.
9. Obtain information related to the patient's social support system, health care insurance coverage, education needs, and needs after discharge. These questions are important in evaluating appropriateness for case management services.
10. Discuss with the patient and family the next step(s) regarding the plan of care and case management.
11. Provide the patient and family, in writing (e.g., on a business card), your name and how you can be reached.

jective and *objective.* The information told by the patient and family makes the subjective data. It is related to the chief complaint and the history of the problem(s) that made the patient seek medical attention in a clinic or an emergency department, or it is the reason for hospitalization. Nurse case managers should be careful when interpreting such data because of its subjectivity. Objective data, however, include the physical exam, laboratory test results, and other diagnostic tests. The objective data are important because they help validate the subjective data and interpret the patient's history more accurately by providing a basis for comparison.

The subjective and objective information nurse case managers collect when interviewing the patient and family, the physical exam, and the laboratory tests make the assessment **database,** which is necessary for better identification of the patient's actual and potential problems. The goal of the "assessment of needs" step of the case management process is to gather and record information that is most helpful in designing the most appropriate plan of care for the individual patient.

Assessment data collection can be extensive, and some of it may not be necessary at times. Nurse case-managers may limit the type of assessment data they collect by answering the following questions. What data should be collected? How should data be collected? How should data be organized for better care planning decisions?

Nurse case managers may elect not to perform a physical assessment of the patient. However, they should review the medical record, particularly the admission history and assessment completed by the primary nurse and the physician. The assessment of needs requires collecting and synthesizing data from multiple sources

across providers and various care settings and/or services, including the patient and family (Strassner, 1996). The initial encounter of the nurse case manager with the patient and family is the beginning of an unwritten contract (Newell, 1996) that dictates the rest of the relationship. It is also essential to the case management process because it helps establish rapport and promote trust in the relationship. This is maximized through the nurse case manager's professional attitude and effective and skillful communication and interviewing techniques. Performing an assessment of needs that is accurate and relevant to the patient's presenting problem(s) requires nurse case managers to possess interviewing and technical skills that are invaluable (Case Manager's Tip 4-1).

Identification of Actual and Potential Problems

A thorough assessment of the needs of the patient and family provides the basis for identifying the actual and potential problems (i.e., nursing diagnoses). Identifying these problems dictates the types of interventions and treatments necessary to achieve the desired outcomes. Accurate and comprehensive identification of these problems has a significant effect on the quality of care, incurred cost, course of care, and length of stay. Nurse case managers are always advised to seek the collaboration of the interdisciplinary team and the patient and family in identifying the actual and potential problems. This strategy improves outcomes and promotes agreement on the plan of care and increases consistency and continuity in the provision of care among the various disciplines involved.

Regardless of the patient's clinical condition, nurse case managers should always identify any needs/ problems the patient and family may have related to health care teaching, discharge planning, and social support systems. The earlier such problems are identified, the sooner they are incorporated into the plan of care. This results in better control over the length of stay and ensures that patients' needs are met. It also expedites the process of resolving the problems.

During the time nurse case managers identify the patient's problems, they elect to reassess the patient's needs to validate uncertain or incomplete areas that existed in the previous assessment. It is important for nurse case managers to be certain of the patient's needs before finalizing the problems list or sharing it with members of the interdisciplinary team.

Interdisciplinary Care Planning

Interdisciplinary care planning helps establish a seamless approach to patient care. It requires the involvement of members of the various disciplines to be caring for the patient. In addition, it is important to involve the patient and family. The first task in this step of the case management process is case conferencing. The nurse case manager presents the findings of the assessment of patient's needs and the identified actual and potential problems to the interdisciplinary team. The team then prioritizes the patient problems, selects appropriate intervention/treatment modalities to resolve these problems, and establishes the expected outcomes of care. During this discussion the plan of care is developed.

A care plan that is interdisciplinary in nature and well developed helps decrease the risk of incomplete tasks or incorrect/inappropriate care. It also provides a seamless approach to care that supports the standards of care of regulatory agencies such as the Joint Commission on Accreditation of Healthcare Organizations (JCAHO). Such plan gives direction to all the disciplines involved in the care of the patient, opens the lines of communication among these disciplines and the patient and family, and ensures continuity and consistency of the care provided.

During this step of the case management process, nurse case managers establish the goals of treatment and the projected/desired outcomes of care. It is important to establish these goals and desired outcomes in collaboration with members of the interdisciplinary team. Interdisciplinary approach to setting the goals and expected outcomes is the key to cost-effective and quality care.

With their assessment skills, clinical expertise, and holistic approach to patient care, nurse case managers ensure that a comprehensive interdisciplinary plan of care is developed and that it is succinct with the patient's and family's goals. They also verify that it contains the identified patient's actual and potential problems, the mutually identified and agreed-on goals with the interdisciplinary team members and the patient and family, the required patient care activities that reflect all the involved disciplines (specifically the nursing interventions and medical treatment), and the preventive measures for complications or undesired outcomes. In addition, the plan should always include patient and family teaching and discharge planning components (McNeese-Smith et al, 1996; Tahan, 1993).

The interdisciplinary plan of care developed is the **case management plan** (CMP) to be followed by all disciplines in the care of individual patients. If a CMP (specific to the patient's diagnosis/procedure) already exists, the nurse case manager presents it to the interdisciplinary team during case conferencing for review and individualization to meet the patient's and family's needs. The CMP then becomes the tool used to identify, monitor, and evaluate the treatments and interventions and the care activities and outcomes. It is constantly evaluated and revised to reflect the changing needs of the patient and family.

Planning an appropriate patient's course of care is a skill required by nurse case managers. To be effective in their role, they should be knowledgeable in the available hospital and community resources necessary for the care of patients, the various care settings, management of resources, cost, and reimbursement (Strassner, 1996), and be clinical astutes.

Implementation of the Interdisciplinary Plan of Care

In this step of the case management process, the interdisciplinary plan of care/CMP is put into action. Each member of the interdisciplinary team ensures that his or her responsibilities, as indicated in the CMP, are met within the projected time frames. Implementation encompasses all the interventions (medical, nursing, and others) that are directed toward meeting the preestablished goals, resolving the patient's problems, and meeting the patient's health care needs and predetermined care outcomes.

Reassessment skills possessed by nurse case managers are the key to success in this role. When reassessing the patient and the care, nurse case managers usually answer some questions such as the following:

- Does the patient have any new needs?
- Does the interdisciplinary plan of care/CMP meet the patient needs?
- Does it need to be revised?
- Are the projected patient care activities indicated in the CMP appropriate and timely?
- Is it possible that patient problems be resolved during this episode of care?

- What is the appropriate time frame for resolving the identified problems?

Answers to these questions help case managers to confirm that the planned interventions remain appropriate to the patient's condition and projected/desired outcomes. When they identify any problems, they are responsible for bringing them to the attention of the interdisciplinary team, discussing them, recommending necessary changes in the CMP, and ensuring that the plan is revised to meet the patient's latest condition.

Nurse case managers are pivotal in facilitating and coordinating patient care activities. They informally direct the work of the interdisciplinary team members in an effort to promote cost-effective and appropriate care and to ensure that services are provided in a timely manner.

Nurse case managers facilitate and coordinate patient care activities related to required tests, procedures, and treatments; patient and family teaching; and discharge planning and the need for community resources. They are responsible for confirming that tests, procedures, treatments, and interventions coincide with those recommended in the CMP and that they are scheduled and completed in a timely fashion. They also make certain that changes in these activities are dictated by the patient's condition and are not arbitrary.

Nurse case managers act as **gatekeepers** of the interdisciplinary teams they belong to. With their continuous follow-up on the implementation of the patient care activities and evaluation of outcomes and reassessment of the patient's condition and needs, they keep all the interventions in order and ensure that what is supposed to occur is taking place. They may remind members of the team of any incomplete or inaccurate activities; expedite tests and procedures; and eliminate or prevent any fragmentation, duplication, or unnecessary services. When nurse case managers identify delays, variations, or deviations in the care from the CMP, they immediately act on the issue and attempt to correct it.

Because of their understanding of the total picture of the care of the patient, they are invaluable in coordinating the scheduling of the different tests and procedures required for a patient's workup and treatment. They ensure that these tests or procedures are not scheduled at the same time. Their careful attention to such situations prevents the occurrence of any delays, duplication, or fragmentation of care. Nurse case managers are also instrumental in facilitating timely reporting of results of the tests and procedures. This function allows the interdisciplinary health care team to make timely decisions pertaining to the appropriateness of care, to change interventions and treatments to more

effective ones as indicated by the clinical status of patients and supported by objective data (i.e., results of tests and procedures), and to validate that the recommended patient care activities outlined in the CMP or interdisciplinary plan of care are achieved in a timely fashion.

Facilitating and coordinating the patient and family teaching activities are important functions of nurse case managers. They are able to manage these activities efficiently and effectively because of their extensive knowledge of the health care system, their clinical experience and skills, and their familiarity with the adult learning theory and the health-belief model. Nurse case managers may be directly or indirectly involved in patient and family teaching. They are more likely to be directly involved in teaching in situations such as the following:

- Patients with complex diagnoses that lead to complicated teaching needs (e.g., patients with multiple problems such as chronic renal failure, diabetes, hypertension, and heart failure). Patients with such conditions require intensive teaching plans. Nurse case managers may elect to develop such plans in collaboration with the interdisciplinary team, including the patient and family and the primary nurse. They may conduct some teaching sessions pertaining to specific topics or needs (e.g., insulin self-injection) or supervise and/or ensure the completion of teaching activities related to other topics (disease process, signs and symptoms, or medications) by the primary nurse or other members of the interdisciplinary health care team.

- Patients with multiple admissions in a short period of time. These patients may have problems that are beyond the understanding of the disease process and signs and symptoms. After careful assessment of the patient's and family's teaching needs, nurse case managers may find that the real problems of repeated admissions are lack of consistent clinic follow-up, noncompliance with the medical/surgical regimen, or an inappropriate social support system. In such situations, active involvement of the nurse case manager is highly essential. The nurse case manager then concentrates on the real issue and works closely with the patient and family to prevent readmission to the hospital and improve compliance with the treatment.

The role of patient and family educator can be challenging to most nurse case managers as hospital **length of stay** decreases and patient acuity increases, and the shift to providing health care services in the home and ambulatory settings is becoming more popular. This role is important in maximizing patient care outcomes, minimizing cost, and promoting the patient/family independence in care (McNeese-Smith et al, 1996). Nurse case managers can function as role models and experts in patient teaching to primary nurses and other members of the health care team. Their responsibility toward patient and family teaching starts at the time of admission in assessing the teaching needs and initiating the teaching plan that helps meet these needs. They also coordinate the teaching activities, based on the plan, to be completed by the different members of the health care team including the primary nurse.

The patient and family education role requires nurse case managers to be astute in assessing patient teaching needs and readiness, identifying any existing barriers and limitations to teaching, and selecting the appropriate methodology. They are also required to be sensitive to the patient condition, culture, values, and belief system. Nurse case managers should demonstrate competency in how to incorporate these factors into the patient and family teaching plan and help members of the interdisciplinary team choose the most effective method and plan for teaching.

Nurse case managers are key people in effective discharge planning. They play an important role in coordinating and facilitating the patient's discharge. Their role in discharge planning starts with admission of the patient to the hospital, or at the time the patient seeks medical attention, and during the first encounter with the patient and family. They are responsible for assessing the patient's needs for safe and appropriate discharge and coordinating the process of getting these services approved and perhaps instituted before the patient is discharged.

Nurse case managers collaborate with the patient and family, physician, primary nurse, social worker, home care planner, and other members of the health care team in establishing the patient's most appropriate discharge plan and work closely with them to achieve this plan. Nurse case managers update and revise the plan as needed based on their ongoing reassessment of the patient's condition and needs. They also discuss and communicate any changes in the discharge plan to the members of the team during case-conference meetings.

Facilitation and coordination of discharge planning activities may require nurse case managers to communicate with external services such as medical equipment providers or home care agencies. They may also need to contact **managed care** organizations to obtain certification for the postdischarge services required by patients. These functions demand that nurse case managers be skillful in negotiation techniques and brokerage of services. They also need to possess excellent communication skills and be knowledgeable in managed care contracts, entitlements, federal and **third-party payors,** reimbursement, regulations, policies, and the variety of available community services and agencies. Seasoned case managers can be found to have established successful business relationships with key people in the different agencies they contact on a regular basis. Such relationships are instrumental in providing nurse case managers with a wide networking circle and expediting the process of approving/certifying discharge services.

Evaluation of Patient Care Outcomes

In the evaluation of the patient care outcomes step of the case management process, nurse case managers evaluate the effectiveness of the interdisciplinary plan of care/CMP and the patient care activities and outcomes. They are also responsible, in collaboration with members of the interdisciplinary health care team, to continuously monitor the patient's condition, responses to interventions, and progress toward recovery. Ongoing communication with the health care team regarding the appropriateness of the plan of care in relation to the patient's changing condition and needs, and whether the plan is realistic, is important for timely revision of the plan and implementation of new interventions and treatments.

When evaluating patient care, nurse case managers should answer the following questions:
- Were the patient care activities accurate and timely?
- Were the goals of the patient and family and the health care team accomplished?
- Have the patient and family needs been met?
- Has the patient's condition progressed toward recovery, deteriorated, or remained the same?
- Which interventions or treatments need to be changed or added?
- Should patient care outcomes, activities, and/or goals be reprioritized?

Answers to these questions by the interdisciplinary team members at case conferences or by nurse case managers when reviewing medical records and evaluating the appropriateness of patient care activities and outcomes help the health care team remain focused and make timely revisions to the plan of care. This function of nurse case managers is important in ensuring that high-quality and cost-effective care is delivered at all times.

Nurse case managers are responsible for monitoring and evaluating **variances** of care on a continuing basis. They identify and track deviations from the CMP (i.e., variances of care) as they relate to the patient (e.g., refusal of test or procedure, deterioration in condition), practitioner (e.g., medication errors, delay in scheduling or performing a certain test, visiting nurse not showing up), or the system (e.g., unable to complete a test because the machine is broken, no physical therapy available on weekends, managed care organization not certifying/approving home care services) (see Chapter 11 for more detailed discussion on variances). They also keep members of the interdisciplinary health care team well informed of the presence/occurrence of variances and together attempt to resolve these variances. Early detection and resolution of such variances are essential to prevent complications or undesired outcomes, delays in the length of stay, increased cost, and deterioration in patient and family satisfaction.

Nurse case managers are also made accountable for evaluating the fiscal, quality, and clinical outcomes of care (Strassner, 1996). These outcomes are interrelated, and a deficit in one usually affects the others negatively. *Fiscal outcomes* are those related to the organizational goals rather than the patient's health. Examples of fiscal outcomes are cost and revenue of care, resource use, length of stay, inappropriate admissions, and system-related variances. However, traditional *quality outcomes* have been those directly related to a patient's health and functioning. Examples of quality outcomes are nosocomial infection rates, independence, health perception, readmissions, inappropriate discharges, complications, and patient and family satisfaction. Moreover, *clinical outcomes* are those directly related to patient care activities, identified proactively by members of the interdisciplinary team and included in the CMP, and expected to be achieved while caring for the patient and family. Some examples are the intermediate and discharge outcomes (see Chapter 11). Through timely facilitation and coordination of patient care activities, patient and family teaching, and discharge planning, nurse case managers are able to maintain a delicate balance of these outcomes.

While monitoring and evaluating care; reviewing medical records; or communicating with the patient and family, primary nurses, members of the interdisciplinary team, and ancillary departments, nurse case managers continually collect data related to variances and outcomes of care. They then aggregate the data based on similarities in issues and diagnoses, conduct a trending and analysis review, and finally generate reports to be shared with appropriate personnel (e.g., quality improvement department, case management department, interdisciplinary team members, chiefs of services/ departments [nursing, medical, and ancillary], and administration). Nurse case managers are instrumental in

their feedback related to the critical issues, particularly system problems that require administrative attention and initiation of quality improvement task forces for resolution.

Throughout the evaluation of patient care outcomes step of the case management process, nurse case managers exhibit certain skills that are essential to the role. These skills are problem solving, decision making, critical thinking, quality improvement, leadership abilities, networking, partnership, collaboration, communication and feedback, and negotiation. It is through these effective skills that case managers are able to make a difference in patient care management and to meet the goals of the case management model and the organization.

Patient's Discharge and Disposition

It is important for case managers to bring their relationship with the patient and family to closure. Discontinuation of case management services, whether it is due to the patient's discharge from the hospital or because case management services are deemed no longer required by the patient, is the last step in the case management process. During this phase case managers hold a "case-closing" conference with the patient and family and the interdisciplinary team, during which the plan of care is evaluated for its completion, particularly the appropriateness of the discharge plan and the effectiveness of patient and family teaching. This is the time when nurse case managers confirm that all postdischarge services required by the patient are in place and the necessary paperwork is completed. If a problem is identified, it should be resolved before the time of the patient's discharge.

Nurse case managers ensure that all discharge activities are completed effectively before the time of discharge. They evaluate the patient's readiness by making sure that the **discharge outcomes** are met and that all the required interdisciplinary activities have been successfully achieved. It is essential to answer the patient's and family's last questions regarding care after discharge and provide them with emotional support. Sometimes it is helpful for them to have the nurse case manager's phone number; this is a safety or reassurance mechanism for patients and families that reduces their anxiety and fear of discharge. It is also important for case managers to provide them with written instructions pertaining to the care after discharge and the scheduled follow-up appointment(s).

Some institutions require case managers to make follow-up phone calls to the patients after discharge and evaluate their level of functioning and adherence to the medical regimen and follow-up and to answer any questions if they exist. This practice may prevent readmissions of patients for the same problems (chief complaint or diagnosis). It also increases the patient's and family's satisfaction and faith in the institution.

Repeating the Case Management Process

Nurse case managers usually repeat the case management process every time they are in contact with the patient and family. This function is not considered a true or direct step in the case management process. Reassessment of patients, ongoing evaluation of patient care activities and outcomes, and constant checking and ensuring that care is delivered as scheduled in a timely fashion are all examples of tasks that require going through the steps of the case management process. Nurse case managers are constantly repeating the process.

Repeating the case management process is one way of ensuring that the provision of care is appropriate, the quality is not compromised in the name of cost containment, and the patient is discharged safely. Nurse case managers have the opportunity and obligation to repeat the case management process every time a task is not completed effectively, a delay in any care activity is identified, or an expected outcome is not met. When repeating the process, they implement new interventions and activities to resolve the identified problem(s). Repeating the case management process functions as a safety net for ensuring that appropriate care is delivered and as a method for developing an action plan for problem solving.

Various Roles Played by Nurse Case Managers

Nurse case managers are involved in many different situations throughout the day. They may provide a patient and/or a family with care instructions and may teach staff members about new trends in patient care. They may also ensure approval/**certification** of services by managed care organizations or negotiate home care services with an agency. The varied scope of roles, functions, and activities they may provide increases their challenge for ensuring that high-quality and cost-effective care has been delivered.

This wide range of responsibilities requires nurse case managers to put more than one role or function into action at the same time. The interrelatedness of these roles is the key to success. Nurse case managers may be found assessing or reassessing patients while monitoring and evaluating outcomes. They may be scheduling a test while trying to resolve delays related to tests or procedures. Their various roles are important for timely patient care delivery and outcomes. The various responsibilities and roles of nurse case managers and their ongoing planning and prioritization of the tasks to be completed require them to be astute in time management, which is integral to the effectiveness of their role (Case Manager's Tips 4-2 and 4-3).

Clinical Expert

Nurse case managers are chosen for their role because of extensive clinical experience and knowledge of pa-

case manager's tip 4-2 — **Time Wasters Nurse Case Managers Should Avoid**

1. Lack of ongoing prioritization and planning
2. Unrealistic goals and time estimates
3. Overambition and desire to impress boss
4. Inattentiveness and insufficient communication and feedback
5. Tendency to be perfectionists
6. Confusion over responsibilities, functions, and boundaries
7. Insecurity, fear of failure, and lack of confidence and self-esteem
8. Failure to follow up on incomplete tasks
9. Ego and feeling of overimportance
10. Sense of unnecessary obligation
11. Inability to say *No* when needed
12. Failure to obtain important information when it is required to do so, or collecting unnecessary information
13. Being an extra "pair of hands" to everyone
14. Inability to delegate
15. Treating every problem as a crisis (overreaction)
16. Procrastination
17. Leaving tasks unfinished
18. Being unaware of importance of things
19. Socializing

tient care. They bring excellence in clinical practice to the role (Case Manager's Tip 4-4). They act as role models and resources to nursing and other staff members. They exhibit clinical competence in the assessment of patient and family needs; establishing the actual and potential health problems, goals for treatment, and desired outcomes; applying the nursing process; planning, implementing, evaluating, and coordinating the care activities to meet the patient and family goals and expected outcomes; using advanced treatment modalities and technologies; and dealing with patients as biopsychosocial systems with the treatment plan directed toward the system as a whole rather than just the disease.

Consultant

Because of their clinical experience and knowledge of the institutional operations/systems, policies and procedures, and standards of care and practice, nurse case managers can be called on as consultants by physicians, nurses, and other case managers and members of the interdisciplinary team. They are helpful in solving clinical and administrative issues when members of the interdisciplinary team are in doubt.

Nurse case managers, particularly those who work in an ambulatory care setting, may provide telephone consultations to managed care organizations or other health care insurance companies, patients and families, and home care agencies.

---

case manager's tip 4-3   **Strategies for Effective Time Management**

1. Set objectives, goals, priorities, and deadlines.
2. Use "to do" lists for the day. List activities in order of priorities/importance based on the number of tasks to be completed. Update your list constantly. Keep your priority list current.
3. Distinguish the urgent from the truly important.
4. Delegate the activities and tasks that can be delegated.
5. Avoid being a perfectionist. Lower your standards to what is reasonable and acceptable.
6. Communicate effectively.
7. Collect appropriate data and necessary information only. Determine what is needed for planning activities, making decisions, and providing feedback.
8. Clarify with your boss your job responsibilities, power, and boundaries.
9. Constantly check progress and follow up on unfinished tasks.
10. Refuse to spread yourself too thin. Say *No,* give reasons, and provide alternatives. You may say, "Sorry, I cannot. I do not have the time, but I have a suggestion . . ." or "Thanks for the compliment, but I am afraid I have to decline."
11. Make no assumptions, and avoid being critical.
12. Recognize that things may take longer to complete than planned. Accept this fact. Impose realistic deadlines on tasks.
13. Seek the help and guidance of your superior as needed. Avoid struggling uncertainties on your own.
14. Avoid socializing, distractions, or unnecessary interruptions.
15. Respect deadlines. Avoid procrastination.

---

case manager's tip 4-4   **Maintaining Clinical Expertise**

1. Become a member in professional organizations and/or nursing societies.
2. Subscribe to journals that pertain to clinical practice.
3. Stay abreast of the health care literature and the changes in technology.
4. Attend organization-base continuing education sessions.
5. Participate in conferences, particularly those related to case management.
6. Seek the help of other experts when faced with a situation that is uncertain or unfamiliar.
7. Make every effort to learn new skills and gain new knowledge when opportunities arise.
8. Participate in clinical activities such as case study presentation, case conference, or clinical research.
9. Spend some time in the library (at least 1 hour a week) searching for new knowledge.
10. Attend medical staff/student teaching rounds.
11. Seek higher nursing education.

case
manager's
tip
4-5   **Strategies for Better Patient Care Management**

1. Maintain constant knowledge of the patient's plan of care. Update your information as indicated by changes in the patient's condition.
2. Prevent delays in patient care activities.
3. Ensure that tests and procedures are prescheduled.
4. Obtain timely results of tests and procedures, and adjust plan of care accordingly.
5. Become knowledgeable of the contracts of managed care companies and federal and third-party reimbursement procedures.
6. Encourage patient's timely discharge.
7. Maximize the use of outpatient testing and same day of admission procedures.
8. Communicate with the interdisciplinary team on an ongoing basis.
9. Ensure the involvement of the members of the interdisciplinary team in patient care–related decisions and problem solving.
10. Maximize the involvement of the patient and family in such decisions.
11. Prevent redundancy, duplication, or fragmentation of patient care activities.
12. Eliminate any unnecessary or inappropriate tests or procedures.
13. Seek administrative support as needed.
14. Seek the guidance of experts when uncertain of a particular situation.

Coordinator and Facilitator of Patient Care

Nurse case managers spend a great deal of their day coordinating and facilitating patient care activities and expediting the completion of tests and procedures. They also ensure that results of the tests and procedures are available within a reasonable turn-around time. This function is important in reducing length of stay and eliminating delays and variances in patient care activities. In collaboration with members of the health care team, they help patients move smoothly and safely through the hospital system.

In this role function, nurse case managers prevent any fragmentation or duplication in the provision of care. Their timely intervention when a patient's condition changes increases the efficiency and effectiveness of care. They coordinate the patient's teaching and discharge plans and ensure that all discharge activities are completed in a timely fashion to prevent unnecessary hospital stay. This role is important in controlling the use of resources and containing cost.

Manager of Patient Care

Nurse case managers function as patient care managers through controlling the use of resources to what is required to achieve the desired outcomes. They act as gatekeepers of the interdisciplinary team to ensure that all patient care activities are accomplished by each team member within the projected time frames. One of their main responsibilities is direct supervision of the process of patient care to ensure quality outcomes. Case Manager's Tip 4-5 lists some strategies for managing patient care.

Educator

The role of educator is twofold. Nurse case managers are involved in patient and family education and staff education. Regarding patient and family, they ensure that all health care needs are met within a reasonable time frame during the hospital stay. They usually incorporate the teaching plan as part of the CMP as early as the time of admission. They may provide direct patient teaching activities or supervise the way they are completed by the primary nurses and/or other team members. Nurse case managers may also be involved in developing patient and family teaching materials and planning and conducting patient teaching classes (Case Manager's Tip 4-6).

Regarding nursing and other staff members, nurse case managers are instrumental in mentoring the less-experienced staff. They participate in inservice sessions related to case management and new trends and advances in patient care. Their staff teaching activities may be done as unit-based sessions or formal classes planned and held in collaboration with staff education departments. Either way, they are actively involved in the dissemination of new patient care knowledge.

Negotiator/Broker

Among the other roles assumed by nurse case managers is the role of negotiator and broker of care. They are instrumental in getting necessary tests and procedures completed on time. They also negotiate the best treatment plan possible with the health care team, patient and family, and most importantly the managed care organization. Nurse case managers also negotiate with

case manager's tip 4-6   Strategies for Effective Patient/Family Education

1. Educate patients and families only when they are ready.
2. Identify the barriers or limitations to learning before you conduct a patient's education session.
3. Maximize the family's/caregiver's involvement.
4. Use visual aids such as handouts, drawings, audiotapes, and videotapes.
5. Ensure the need for low-level reading skills, at the same time avoiding being "cutesy." If that is the case, adult learners might feel insulted.
6. Apply the concepts of adult learning theory in your teaching sessions/activities.
7. Encourage the patient's/family's participation in the decision-making process regarding learning needs.
8. Include return demonstrations or verbalization of material taught.
9. Adapt the teaching strategy to the patient's level of understanding, capabilities, or preferences.
10. Involve other professionals (e.g., pharmacists, staff nurses, clinical nurse specialists) in educating patients/families.
11. Limit the material to be taught to what the patient is able to grasp in one session.
12. If possible, schedule the next teaching session with the patient/family.
13. Evaluate the ability of the patient/family to retain the information taught.
14. Be consistent in the information provided, especially if other professionals are involved in teaching or reinforcing patient/family education.
15. Put special emphasis on the care needs of patients after discharge.
16. Conduct small group education sessions when appropriate.
17. Allow for questions and answers.
18. Avoid the use of medical jargon. Speak a language the patient understands.
19. Clearly indicate the patient's teaching plan in the medical record.

health care agencies for community services, such as home care, needed for patients' support after discharge from the hospital. In addition, they negotiate with managed care companies for approval of the patient's hospitalization, the need for durable medical equipment, or the necessary services needed after discharge. Case Manager's Tip 4-7 lists strategies for effective negotiation.

Patient and Family Advocate

One of the important responsibilities of case managers is the patient and family advocacy (Case Manager's Tip 4-8). Case managers assume a liaison role between the patient and family and the health care team. With their relationship with the patient and family at the time of admission, nurse case managers are able to build trust and establish rapport to help facilitate the implementation of the plan of care. They keep the patient and family constantly informed of the plan of care, tests and procedures, and condition, which makes them the best vehicle through which the care is advocated, negotiated, agreed on, facilitated, and coordinated.

Nurse case managers advocate for patients in case conferences and health care team meetings held throughout the patient's hospitalization, during which they communicate the needs and wishes of the patient and family. They also advocate for the patient when ne-

gotiating with agencies for community services or informing them of a patient's care needs after discharge.

Outcomes and Quality Manager

Monitoring and evaluation of patient care quality and outcomes are integral to the role of nurse case managers. They are important because they link case management to quality improvement and evaluate whether the patient and organizational goals are met. Nurse case managers monitor the occurrence of variances and outcomes of care as they relate to the CMP. The results of this monitoring process are essential in providing data for quality improvement efforts and in evaluating the effectiveness and efficiency of the case management model and the use of CMPs. Nurse case managers also participate in investigating the reasons of variances and attempt to resolve them as soon as they are identified.

Nurse case managers communicate variances, delays, and undesired patient care outcomes to members of the interdisciplinary health care team so that the team can revise the CMP as necessary. Together as a team, they are better able to convince administration of the need for quality improvement task forces to have a closer look at certain system issues, particularly those that require immediate attention. Case Manager's Tip 4-9 lists actions to help improve patient care quality.

case manager's tip   4-7   Successful Negotiation

The strategies discussed in this section could be applied when the nurse case manager negotiates services with outside agencies, physicians, consultants, and professional and ancillary staff, as well as when attempting to facilitate and coordinate patient care activities and prevent delays in patient care within and outside the boundaries of the institution.

1. Separate people from positions.
2. Negotiate for agreements—not winning or losing.
3. Establish mutual trust and respect.
4. Avoid one-sided or personal gains.
5. Allow time for expressing the interests of each side/party.
6. Listen actively during the process, and acknowledge what is being said.
7. Use data/evidence to strengthen your position.
8. Focus on interests—patient care interests.
9. Always remember that the process is a problem-solving one, and the benefit is for the patient and family.
10. Never forget that patient care is the priority.
11. Avoid using pressure.
12. Be knowledgeable of the institutional policies, procedures, systems, standards, and the law. Apply this knowledge in the process.
13. Try to understand the other side well. Ask questions and seek clarifications when unsure or uncertain.
14. Avoid emotional outbursts. Do not overreact if the other party exhibits such behavior.
15. Avoid premature judgments.
16. Be concrete and flexible when presenting your stand.
17. Use reason and be reasonable.
18. Be fair.

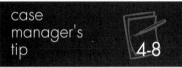

case manager's tip   4-8   Advocating Effectively for Patients/Families

1. Know the plan of care of your patients well, including the minute details.
2. Spend enough time discussing the care with the patient and family, and understand their concerns.
3. Be familiar with the patient's bill of rights.
4. Be knowledgeable of the law and the standards of regulatory agencies regarding certain patient care issues such as informed consent and do not resuscitate.
5. Be honest with the patient and family. Admit when you do not know the answers to their questions.
6. Convey patient/family concerns to the appropriate personnel, obtain answers, and report results back to the patient and family.
7. Identify ethical dilemmas and refer them to the ethics committee in a timely fashion.
8. Provide the patient and family with emotional support as needed. Alleviate their anxieties and apprehension.

Scientist/Researcher

Research has been made a part of the nurse case manager's role in institutions where the required educational background of case managers is Master's Degree in Nursing. In this role, nurse case managers are expected to participate as active members of institution-based research committees. They are also expected to write grant and research proposals, collect research data, and evaluate patient care activities. They are excellent at nursing knowledge development and dissemination and research utilization. Nurse case managers help nursing departments establish a research-based clinical practice,

policies, procedures, and standards of care. Case Manager's Tip 4-10 lists some strategies to help in becoming involved in research.

Risk Manager

Because of their proximity to the bedside and involvement in direct patient care activities, nurse case managers are at the forefront of identifying patient care issues that are considered legal risk. They are good at ensuring that the care delivered is in compliance with the standards of regulatory agencies, such as the U.S. Department of Health and the JCAHO, and the internal/

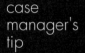

case manager's tip   4-9

Strategies for Improving Patient Care Quality

1. Focus on the process, not the people.
2. Listen to the patient and family concerns.
3. Identify patient care problems (variances and delays) early and attempt to resolve them in a timely fashion.
4. Attend as an interdisciplinary team, rather than individually, to the patient problems.
5. Keep lines of communication open at all levels. Discuss the issues as they arise with the patient/family, superiors, subordinates, and whoever is deemed appropriate.
6. Ensure that the desired/projected outcomes of care are met.
7. Ensure patient's safe discharge.
8. Provide care that is patient focused.
9. Attend customer-relations classes. Apply strategies learned to practice.
10. Obtain and read the results of patient satisfaction surveys and quality improvement monitors. Change behavior and practice as indicated by the results.
11. Conduct concurrent or retrospective chart reviews on an ongoing basis.

case manager's tip   4-10

Strategies for Getting Involved in Research

1. Learn the research process. Take courses in research or seek the help of research experts.
2. Apply research outcomes to practice.
3. Conduct research.
4. Obtain funding; write grants.
5. Participate in institutional research efforts—collect data, identify potential subjects, and so on.
6. Become a member of the research committee.
7. Get involved in research utilization and dissemination programs.

institution's policies, procedures, standards of care, and standards of practice. Their role in assessment and monitoring of the delivery of patient care activities and evaluation of outcomes makes them crucial in identifying risk management issues and bringing them to the attention of the legal department in a timely fashion.

Nurse case managers are able to establish a trusting relationship with the patient and family. Because of this relationship, they are able to prevent the problems from escalating and becoming potential legal risk issues (Case Manager's Tip 4-11). Their advocacy of patient care helps them reduce the seriousness of the problems and makes patients view them as "God-sent angels." They are also helpful to members of the health care team. They provide them with answers to their clinical dilemmas and act as resource people to the team when faced with administrative problems. Nurse case managers are excellent in this role because of their knowledge of the institution's administrative and clinical policies and procedures.

Change Agent

Nurse case managers are the *champions of change.* They are the most helpful change agents an institution may have while implementing a new case management model (Case Manager's Tip 4-12). Nurse case managers act as role models and resource people and experts in case management to all staff during the transition into case management and thereafter. They are knowledgeable in the subject matter, which makes them well versed in case management and able to educate other staff members such as physicians, staff nurses, and ancillary staff.

In their training, nurse case managers are prepared to handle resistance to change and resistant people. Their coaching, mentoring, and teaching approach to staff when facing resistance makes them able to conquer the problems. They are well aware that resistance is a normal method some people choose to follow when experiencing change. Their professional and mature approach to such situations makes it easier to convince staff to support the change. Nurse case managers are

case manager's tip 4-11

Reducing Legal Risk

1. Always know the law. Seek the help/advice of the legal and risk management department in your institution when uncertain.
2. Familiarize yourself with the standards of care and practice of regulatory agencies.
3. Familiarize yourself with institutional policies and procedures and standards of care and practice.
4. Refer to the experts or the available reference manuals when unsure of a situation or a decision.
5. Attend to problems immediately as they arise. Do not wait for them to escalate.
6. Do anything possible to prevent problems from occurring.
7. Advocate for patients/families as opportunities arise.
8. Know the details of the patient's bill of rights. Ensure that patients are also educated about their rights.
9. Obtain knowledge of the requirements of federal and third-party payors.
10. Understand well the managed care contracts and their impact and relation to patient care.
11. Monitor and observe patients constantly. Make sure you are aware of the latest changes in your patient's condition.
12. Communicate changes in the plan of care to the patient and family in a timely fashion.
13. Apply the scientific method to the development of CMPs.
14. Base CMPs on the latest therapies, research outcomes, expert opinion, and recommendations/standards of professional societies.
15. Use CMPs as standards of care. Develop and apply one CMP for each diagnosis or procedure.
16. Include a disclaimer in the CMP explaining that it is only a recommended treatment plan and needs to be individualized to the patient's needs when applied. For example, a disclaimer might read: *"This case management plan is a suggested interdisciplinary plan of care. It is a guideline that may be changed and individualized according to patient condition and needs."*

case manager's tip 4-12

Instituting Effective Change

1. Become familiar with change theories and processes.
2. Recognize and foster the attitude that change is inevitable.
3. Learn the goals and objectives of the change happening at your institution. Communicate them to all those involved.
4. Give special consideration to all the aspects of change: physical, emotional, conceptual, perceptual, individual, and organizational.
5. Acknowledge the fact that an organization cannot change unless all staff buy into the change.
6. Reduce turf battles.
7. Educate all staff about the change, reasons, goals, the new processes/systems, mission, and philosophy.
8. As a nurse case manager, act as a change agent, champion, coach, or mentor.
9. Identify and communicate the benefits of change.
10. Avoid surprises. Be as open as possible.
11. Keep lines of communication open. Invite questions, and provide answers.
12. Invite participation of all those interested. Encourage and support them in promoting the change.
13. Admit to difficulties.
14. Attend to those resistant to change. Investigate their reasons and concerns. Consider their recommendations for improving the situation.
15. Recognize and reward everybody's efforts regardless of their position in the organization or degree of participation. Every little effort is important.
16. Involve informal leaders and those who are powerful.
17. Maintain ongoing follow-up and reinforcement.
18. Establish/clarify new policies, procedures, and standards.
19. Establish an open forum for communication and dissemination of information.

also trained in problem solving, conflict resolution, and negotiation. These skills help improve their outlook on things and their strategies for preventing resistance. They also help them build a better response to staff concerns.

Nurse case managers are the main advocates for case management systems an institution is lucky to have. Their commitment to their role and their hard work make them successful and help them attain excellence in their practice.

case manager's tip 4-13 Providing Holistic Patient Care

1. Deal with the patient as a biopsychosocial being.
2. Develop an action plan that meets all of the patient's symptoms and needs rather than just the disease.
3. Attend not only to the patient's actual needs but also to the potential ones.
4. Educate the patient about health-promotion activities and strategies for risk reduction of diseases.
5. Promote a healthy life-style.
6. When dealing with the patient, do not forget about the family or the caregiver.
7. Evaluate the impact of the patient's illness on the patient-family system and relationship, not just the patient.
8. Encourage a healthy adjustment to illness (patient and family related).
9. Include health-promotion activities in the CMP.

case manager's tip 4-14 Effective Counseling

1. Evaluate the patient's and family's ability to cope with and respond and adjust to illness.
2. Alleviate anxieties and apprehension.
3. Address the patient's and family's spiritual, emotional, and psychological needs.
4. Conduct therapy sessions.
5. Communicate therapeutically.
6. Allow for questions; provide answers.
7. Attend to patient and family concerns.
8. Alleviate the patient's fears and concerns regarding care after discharge.

Holistic Care Provider

Nurse case managers attend to their patients as whole systems (i.e., biopsychosocial systems). They assess patients and families for any actual or potential health problems regardless of the chief complaint or the disease for which they are admitted to the hospital (Case Manager's Tip 4-13). They are savvy in their evaluation of the patient's condition; they identify the physical, psychological, and spiritual needs and make sure that these needs are incorporated into the CMP/interdisciplinary plan of care. For example, when a patient is admitted to the hospital for uncontrolled diabetes, case managers not only assess dietary habits, blood glucose levels, and compliance with insulin and follow-up visits but also assess the patient for complications of diabetes such as deficiency in vision and foot ulcers. They also assess footwear, skin care, support system, and adjustment to the disease.

Nurse case managers ensure that disease prevention and life-style changes are addressed with their patients and families during hospitalization. They work with them closely to identify the best strategies to improve compliance with medical/surgical regimen and disease risk reduction. For example, they may counsel a cardiac

patient on strategies for quitting smoking or drinking alcohol or beginning a physical exercise program. They may provide patients and families with important information regarding community services and support groups for the same purpose.

Counselor

Another characteristic in the role of nurse case managers is counseling and support of patients and families (Case Manager's Tip 4-14). Case managers are attentive to the emotional and spiritual needs of patients. They are astute at providing patients with emotional support, and they counsel them regarding adjustment to the hospitalization and their coping skills and mechanisms with the disease—particularly if they are suffering from a chronic disease that requires frequent hospitalization, such as cancer.

Nurse case managers may also work closely with victims of domestic violence and sexual and physical abuse. Their counseling skills and emotional support to these groups of patients are highly appreciated. They also ensure that these patients are well educated regarding availability of crisis teams and how they can be accessed, and they direct them to local agencies or support groups for further follow-up and support after discharge from the hospital.

In these various roles, functions, and responsibilities, it is highly important for nurse case managers to be able to work efficiently and effectively with the interdisciplinary team members. Teamwork is essential at all times and in all situations. In addition, nurse case managers are expected to be skilled in time management, organi-

zation and prioritization of work and responsibilities, and follow-up on issues continuously until closure or resolution. Their role is a challenging one, especially when their priorities are always changing throughout the day as a result of changes in patients' conditions or priorities of the interdisciplinary team.

Box 4-2 provides an example of a day in the life of a nurse case manager. This example is a concise version

---

box 4-2

A Day in the Life of a Nurse Case Manager

To be able to provide efficient and effective case management services for an entire group of patients, nurse case managers may elect to follow the daily routine presented here.

This routine is only one example of how a nurse case manager may spend his or her day to ensure that the important tasks for the day are completed. When adopting this schedule of activities, one should be careful not to be rigid about the time frames suggested. One should be able to adjust this schedule to the specific organization, area of practice, specialty, and responsibilities of the role as delineated in the nurse case manager's job description of the individual institution.

An important function of the nurse case manager is priority setting. This function is essential for time management, organization of activities and responsibilities, and completing the most important tasks first. Nurse case managers adopting this schedule of activities should factor in the need to constantly revise their "to do" lists based on the significant changes in the conditions of their patients and the constantly changing priorities. They ought to understand that the key here is flexibility and fluidity.

07:30 - 08:30

1. Obtain informal report from night staff regarding significant changes in patients' condition, new admissions, and new referrals.
2. Review medical records of new admissions and screen potential patients requiring case management services.
3. Identify/make a list of patients to be seen before discharge.

08:30 - 09:30

1. Participate in interdisciplinary rounds.
2. Check on all patients scheduled for discharge and ensure that all discharge planning activities have been met (e.g., patient teaching, home care services, follow-up appointment).
3. Conduct case conferencing with the interdisciplinary team, and communicate patients' needs.

09:30 - 11:00

1. Complete the assessments of those patients who meet the criteria for case management services.
2. Confirm, finalize, and follow up on or update the plans of care/CMPs of those patients who are a part of the caseload.
3. Facilitate and coordinate patient care activities (e.g., call ancillary departments and expedite scheduling of tests

and procedures, obtain results), investigate and attempt to resolve delays in the provision of care, and initiate appropriate consults and referrals—particularly those necessary for timely discharge planning.

11:00 - 12:00

1. Communicate with managed care insurance companies regarding appropriateness of and necessity for continued patients' hospitalization.
2. Follow up on the patients scheduled for discharge and verify that discharge has occurred.
3. Start documenting in patients' medical records.

12:00 - 13:00

Lunch break.

13:00 - 15:00

1. Perform/reinforce appropriate patient/family teaching (e.g., preoperative and postoperative teaching, discharge teaching).
2. Meet with patients and families to discuss the plan of care, answer questions, and provide emotional support.
3. Complete necessary paperwork for patients' discharge. Continue documenting in patients' medical records.
4. Attend to any consultations called for by primary nurses or other case managers.

15:00 - 16:00

1. Review scheduled discharges for next day, and ensure patients are ready.
2. Follow up on tests that are not completed. Ensure tests/procedures that were discussed in morning rounds are scheduled appropriately.
3. Continue documenting in patients' medical records.

In addition, nurse case managers conduct patient care rounds informally with the attending physicians when they visit their patients, and they discuss the plans of care. They attend to emergency situations as they arise. They also collect/track patient care variances and follow up on resolutions of problems identified. Nurse case managers are also expected to collaborate with other disciplines (e.g., utilization review, social work, nutrition, physical therapy) as needed. They may also attend certain meetings (e.g., patient/family teaching committee, CMP development teams) and conduct staff inservice education regarding case management.

of what needs to be accomplished daily by case managers. It can be used especially by those who are struggling with how to survive their busy day, as a structure for prioritizing what needs to be done on a certain day, and as a tool for time management and improving productivity. When electing to apply this example in their daily activities, nurse case managers are advised to adjust the example to meet the constantly changing needs of their patients. In addition, they are urged to reprioritize their task lists to meet the changing demands of their patients.

The role of nurse case managers is essential to the success of the case management system. It is the key to ensuring that cost-effective and high-quality patient care is provided. This role is designed to maximize collaboration among all members of the health care team; integration of the services required for the care of each patient; coordination and facilitation of tests, procedures, and other patient care activities; continuity and consistency in the provision of care across care settings and services; and most importantly the openness of lines of communication among all disciplines and on all levels.

The nurse case manager's role is successful only when full support and commitment of hospital and nursing administrators are evidenced and their belief in case management becomes part of the culture and values of the institution. The description of the role presented in this chapter is extensive and could seem to be overwhelming in terms of the amount of responsibilities put into the case manager's role. It is important, however, to keep in mind when studying this role description that it is a thorough approach to the functions and responsibilities of case managers. Health care administrators are urged to evaluate this description and only adapt to their institution what seems to be appropriate to their needs based on their procedures, policies, standards, operations, financial status, care settings, and most importantly, the goals of their case management system/model and what they are attempting to achieve through this role.

KEY POINTS

1. Nurse case managers function as an integral part of the interdisciplinary health care team.
2. Nurse case managers usually manage, coordinate, and facilitate patient care. They ensure timely patient and family teaching and discharge planning.
3. Nurse case managers have many different roles and responsibilities, which are defined differently in each institution. Sometimes their responsibilities cross the boundaries of a particular care setting.
4. Today, nurse case managers work in all patient care settings. They are found to be effective in reducing length of stay and health care cost and improving quality and patient and family satisfaction.
5. Nurse case managers should be clinically competent and astute in time management, problem solving, negotiation, and teamwork.

References

Bower KA: *Case management by nurses,* ed 2, Kansas City, Mo, 1992, American Nurses Association.

McNeese-Smith D et al: Roles of the professional registered nurse in case management and program director. In Flarey DL, Smith-Blancett S, eds: *Handbook of nursing case management,* Gaithersburg, Md, 1996, Aspen.

Newell M: *Using nursing case management to improving health outcomes,* Gaithersburg, Md, 1996, Aspen.

Strassner LF: The ABCs of case management: a review of the basics, *Nurs Case Manage* 1(1):22-30, 1996.

Tahan HA: The nurse case manager in acute care setting: job description and functions, *J Nurs Admin* 23(10):53-61, 1993.

CHAPTER 5

SKILLS FOR SUCCESSFUL CASE MANAGEMENT

Professional nurses have traditionally been key advocates in the provision of quality health care. Their broad skills and training allow them to assess patient's needs and work with families and other members. Negotiating, communicating, team building, preceptoring, educating, and consulting are the basis of what a successful nurse brings to the care setting each day.

The application of the nursing process is concerned with the whole person and the full range of patient needs. This clearly leads to comprehensive and consistent care. Much has been written about the nursing process and its unique qualities. Yura and Walsh (1983) noted the following, which is still applicable today: in contrast to the goals of the other members of the health profession, the nurse is involved with human needs that affect the *total* person rather than one aspect, one problem, or a limited segment of need fulfillment.

Nursing case management, therefore, is no different in its approach to successful coordination of patient care. The role of the **case manager,** by its definition as outlined in the *Case Management Society of America Proposed Standards of Practice* (1994), upholds and expounds on the nursing process. **Case management** is a collaborative process that assesses, plans, implements, coordinates, monitors, and evaluates options and services to meet individuals' health needs through communication and available resources to promote quality, cost-effective **outcomes.**

The case manager's expertise is the vital line between the individual, the provider, the payor, and the community. Successful outcomes cannot be achieved without utilizing all of the specialized skills and knowledge applied through the nursing process. It must be emphasized that the skills necessary to be a successful case manager are not possessed by everyone. Case managers need to be clinically astute and competent in all areas. It is very important for case managers to be astute in the nursing process, to acquire the best assessment skills that make them better able to identify the patient's actual and potential health problem, to implement the required interventions to successfully resolve these problems, and to evaluate the outcomes of care and responses to treatments (Bower, 1992).

Not all nurses acquire the professional credentials, education, and expertise in the application of the nursing process to succeed as a case manager. Case managers are notoriously the consummate organizers, paid to be in control of what many would regard as sheer chaos. Does their skill for organization derive from a compulsive personality, years of experience, mastering the nursing process, or a balanced blend of all of these components? One would believe the latter to be true. As long as there is a subtle balance of the dynamics a case manager possesses, there will be a positive effect.

How does this overview translate and apply to the required skills necessary for today's successful case manager? The section that follows categorizes and details each function and skill that becomes a critical element when providing the services of an effective case manager (Box 5-1).

NURSING PROCESS
Assessment

Assessment is an ongoing continuous process occurring with all patient/case manager interactions. It is during the assessment phase that the case manager seeks a better understanding of the patient, the family dynamics, and health care beliefs and/or myths. An assessment generally involves three phases, which at times seem inseparable: gathering data, evaluating the data, and determining an appropriate nursing diagnosis. A multifaceted subgroup of skills (Rorden and Taft, 1990) is utilized to assess a patient's needs accurately:

- Interview skills that include the ability not only to listen but also to formulate insightful questions.
- Interpretation skills that allow the case manager to understand what patients say about their concerns and symptoms and transmit them in concise, appropriate terminology to other **caregivers.**

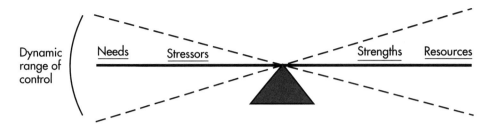

Fig. 5-1 The health balance model. (Redrawn from Rorden JW, Taft E: *Discharge planning guide for nurses,* Philadelphia, 1990, WB Saunders.)

---

box 5-1

Functions and Skills for Effective Case Management

NURSING PROCESS

1. Assessment
2. Planning
3. Implementation
4. Coordination
5. Evaluation

LEADERSHIP SKILLS

1. Patient advocate
2. Facilitator
3. Negotiator
4. Quality improvement coordinator
5. Utilization manager
6. Educator
7. Financial analyst/consult
8. Decision maker
9. Critical thinker

COMMUNICATION/INTERPERSONAL SKILLS

1. Team building
2. Customer relations
3. Public speaking
4. Conflict resolution
5. Delegation
6. Information sharing

- Nonverbal communication skills that permit the case manager to recognize responses to treatments that reflect the patient's moods, attitudes, and psychosocial needs.
- Relationship skills that cut across potential social and cultural barriers to promote trust with patients, family members, and professional colleagues.
- Observational skills that allow the case manager to distinguish normal from abnormal functioning and to recognize changes in patients' responses to treatments.
- Evaluation skills that permit the case manager to consider the facts about a patient's condition, as

well as the interconnections and balance between strengths and weaknesses.
- Goal-setting skills that help the case manager see beyond the immediate needs, to identify intermediate and long-term goals of care.

As an assessor, the case manager must obtain relevant data through skillful investigation. All of the information related to the current plan must be evaluated with a critical eye to objectively identify trends, set and reset realistic goals, and seek viable alternatives as necessary.

Part of being a successful assessor is to find a delicate health balance for each patient. Needs and demands are balanced by strengths and resources. When there is a balance between these factors, there can be positive movement. When a patient is in acute distress, patient needs may be only the obvious; however, if a health balance is to occur or be restored, the case manager must uncover factors that influence the relationships between needs, strengths, and resources. A representation of this health balance model is shown in Figure 5-1 (Rorden and Taft, 1990). Case Study 5-1 presents an example of using the health balance model when assessing a patient.

Planning

Planning is the next step in managing the patient's care. This is accomplished by planning the treatment modalities and interventions necessary for meeting the needs of patients and families. The planning phase determines, in collaboration with the other members of the health care team, the goals of treatment and the projected **length of stay,** and it initiates the discharge plan of care immediately on admission. This becomes vitally important as it provides a clear time frame for accomplishing the care activities needed (O'Malley, 1988). This is done by identifying immediate short-term and long-term needs, as well as where and how these needs will be met.

Planning is initiated as the patient is admitted or before admission to any health care setting. The case manager's clinical expertise is quickly tapped into when establishing whether the treatment plan and interventions

case study
5-1

Assessment and Health Balance

Ms. J. Mazure is a 50-year-old professional career woman. She recently noticed excessive vaginal bleeding. A pap smear revealed a malignancy leading to the need for a hysterectomy. From this you must begin to assess the health needs of the patient and work toward the balance.

You will use a range of skills to help to identify the changes in this patient's health balance as a result of her hysterectomy.

You must also explore the patient's strengths and resources, such as insurance benefits and employee sick leave, as well as evaluate stresses and demands such as the self-imposed pressure of missing work, work responsibilities piling up in her absence, or familial obligations that she temporarily will not be able to handle. By using the health balance, you can connect the physical and the psychosocial aspects of the patient's care.

case study
5-2

Planning

Mrs. Smith is a 25-year-old married woman with a history of miscarriage and no living children. She is now hospitalized for the second time in her pregnancy. She is admitted with a diagnosis of preterm labor at 30 weeks gestation with a low-lying placenta. Mrs. Smith was home only 2 days between hospitalizations when cramping and vaginal bleeding began. She is very anxious about delivering early. She lives in an upstairs apartment and has no family support to help her. You have assessed her needs to include the following:

- Preterm labor requiring medical intervention
- Teaching about her preterm labor to reduce her anxiety
- Motivation to comply with the probable bed rest regime that is ahead of her

- Investigation of the need for home care to follow her pregnancy and medical regime while at home

You quickly establish that the patient's apartment is a problematic setting and determine the need to put home care into the plan, because visits to the physician's office would need to be minimized and bed rest maximized. You also educate Mrs. Smith's husband about preterm labor and the importance of his wife maintaining bed rest. The overall plan includes the patient's goal of returning home as soon as possible. You plan clear guidelines for patient compliance and establish community resources to meet the goal of leaving the hospital. By utilizing a step-by-step planning process, and going beyond the walls of the acute care setting, you are able to meet the needs of this patient while maintaining quality, safe care.

are appropriate. Data are assimilated and a multidisciplinary plan of care begins to unfold.

Throughout the acute hospital, subacute, or home care stay the case manager monitors and reevaluates the plan for accuracy as the patient's condition changes. As a planner, the case manager identifies a treatment plan while remaining cognizant of the patient outcome and minimization of payor liability. The case manager must include the patient and family in decision making and considers the patient's goals as an integral part of the care plan. Alternate plans must always be incorporated, in anticipation of sudden shifts in the treatment process or in response to treatments yielding complications. Case Study 5-2 illustrates the principles of successful planning.

Implementation and Coordination

Implementation and *coordination* involve building the plan, determining the goals of patient care, and deciding what needs to be accomplished to make a viable and realistic plan move to completion. The aim of the case manager at this point is to give the patient and family the knowledge, attitudes, and skills necessary for the

implementation of the established plan. Through communication, collaboration, and teaching the case manager works with the multidisciplinary team to motivate the patient to succeed in fulfilling the plan of care determined by all of the participants. Abraham Maslow (1970), in his theory of hierarchy of needs, suggested that everyone seek fulfillment of general needs. These needs motivate behavior. At a time of high stress or ill health, people experience needs in a more basic fashion, such as survival and safety. The higher needs of self and creativity do not seem as much a priority at this time (Maslow, 1970). The case manager needs to be aware of this motivational factor when trying to illicit decisions about discharge planning or future goals for a patient. The patient and family must first reach an awareness level to be able to focus on the goals of the care plan. The patient and family must then reach an understanding level in which they learn in greater depth what the patient's needs and the available options are, the likely consequences of these options, and what aspects need to be learned. It is at this juncture that motivation will take place and the implementation of the plan will come to fruition.

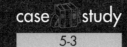

case study
5-3

Implementation and Coordination

You recently thought all steps were taken to provide a safe discharge plan for your cardiac patient. The patient's plan included an ambulance to bring the patient home from the hospital, because he had no family support or means of transportation. Shortly after his departure from the hospital, the ambulance driver called the medical unit rather displeased with the lack of assessment and planning done for this patient. Apparently the address given for the patient's home did not exist and was a vacant lot. After investigating the situation further it was discovered that the patient's medical record had an address from a previous hospitalization that was no longer valid. No one had verified where the patient lived or reconfirmed his address during the assessment or planning phase. This situation could have been avoided by following the simple steps to implementation, thus avoiding a distressful and embarrassing situation for the patient, you, and the hospital.

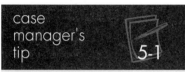

case manager's tip | 5-1 | The Importance of Confirming the Plan

Taking the time and making the effort to confirm the plan greatly increase the probability of the plan's effective and efficient implementation. Follow-through will help ensure that the goals are met.

As the patient nears discharge, there are several actions that improve the chances of effective implementation of the case manager's plan. These involve communication activities whose goal is to improve the whole plan with the objective of clarifying the transfer of responsibilities of care, reviewing the plan to ensure that nothing has been overlooked, and making last-minute alterations and arrangements for the immediate discharge period. Following these steps will confirm the plan for continuing care (Case Manager's Tip 5-1). Case Study 5-3 presents an example of what can happen to implementation if a step-by-step approach of assessment, planning, and coordination does not take place.

Evaluation

The final step in the nursing process, *evaluation,* is designed to measure the patient's response to a formulated plan and at the same time ensure the appropriateness of the care plan and the quality of the services and products being offered to the patient.

To achieve successful evaluation criteria, the case manager must routinely assess and reassess the patient's status and progress toward reaching the goals set forth on the care plan. If the situation is at a halt or regressing rather than moving forward, the case manager must then make appropriate adjustments and alter the plan accordingly.

The following important questions must be asked as the evaluation proceeds:

- Were the patient's needs identified early in the hospital stay?

- Were learning goals identified and teaching documented?
- Were referrals complete and timely?
- Was the patient clearly able to verbalize the goals of the care plan?
- Did the patient seem satisfied with the plan and the decisions surrounding the plan?
- Did the patient comply with medical advice and follow the recommendations of the case manager?

These questions will help in determining if the overall discharge plan for a particular patient was effective and will assist in quality improvement efforts for future patients. This information also be valuable when evaluating the facility's total case management program. Throughout the evaluation process, all participants in the interdisciplinary team will identify system, process, clinician, and patient **variances** and trend them. These trends will be further analyzed in continuous quality improvement teams to improve, fine tune, revamp, and reorganize the current process.

The case manager must use many skills and functions of leadership to effectively master the nursing process (Case Manager's Tip 5-2). A more specific and comprehensive breakdown of these skills will add to the role dimensions of the case manager.

LEADERSHIP SKILLS AND FUNCTIONS

Because case managers function as members of the multidisciplinary health care team, they should be highly skilled in various leadership qualities. Nursing

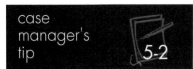

Applicability of Skills to Different Settings

Keep in mind that all the skills delineated in this chapter are applicable to all forms of case management, including acute care, subacute care, home care, or insurance case management.

case managers must be adept at negotiation and contracting and be capable of making sound decisions and resolving conflicts. To do this successfully, they should acquire critical thinking and problem solving skills. Because of their managerial responsibilities, case managers must be involved in quality improvement efforts, speak publicly, and write for publication.

The case manager's work as an *advocate* for the patient is one of the most critical elements of the role. The patient/case manager relationship is built on the ability of the case manager to be trusted; have mutual respect between patient and case manager; and establish a rapport that facilitates communication among the family, care givers, payors, and other health care team members. As the case manager gains a clear understanding of the patient's needs, care desires and goals can be communicated effectively to the members of the health care team and perhaps impact the course of treatment to effect an earlier discharge or negotiate better fees for medical supplies or equipment or more efficient home care. As a *facilitator,* the case manager can be a catalyst for change by empowering the patient or family members to seek solutions throughout the acute care phase and beyond the hospital setting. The case manager is always on the lookout for quality improvement that could result in potential cost savings or possibly prolong the health care benefits of an individual.

The patient's best interests are always the focal point for the case manager's advocacy efforts, whether for needed funding, treatment options, appropriate and timely home health services, or reassessment and evaluation of goals. Case managers are concerned with every detail, sifting through the complex array of paths that can easily lead to confusion for any patient. The case manager's skills in decision making must work through the confusion for the patient and answer certain questions, such as the following. Will the electricity in the home support a ventilator? Does the patient have access to a bathroom on the main floor? Is it worth the hospital's financial support to fly a patient home to Florida rather than incur extended length of stay? Is the family capable of learning how to perform endotracheal suctioning so their loved one can go home with them rather than to an extended nursing facility? Answers to these questions influence the type of care a patient will

receive and how it will be accomplished to ensure the best possible outcome for a patient in the most cost-effective manner. If critical thinking is used in the decision-making process efficiently, the patient and family will receive the necessary support, potential obstacles to the treatment plan will be avoided, the potential for readmission will decrease, the educational component of care will be reinforced, and a positive outcome and promotion of health will take place.

Negotiation and Financial Analysis

Negotiation and financial analysis are two areas that are not primarily taught in nursing. Time management is so important in today's health care arena that entire management courses are devoted to it. Along with managing their own time, case managers must learn to determine what work others can and should do in assessing a patient's needs when preparing a patient's plan.

Negotiation is a skill used with payors and providers, with vendors for durable medical equipment, or even with physicians reluctant to opt for a home care discharge plan. The art of fair negotiation uses strategies of trust and rapport and never offers anything but complete honesty regarding a patient's care needs. Successful negotiation will be achieved by being well prepared to present the facts clearly and succinctly. To know if you have negotiated your case well, you must be a good listener who tunes into verbal and nonverbal cues, or windows of opportunity could be missed. On the financial side of the equation, we know all too well that health care environments are committed to doing more with less and at less cost. A case manager's financial prowess is a must in these times of cost containment. Case managers must work with the financial support personnel to assist them in keeping abreast of a patient's insurance **health benefit plan** or no-fault coverage or lack of finances that could lead to Medicaid eligibility.

Case management plans can be useful tools when determining the allocated resources for a particular diagnosis. Variance analysis or **comorbid** conditions can help a case manager anticipate extra costs, such as the need for expensive antibiotic treatment or pain management therapy.

Working alongside the hospital's controller to review the expenses incurred for various diagnoses will serve as a checks-and-balances system of appropriate allocation of funds. The case manager has a key role in being able to communicate the overutilization of laboratory tests, repetitive diagnostics, or underutilization of a less-expensive antibiotic. Thus the case manager can have a major impact in providing the same quality care that an institution is accustomed to while being more cost efficient in the process.

Another way in which case managers affect the financial balance of an acute care setting while monitoring quality is through **utilization** review. Participation in a hospital length-of-stay committee is one way to monitor utilization. The health care team can then be alerted to an inappropriate admission, an unusual length of stay for a given patient, a planned premature discharge with no clear discharge plan and with potential readmission risk, or inappropriate use of resources. It is case managers who will be charged with monitoring these potentially financial drains on the hospital. It is their high-quality efficiency that will provide the hospital with a safety **gatekeeping** mechanism to avoid potential utilization problems. Utilization knowledge will also be effective in subacute, home care, or insurance arenas to justify or nullify care requested.

In this ever-shrinking resource environment it becomes more and more prudent for the case manager to be an instrumental participant in payor contract negotiation, resource management teams, clinical pathway development committees, and any groups designed to promote quality care at less cost but high efficiency. It is the driving force behind every great case manager to maximize patient outcomes and quality of care while being ever cognizant of the dwindling resources to provide that care.

One of the last but certainly not least leadership skills is that of educator. This is a large responsibility within the case manager's role, because it covers a broad scope of functions. Being a facilitator of both the patient sector and the staff is at times a monumental task that brings with it times of extreme challenge. A good principle to follow is to begin with the end result in mind. First there is the mental picture of the outcome of your patient's plan of care. Then you begin to formulate the blueprints and develop your construction plan to get the patient and family to the projected outcome. This idea

can be conveyed by using the analogy of constructing a house. The blueprint for the house is meticulously designed well before any physical creation of the house is begun. Without a developed blueprint, the physical creation will undoubtedly have expensive changes that could double the cost of the house. The case manager, much like the carpenter, must make sure the blueprint (patient's plan of care) includes everything needed and that everything has been thought through (Covey, 1989).

Educating the patient and family is part of the blueprint for success. The clearer the understanding of the disease process and the course of the acute level of care, the better the plan will be. Of utmost importance is that the case manager consider educating in language that is understood, with consideration for cultural diversity and health care beliefs. In our constant awareness of pressures to reduce length of stay, education is sometimes elected to take a back seat. Timely education is crucial, especially as patients experience shorter hospital stays. Placing education at the bottom of the priority list can have devastating effects on outcomes. For example, a family decides to take their loved one, who is ventilator dependent, home. All plans appear to be in place: the respiratory company has been arranged, the home is prepared, and the nursing visits are on standby. Everything seems to be ready, but a crucial element is missing. No one thought about the necessity to teach the family how to care for their family member at home, including expertise in ventilator function and resuscitative measures. Without this most important step of early education, the discharge plan runs the risk of failure, costly extra days in the hospital, or potential rehospitalization of the patient due to lack of knowledge of the family members.

Do the patient and family respond better to verbal or nonverbal communication, audio or video, written word or pictures, discussion or demonstration? It is the case manager who can impact the education process by serving as the resource for staff to develop or select supporting educational materials and define the best method of conveying the information (Case Manager's Tip 5-3). The case manager may also serve as a member of patient teaching committees responsible for patient and family teaching materials or documentation tools such as the one shown in Figure 5-2.

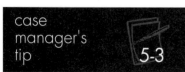

case manager's tip 5-3 **Assessing for Readiness to Learn**

The case manager must use every possible means of assessing for readiness to learn or potential barriers to learning. The method of education must be determined.

MOTHER / BABY NURSING EDUCATION RECORD / DISCHARGE SUMMARY (PAGE 1)

MERCY MEDICAL CENTER
1000 NORTH VILLAGE AVENUE
ROCKVILLE CENTRE, NEW YORK 11570

Interview Date:

Person Involved in Patient Teaching/Relationship:

Lives with Patient: ☐ Yes ☐ No

Primary Language Spoken:

Preferred Learning Method: ☐ Listening ☐ Demonstration ☐ Reading Pictures ☐ Other

Identified Barriers: ☐ Auditory ☐ Visual ☐ Cultural/Religious ☐ Other

Comments:

ADDRESSOGRAPH

OUR NURSING STAFF WISH TO GIVE YOU THE INFORMATION YOU WANT AND NEED MOST DURING YOUR STAY WITH US.
PLEASE LOOK OVER THE FOLLOWING LIST OF EDUCATIONAL TOPICS AND COMPLETE THE FORM BY PUTTING A CHECK IN THE COLUMN THAT MOST APPLIES TO YOU, USING THE FOLLOWING SCALE:
1 = MOST IMPORTANT TO LEARN BEFORE I GO HOME   2 = I WOULD LIKE TO REVIEW   3 = I ALREADY KNOW OR AM COMFORTABLE WITH

SELF ASSESSMENT CHECKLIST	1	2	3	Date Time	Nurse Initial	Mode	Code	Date Time	Nurse Initial	Mode	Code	Nurse Initial	Signature
BABY CARE													
DIAPER CHANGE													
BATH SPONGE / TUB													
TEMPERATURE													
DRESSING													
CORD CARE													
SKIN CARE / RASH													
JAUNDICE													
CIRCUMCISION CARE													
UNCIRCUMCISED BABY CARE													
BULB SYRINGE / CHOKING													
CRYING AS COMMUNICATION													
CAR SEAT													
WHEN TO CALL THE PHYSICIAN													
NOTIFY M.D. FOR SIGNS OF INFECTION													
SLEEP POSITIONS													
OTHER													
BREASTFEEDING													
LATCHING ON													
POSITIONING MOM / BABY													
FREQUENCY & LENGTHS OF FEEDINGS / BURPING													
CARE OF BREASTS / NIPPLES													
BREAST PUMP / PUMPING STORAGE													
WHEN TO CALL THE PHYSICIAN													
BOTTLE FEEDING												**Comments**	
LATCHING ON													
POSITIONING													
FREQUENCY & LENGTHS OF FEEDINGS / BURPING													
FEEDING WATER													
FORMULA PREPARATION													
WHEN TO CALL THE PHYSICIAN													
MOTHER CARE													
VAGINAL DISCHARGE / BLEEDING													
INCISION CARE / EPISIOTOMY CARE													
BREAST CARE-WHEN NOT BREASTFEEDING													
BLADDER / BOWEL FUNCTIONS													
ACTIVITY / REST													
NUTRITION / DIET													
EMOTIONS													
MEDICATION													
WHEN TO CALL PHYSICIAN													
OTHER													

PATIENT EDUCATION DOCUMENTATION

TEACHING MODES: D = DEMONSTRATION   R = REINFORCEMENT   B = BOOKLET   H = HANDOUT   A = AUDIOVISUAL   MT = MEDICATION TEACHING RECORD
I = ICN / NBN DISCHARGE PLANNING FORM

EVALUATION CODES: 1 = UNABLE TO PERFORM / UNABLE TO UNDERSTAND*   2 = NEEDS REINFORCEMENT AND / OR PRACTICE   3 = PERFORMS / VERBALIZES UNDERSTANDING

MB-100A/95

#22110 MBS 11/96

Fig. 5-2 Mother/baby nursing education record/discharge summary. (Courtesy Mercy Medical Center, Rockville Center, New York.)

Fig. 5-3 Diagram of the communication model. (Redrawn from Rawlins C: *Harper Collins college outline—introduction to management,* New York, 1992, American Book-Works.)

Ensuring compliance with standards of patient and family teaching as outlined by regulatory and accreditation agencies is also a required facet of the case manager's role. Case managers are involved in nursing staff development by enhancing and disseminating new knowledge and skills. They act as mentors and preceptors of less senior staff. The knowledge of case management itself must also be conveyed across professional lines and levels of hierarchy. The community is also in need of hearing more and learning more about case management; if hospitalized or offered the option of home care, a person will have an appropriate expectation of case management and how the case manager will be involved in the plan of care.

Communication and Other Interpersonal Skills

Communication and other interpersonal skills are the lifeline that connects each individual in any walk of life and in any organization. As our technological world moves faster, quality communication becomes essential. Many would claim that communication is the core of leadership and decision making; thorough communication is the core managerial function. Therefore, as managers and leaders, case managers must master effective communication to be successful. Communication is the transfer of information, ideas, understanding, or feelings. Managing is working with and through others; communication is necessary so that each person knows his or her role in the process of accomplishing goals. Communication can be defined as follows (Dash et al, 1996):

• A complex, dynamic interchange of verbal and nonverbal messages and meanings between people, the means by which information is transferred
• The process of imparting knowledge
• A social process
• Something continuous and fluid

We take communication for granted, but in the case of quality job performance—as in the role of a case manager—it should not be treated lightly. A miscommunication or a barrier to effective communication could lead to expensive hardship for a hospital, payor, or family. In fact, it is easier to miscommunicate than to communicate clearly. At any stage in the process of communication something can interfere with its effectiveness, clarity, or accuracy. This interference is called *noise.* Noise can be physical, such as a cardiac monitor beeping in a patient's ear; psychological, such as fear or anxiety of being hospitalized; or anything else that keeps the message from getting from sender to receiver.

A communication model has at least four elements (Figure 5-3). The first is the *sender,* as in the case manager, who transmits the communication message. The second element is the *message,* which includes the verbal and nonverbal, as well as facial expressions and body language. The third component, the *receiver,* is the person to whom the message is sent. If all goes well, the intended message sent will be the correct message received. The fourth component, the *context,* is the surroundings in which the communication takes place. The environment is identified by such factors as patient's condition, cultural background, health beliefs, and values (Dash et al, 1996).

The *channel* one chooses is also a key to effective communication and must be individualized to the patient's readiness to learn and preferred method of communication (e.g., face-to-face, group meeting, or written information). The listener's receptivity must also be established and maintained if quality communication is to take place.

Because barriers to communication are the pitfalls for any case manager to try to avoid, it is helpful to review some examples in depth.

Physical interference. The first and most important step in improving communication is to make sure that your intended receiver receives the message. The sender (case manager) must take full responsibility for seeing that the physical barriers to communication are reduced. Case Study 5-4 provides an example of such a situation.

Psychological noise. The root cause of this interference is distraction (thinking about something else). Accuracy is

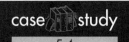

case study
5-4

Dealing With Physical Interference

You enter room 410 to speak to Ms. Blondin about her discharge plan. The first thing you notice is that her television is on, she has two visitors by her bedside, housekeeping personnel are emptying the garbage, and the lunch carts are arriving in the hallway. Obviously, very little effective communication will occur unless the physical barriers are reduced. First, ask the patient's permission to turn off the television; next, invite visitors to participate in the meeting if agreeable to the patient and appropriate to the purpose of your meeting. Then explain why you are there and make eye contact. If distractions are still evident, wait until the housekeeper has left the room and the dietary cart has passed in the hallway. Then you can proceed because you have taken control of the physical environment and have reduced the physical interference that would have certainly had a negative effect on your communication effort.

case study
5-5

Dealing With Psychological Barriers

You approach Mr. Tumbie, an 80-year-old frail looking man admitted for dehydration and intractable diarrhea. Your first question, "How are you today, Mr. Tumbie?" gets a nonverbal response of sighs and wringing his hands but a verbal response of feeling fine. Mr. Tumbie's expressions and actions do not match his verbal reply, and you interpret this as anxiety. As you probe further into his apparent anxiety, you learn that he is very tired and is preoccupied with his daughter and son-in-law who are "after his money."

Your original goal of offering Mr. Tumbie some discharge planning options may be too premature in light of the fact that there is a clear psychological barrier that must be tackled first: his relationship with his daughter and son-in-law. It may also be a belief of this patient that personal or family problems are inappropriate to discuss with a nurse. You may first need to establish a trust to make the patient feel more comfortable before discussing his personal life. Beginning with a less emotionally charged topic would be advantageous in building a rapport and becoming better informed about the patient. You will no doubt be more successful when approaching this sensitive subject in the future.

 case manager's tip 5-4

Information Overload and Quality of Communication

Too much information delivered too quickly will result in a poor-quality communication effort.

at stake here. Hunger, anger, depression, medication, and fear all have a different impact on the way the receiver understands. Asking for feedback, providing feedback, and verifying the accuracy of the message helps identify the existence of a psychological barrier. See Case Study 5-5 for an example.

Information processing barriers. Our brains have the miraculous ability to take in enormous amounts of data but can only process consciously one thought at a time. If information is being sent too fast, the brain and therefore the receiver have trouble taking it in (Case Manager's Tip 5-4). *Communication overload* is a classic example of a processing barrier. This refers to a case where too much information is being sent and the receiver cannot process all of it. The receiver then becomes overwhelmed and shutsdown. You have probably seen this occur numerous times. Picture yourself giving a patient instructions on how to test his own blood sugar. You go on and on reciting the steps of pricking his finger, dabbing a drop of blood on the glucose test strip, and preparing the machinery to accept the strip for reading. When you suddenly try to make eye contact, what you see is a face staring back at you blankly. The patient is overwhelmed by your instruction, is overloaded, and has shut down.

Perceptual barriers. Individuals bring a unique set of past experiences to a communication. These experiences, good or bad, will influence how a person perceives the meaning of your communication. Perception is greatly influenced by our value system. We interpret everything

case manager's tip   5-5

Limiting the Chain of Communication

The fewer people to whom messages must be relayed, the more effective the communication.

case manager's tip   5-6

Power and Communication

Always keep yourself focused on the goals of your communication, and do not get intimidated by hierarchical status when quality patient care is at stake. Seeking feedback and verifying the information conveyed will help you maintain power.

case study
5-6

Appropriate Use of Power on a Patient's Behalf

Mrs. Rose is a resident of Florida who came to visit her elderly sister in New York and became ill, requiring hospitalization. The patient has remained hospitalized for 20 days and is now essentially ready for discharge. In the course of the hospitalization, the patient's functional status has deteriorated and the likelihood that she can remain home alone is slim. The patient requires oxygen and a wheelchair. The dilemma becomes how to get the patient discharged when she refuses nursing home placement and wants only to return to Florida where her friends could help her. Many contacts and more hospital days later, it becomes clear to you that it would be less expensive to arrange for medical air transport to Florida than to continue her hospitalization.

The case manager in this scenario has the ability to affect the outcome of this patient's hospitalization by utilizing directive power and educating the hospital's administrative body. It would be soon realized that it is financially more prudent to send this patient back to Florida rather than keep her hospitalized indefinitely. The case manager needs to clearly communicate to the hierarchy holding the purse strings the cost of a few days in the hospital vs. the cost of an ambulance and medical air transport.

we experience through mental images. We tend to assume that the way we see things is the way that they really are and the way everyone else sees them.

Structural barriers. There are aspects of organizational structure that can affect the quality of communication. These next barriers to communication, as with all those previously mentioned, can be applied not only to a case manager's patients but also to a case manager's peers, other members of the multidisciplinary team, payors, and upper administrative management.

The more people who are involved in a chain of communication, the greater the likelihood that message interruption can occur (Case Manager's Tip 5-5). You may remember an old game of telephone in which a message is whispered into the ear of a line of people. By the time the message reaches the last person in the line, that final message will be substantially different from the initial message. Usually the important details such as times, dates, and names become confused.

If communication must take place on various levels of authority or power, the differences in *status* can result in poor-quality communication. This is known as information processing or filtering. Overcoming the communication barrier imposed by status differences is mostly a matter of realizing that they can occur (Case Manager's Tip 5-6).

There are generally two types of power: (1) *directive power,* or power used to affect the behavior of others with the intent of satisfying personal needs; and (2) *synergistic power,* or power used to increase the energy and creativity of all participants with the intent of satisfying the needs of all participants. Knowing how and when to enforce power appropriately along with the components of a trusting relationship will result in a shared sense of responsibility and better outcomes. Possessing a solid power base is crucial, and its appropriateness is essential. As an expert case manager, you must be willing to share expertise, issue directives, follow up on compliance, and attempt to influence as occasions arise (Bass, 1985). Case Study 5-6 provides an example.

Lack of trust and stress are additional structural barriers to communication. They both interfere with accurate, clear communication, and they both affect the ability to express needs and information openly. Building rapport and a trusting relationship usually has the added bonus of reducing stress, thereby increasing the chances of accurate communication.

The following sections outline the four basic qualities a case manager should use to initiate a patient–case manager or case manager–colleague relationship in which trust can be developed.

Warmth. This quality helps others feel accepted. Nurses who are willing to extend themselves with openness rather than cold, expressionless, disapproving behavior will gain trust more quickly. Warmth reflects self-respect, self-acceptance, and genuine concern for others. People respond to this type of behavior favorably.

Respect. Treat others as you would want to be treated; take into consideration personality, culture, opinions, and beliefs. To respect does not necessarily mean that you must like but that you must accept and value the other human being. This becomes important to a case manager when a family or patient's decisions regarding a discharge plan are not in full agreement with your recommendation. Keeping patients informed about their care gives patients the feeling that they are respected as individuals not a bed number or a disease entity.

Empathy. Helping people feel understood means actively tuning into feelings and thoughts and letting go of stereotypes and prejudices. This is an essential ingredient in trusting relationships. You must really hear, without demanding that someone feel as you think they should in a given situation (Rorden and Taft, 1990).

Genuineness. This final component in verbal communication enhances the trust relationship. This quality allows people to feel they are interacting with a "real" person who is interested in their well-being. Consistency is another facet of being genuine. If there is inconsistency between verbal and nonverbal behavior, communication will break down (e.g., the case manager who voices concern about a patient's situation but fails to make eye contact will surely be judged as "put on"). Keep in mind that people who are already stressed by their situation will be more astute to false behavior and inconsistent communication. Armed with the knowledge of the many barriers to communication and ways in which to avoid or minimize them, you must now become versed in types of communication channels for effectively bringing your message from sender to receiver. The path a communication takes, whether it be formal or informal, has an effect on the communication itself (Rawlins, 1992).

Formal communication takes two forms: downward and upward. Downward communication is communication about what to do, how to do it, and when it is to be completed. This is usually delegated to subordinates. To delegate effectively, all of the aforementioned barriers should be avoided. An example of upward communication is speaking with a CEO for financial approval, as in the previously discussed scenario of flying a patient back to her home rather than incurring an extended hospital stay. The result is a more accurate managerial process, greater participation, and interactive control of the positive destiny of an organization.

Informal communication usually takes place between smaller groups, such as the case manager and the social worker. Managers of these two departments may get together after a more formal meeting to discuss a policy that may affect both of their departments. This type of communication must be based on mutual trust, or a more formal communication will need to follow.

In addition to becoming aware of typical barriers to effective communication and channels of communication, case managers can take additional steps to improve communication competency. How colleagues work together as a team can determine the success or failure of any work environment. Good relationships are fostered by being respectful to each other's job duties. There is a great difference between an effective team and a group of people who have been thrown together with no clear goals (Haase, 1992).

There are generally 10 elements of an effective team. While reviewing these elements, think about the members of your organizational team, whether it is social work, discharge planning, utilization review, nurse managers, payors, or physicians. Rate the effectiveness of your team effort toward a productive case management program and better patient outcomes. You will begin to see that many if not all of the elements incorporate the communication and interpersonal skills discussed throughout this chapter (Haase, 1992).

1. Team members communicate openly and honestly. They listen with understanding.
2. Team members have common goals and a clear idea of the team's mission.
3. Team members support each other. They have assigned duties and are not engaged in turf wars.
4. Team members take pride in their group's efforts and results.
5. Team members help make decisions on important issues but are willing to look for guidance, when necessary, for final decisions.
6. Team members feel comfortable expressing ideas, opinions, and disagreements.
7. Team members are encouraged to make the development of new skills a way of life.
8. Team members are encouraged to use their unique skills and talents.
9. Team members realize that conflict is normal and that working out differences can lead to new points of view and creativity.

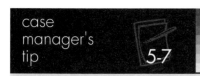

5-7 Positive Effects of Conflict

If conflict is well managed, it can actually increase the effectiveness of an organization.

---

10. Team members value appropriate humor. Having fun increases openness, enthusiasm, and energy. These ten elements involve potential attitude adjustment, releasing of power, respect, compromise, and conflict resolution.

Keep in mind that conflict is inevitable. It is also not a negative occurrence as it was once believed. Conflict is merely individuals or groups experiencing differences in views, goals, or facts that place them at opposite poles. It usually involves areas of differing expertise, practice, or authority. In most situations conflict falls into one of three categories: *perceived* conflict, the thought that conditions exist between groups that cause the conflict; *felt* conflict, when the conflict evokes feelings of threat, hostility, fear, or mistrust; and *expressed* conflict, which takes the form of debate, assertion, competition, or problem solving. The most often used tactic to resolve conflict is the win/win resolution. Groups usually identify solutions that will allow each to maintain their goals and ultimately create a resolution that they can live with (Kirsch, 1988).

The ability to successfully manage conflict is an important skill for the case manager to master. It can help the case manager increase the total benefits of the group efforts by becoming more innovative and creative, with the overall outcome of increasing productivity and goal achievement (Case Manager's Tip 5-7).

One member of the multidisciplinary team, the physician, is a vital communication source. If there are conflicts or obstacles to the case manager–physician communication, then quality patient care will suffer. Professional and up-front communication regarding the case manager's role is a good place to start in building an effective team between the disciplines. Case managers must initiate positive dialogue with physicians and address the stereotypes and stresses of a shifting health care system (Mullahy, 1995). Despite the common goal of the patient's well-being, physicians and case managers can easily become adversaries when distrust surrounding the case manager's intentions is raised. Comments such as "Case managers are the police who work with the insurance payors to deny care" misguide physicians into perceiving case managers as a threat to their medical judgment and their income. Due to the changing working relationship between case managers and

physicians (nurses, social workers, utilization coordinators, discharge planners), the transition to a full cooperative relationship is at times awkward and frustrating. Being caught up in past traditional roles hinders the establishment of a collaborative alliance necessary to achieve success in the health care of the twenty-first century.

We must constantly remind ourselves that we are all here for the patient and must remain focused on that goal. Case managers need to be especially clear on this point—that their interest is in ensuring better quality of care and the best possible outcomes. The physicians (social workers, utilization coordinators, discharge planners) must be reassured that the case managers are not there to control or dictate but are instead there to foster effective, quality communication between members of a multidisciplinary team.

Today's case managers face the challenge of dealing with a diverse customer population. The case manager of today must be astute to incorporate the communication techniques and skills reviewed in this chapter when communicating with such a diversity of groups involved in patient care. For example, a group of growing prominence involved in patients' care is the payor source or insurance company. The case manager must listen closely to what the payor is requesting and must clarify any vague communication at the onset. The case manager should not assume that the insurance claims department has all the knowledge necessary regarding a patient's discharge plan. The case manager, as educator, becomes vital to the success of the patient's outcome by sharing medical knowledge of what the patient needs. Case managers must keep in mind that they are the problem solvers and cannot easily accept a simple *"No"* or "We don't do that." Case managers must be risk takers when communicating with the payor members of the team, or patients could suffer the consequences. The communication with external members of the multidisciplinary team (payor, community resources, family members) becomes just as important to the success of the patient's outcome as to the internal members of the team.

Much of this chapter has been devoted to communication, because it is perhaps the most vital skill a case manager must master. It is the flow of information from

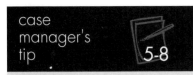

case
manager's
tip 5-8   ## Improving the Effectiveness of Communication

In addition to improving basic communication skills of reading, writing, listening, and speaking, case managers can improve communication effectiveness by withholding judgment, avoiding inconsistencies, and valuing all members of the team inclusive of patient and family.

one to another. However, psychological, physical, and structural barriers can cause turbulence in the information flow. Effective case managers will work fiercely to reduce these barriers. The more rapidly they receive information, the better-quality decisions they will make (Case Manager's Tip 5-8).

SUMMARY

Successful leaders possess quite an extensive list of skills. This is especially true of case managers as leaders. They must be able to incorporate all of these skills into their day-to-day functions with the gracefulness of a gazelle.

As stated earlier, not everyone can be or aspire to be a case manager, even with proper education and development. Successful case managers are likely to demonstrate special ability to operate in peer relationships, to lead others in subordinate relationships, to resolve interpersonal and decisional conflicts, to communicate in the verbal media, to make complex interrelated decisions, to allocate resources (including their own time), and to innovate (Mintzberg, 1973). This idea should be slightly altered to read as follows: successful *leaders,* not *managers.* Leadership is not management. Management has a more narrow focus: How can I accomplish certain things? Leadership, on the other hand, deals with the broader picture: What are the things that I need to accomplish? In the words of Peter Drucker and Warren Bennis, management is doing things right, whereas leadership is doing the right things. Management is efficiency in climbing the ladder of success; leadership determines whether the ladder is leaning against the right wall (Covey, 1989).

You can quickly see the important difference between the two if you envision a group of new graduate nurses cutting their way through a jungle. In the front will be the workers cutting through the undergrowth, cleaning it out. The potential managers will be behind them, sharpening their machetes, writing policy and procedure manuals, holding development programs, and setting up work schedules. The potential leader (case manager) is the one who climbs the tallest tree,

surveys the entire situation, and yells, "Wrong jungle!" (Covey, 1989).

The metamorphosis taking place in almost every industry, including the health care industry, demands professional leadership first and management second. All that has been conveyed in this chapter clearly depicts qualities of a leader in today's health care arena. Although the title has generally become associated with management, leadership more fully and accurately defines the role of the case manager. Efficient management without effective leadership is "like straightening deck chairs on the Titanic" (Covey, 1989).

Effectiveness does not depend solely on how much effort we expend but whether or not the effort we expend is in the right place. It is irrelevant if a case manager spends days on a discharge plan, expending much energy, only to find out that due to poor leadership vision the plan was not the right blueprint for the patient.

The pressure for change within our health care industry will most definitely intensify rather than diminish in the coming years. This pressure will require nurses to respond with new dynamic transformational leadership to cope with future changes. The transformational leader approaches leadership from an entirely different perspective or level of awareness. The transformational leader, as defined by Bass (1985), is one who does the following:

- Raises levels of consciousness about the importance of certain goals or actions
- Encourages subordinates to transcend self-interests for the good of the team

House (1971), who developed the path-goal theory in the 1970s, depicts the qualities of a transformational leader as someone who does the following:

- Serves as a role model
- Builds an image
- Articulates goals
- Sets high expectations

Although these theorist's research goes back a number of years, perhaps they were ahead of their time, because the case manager of the 1990s and beyond characteristically fits into all of these categories. Any organization setting out to begin a case management program should heed these role characteristics to start a program with a solid foundation of leaders called case managers.

Key Points

1. Utilization of the nursing process—assessment, planning, implementation, coordination, and evaluation—is vital to a successful case manager.
2. Assessment will connect the physical and the psychosocial aspects of a patient's care.
3. Planning will determine the treatments and interventions necessary for meeting the needs of patients and families.
4. Implementation/coordination will build on the plan and determine the goals of patient care, moving the plan to completion.
5. Evaluation will measure the patient's response to the case management plan.
6. Leadership and communication skills such as facilitation, negotiation, utilization management, education, team building, and conflict resolution must be added to the case manager's repertoire throughout the day-to-day function.
7. Teamwork is essential to the success of any patient plan. Learn who the members of the team are and develop effective relationships.
8. Acquired skills are applicable to all forms of case management, including acute, subacute, home care, and insurance case management.

References

Bass B: Leadership good, better, best, *Organiz Dynam* 13:26-40, 1985.

Bower XA: *Case management by nurses*, ed 2, St Louis, 1992, American Nurses Association.

Case management society of America proposed standards of practice, *Case Manage* St Louis, 1994, Mosby.

Covey S: *The 7 habits of highly effective people*, New York, 1989, Simon & Schuster.

Dash K et al: *Discharge planning for the elderly*, New York, 1996, Springer.

Haase J: The 10 elements of an effective team, *Home Care* 38:236, 1992.

House R: A path-goal theory of leadership effectiveness, *Admin Q* 16:321-338, 1971.

Kirsch J: *The middle manager and the nursing organization*, E. Norwalk, Conn, 1988, Appleton and Lange.

Maslow AH: *Motivation and personality*, ed 2, New York, 1970, Harper and Row.

Mintzberg H: *The nature of managerial work*, New York, 1973, Harper and Row.

Mullahy CM: *The case manager's handbook*, Gaithersburg, 1995, Aspen.

O'Malley J: Dimensions of the nurse case manager role, *Nursing case management* (Part II), Gaithersburg, Md, 1988, Aspen.

Rawlins C: *Harper Collins college outline—introduction to management*, New York, 1992, American Book-Works.

Rorden JW, Taft E: *Discharge planning guide for nurses*, Philadelphia, 1990, WB Saunders.

Yura H, Walsh M: *The nursing process*, E. Norwalk, Conn, 1983, Appleton-Century-Crofts.

CHAPTER 6

HIRING CASE MANAGERS: ROLE OF THE CANDIDATE AND THE INTERVIEWER*

Interviewing or being interviewed for a job is something nearly everyone has to do at one time or another during one's career. It is probably the most important, intimidating, and demanding task one will ever be involved in. The reward of interviewing well is getting hired for the job. Candidates for the **case manager** role face a challenging task. They need to prove to their prospective employers, on paper and in person, that they are the *best candidates* for the role.

The number of experienced candidates for the case manager's role has been increasing, because restructuring and redesigning of patient care delivery have resulted in case management systems being identified as key delivery models in most institutions. Given this demand, many nursing schools are now including training and education for case management. This change has increased competition as recruiters and potential employers select the best candidate for the nurse case manager's role. This chapter discusses the interview process of nurse case managers. It discusses the roles of the candidate and the interviewer. In addition, it provides some tips for success in both roles.

CANDIDATE

Candidates for the nurse case manager's role are selected based on their clinical and leadership skills and knowledge in case management. The criteria considered in the potential candidate include resourcefulness, flexibility, adaptability, tolerance to stress and hard work, teamwork, dependability, truthfulness, reliability, effectiveness, perseverance, and ability to manage change and conquer challenge.

To be hired for the case manager's position, potential candidates should prepare themselves to be "The Candidate." Their responsibilities are beyond the "at-

tractive" resume. They need not only be able to intelligently market themselves on paper but also to sell themselves even more carefully during the job interview. This task can be quite intimidating and requires high-level written and verbal skills.

Preparing the Resume

Today's advertisements (ads) no longer include the telephone numbers of the recruiter or recruitment office; instead a mailing address and/or a fax number are provided. This change in advertising makes the resume extremely important. The resume becomes the only compelling source of information available to prospective employers for targeting candidates for interviews. It should summarize the candidate's best attributes, including the following:

- Career objective(s)
- Employment history, highlighting the most recent experience
- Education
- Licensure, certifications, awards, and honors
- Previous research, public speaking activities, and citations of published materials
- Professional organizations or societies
- Volunteer work or community services
- Other skills (e.g., different languages spoken, computer skills)
- Available references

The resume is a special type of writing that may not conform to the rules of grammar or punctuation, which makes it easier to write. When preparing their resumes, candidates for the case manager role may face some challenges in articulating their previous experiences or conveying the extent of the skills they possess. To overcome this challenge, they may seek the help of professional agencies that are specialized in writing resumes, or they may refer to books on business writing (i.e., how to write resumes and cover letters). Such books can be found in public and private libraries and in the business sections of bookstores. Today, similar information can

*This material first appeared in *Nursing Case Management* 2(2), 1997, Lippincott-Raven, Philadelphia, PA.

be found on-line (i.e., the Internet). However candidates may seek help for writing the resume, it is important that they make sure the final product provides the potential employer with a comprehensive profile of oneself, stressing what contributions the candidate offers the institution.

The length of the resume should not exceed three pages. The work history and experience consume most of the resume's length. Candidates may highlight their work experience and skills following either a reverse chronological format or a grouping of tasks and skills. Either format is equally appropriate. In the reverse chronological history, the work history is listed starting with the latest job held first. In contrast, the grouping of tasks and skills format requires a synthesis of the categories of these tasks and skills based on all the previous jobs held. The advantage of the latter format is that the candidate has the flexibility of highlighting the skills, tasks, and qualities most appropriate to the case manager's role regardless of the time they were acquired, performed, or applied. Candidates for the case manager's role who do not have case management experience are advised to prepare their resume following the grouping of tasks and skills format. This format will clearly show the qualities that make them the best candidates for the job.

Box 6-1 presents an excerpt from an ad for a case manager position one may come across in newspapers, professional nursing journals, or recruitment newsletters. Potential applicants should study the ad carefully and be able to identify the qualities, skills, and qualifications the organization is looking for in the candidate (i.e., the bolded areas in Box 6-1). These qualities and skills may not be clearly stated in the ad. It is the responsibility of the candidate applying for the job to syn-

thesize the desired qualifications. The resume should then be written in a way that addresses the identified characteristics of the job.

Cover Letter

A cover letter explaining the candidate's intent for applying for the job is important to have attached to the resume before mailing or faxing the application. In the letter, candidates should indicate the specific ad they are responding to (i.e., specify the job title and the source of the ad). The letter should also include the career objective(s) of the candidate and highlight the acquired qualities and skills that meet the job requirements. For example, if you are responding to the ad presented in Box 6-1, it is important that you describe your skills in communication, teamwork, negotiation, brokering, facilitation and coordination of patient care activities, and evaluation of care outcomes. Your knowledge of the health care reimbursement systems, managed care organizations, and patient and family satisfaction issues is important to highlight. It is also beneficial to identify your clinical and leadership skills as they relate to the advertised job.

Because there will be no personal contact with the recruiter or prospective employer to discuss the job, you should put special efforts into writing the best resume and cover letter possible to increase your chances for an interview. The resume and the cover letter are your selling tools. They reflect one's marketability, and they should "paint a picture" of one's potential for success in the job. Review them carefully for any typographical or spelling errors, long or run-on sentences, and appropriateness of the adjectives used to describe yourself. Always remember to be concise, clear, and direct.

In the letter, candidates should indicate how their skills and previous experiences can be used in the prospective job or for the benefit of the institution. The style applied in the cover letter should appeal to the recruiter or the prospective employer. Avoid being overly clever or too wordy. Try to be honest and sincere. Use phrases that will increase the interest in you, and emphasize those aspects of yourself that you think will meet the case manager's role and make you look attractive. The cover letter should not be too long or boring to read. It should urge the prospective employer to review the resume and call you for an interview.

Looking Your Best

The interview is the opportunity to prove yourself. It is an act of validating that a potential candidate is the best fit for the job. The interview process should validate to the interviewer that your description of your qualifications and skills, evidenced in the resume and cover letter, is ac-

---

box 6-1

Excerpt from an Ad for a Case Manager's Job

In this position as a case manager you will be responsible for **working with an interdisciplinary team** of health care providers and **managing the care** of a select group of patients with complex diagnoses and needs. You are expected to achieve **high-quality care outcomes** in a **cost-effective** manner. You will act as a **patient and family advocate** and a **consultant** for members of the health care team within the institution and externally for **managed care organizations** and **community resource agencies.** The ideal candidate will possess a minimum of **4 years clinical nursing experience** and a current license as a registered professional nurse. A bachelor's degree is also required. Excellent **verbal and written communication skills,** case management experience, and certification are a plus.

curate. Your responses to the interview questions should strongly support what you have written in the resume. You should be at your best and look your best.

One way of improving the chances of being hired for the job is by familiarizing yourself with the role you are interviewed for. It is important for any case manager candidate to keep abreast of the latest changes occurring in the health care industry. A little over a decade ago, case management models were strange to hospitals and health care organizations. Training of case managers was held in the health care organization itself as part of the orientation to the new work environment and the role. However, because of reengineering and redesign of patient care delivery systems, today these models and roles are more popular, and training in case management has become available in schools of nursing as certificate and degree programs. This shift into case management has increased the competition among the candidates for the case manager's role and helped prospective employers in selecting the best-prepared candidate for the job.

The health care–related literature contains a substantial amount of information on case management models and roles. It is important for potential candidates to become knowledgeable in this field before applying for the role, especially if they have not had any prior training or experience in case management.

The case manager's role varies from one institution to another. One's experience as a case manager in one institution might not be transferrable. It is important, however, for the candidates to evaluate their previous experience in relation to the skills and qualifications required for the job and to proactively determine how to maximize the benefit of this experience for the interview.

It is important for candidates to obtain the job description of the advertised role and the mission and philosophy statements of the institution or its nursing department before the interview and to study them carefully. These documents are invaluable for candidates who are preparing for the interview process. They are instrumental in familiarizing the candidates with the potential work environment; expectations of the role; and the institution's culture, values, and beliefs. Candidates may ask for this information in advance through a personal letter or a fax addressed to the recruiter at the address/fax number available in the ad. They may ask for these documents in the cover letter attached to the resume, at the time it is sent to the recruiter or the prospective employer, or when the candidate is contacted to set up a date for the interview. Either way, it is important for candidates to obtain and review these documents before the interview.

Candidates must provide evidence to the interviewer that they possess the qualities, skills, and attributes necessary for the position. Sometimes it is helpful to maximize the use of real examples related to previous experiences to convince the interviewer that you are "The Candidate."

Potential case managers should be able to convince their prospective employers that they are the *right* candidates for the job and the organization. One way to accomplish this is by conveying a sense of professionalism. You should clearly articulate your strengths and weaknesses as they relate to the job. You should also explain your willingness to learn and improve in the areas in which you lack experience. The interviewer expects a candidate to be lacking knowledge or experience in some aspects of the job. Candidates who recognize or address these issues demonstrate a clear understanding of the job requirements and willingness to learn. It is also important that you make the interviewers aware of your potential. Explain to them what it is that you are able to bring with you that is considered beneficial to the institution. Concentrate on meeting the organization's mission statement and philosophy. Make an effort to discuss your transferrable skills (i.e., the skills you can carry with you to any job or organization).

The outer appearance of potential candidates for the case manager's role is important. It is the first impression you leave with the interviewer/prospective employer. The way you are dressed should create a positive and professional image. This image plays a crucial role in setting the tone for the rest of the interview. You should make an effort to look professional even if you know the prospective employer has a relaxed dress code. You should *dress for success*.

During the interview, candidates should be extra careful in how they respond to the interviewer's questions. They should not appear to be rigid, indifferent, or inflexible. Candidates should avoid using statements that begin with "I never . . .," "I don't like . . .," or "It is impossible to. . . ." The following examples illustrate this point.

Do not say: "In my previous job I never attempted to call the private physicians myself because it makes them angry. Instead, I always asked the nurse manager to do that."

It is better to say: "In my previous job I was not expected to contact the private physicians myself, but I understand the importance of discussing a particular situation with them directly. I am willing and have no problem doing that in this position."

Do not say: "In the past, I found it impossible to discuss the plan of care of each patient with the various health care providers."

It is better to say: "It is a great challenge to discuss the plan of care of each patient with the various health care providers, and I understand its importance in improving the quality of care. I will do the best I can in this area."

Do not say: "Why should I keep pushing for rescheduling a procedure that is canceled. It is not my responsibility to do it. It is the responsibility of the department canceling the procedure."

It is better to say: "I understand how difficult it can be to ensure that a procedure is completed as scheduled. It is important not to delay the completion of a procedure. Otherwise, the patient and the institution suffer (or the cost and quality of care are compromised)."

In their answers to interviewers' questions, candidates are encouraged to use statements that convey an understanding of the case manager's role, flexibility in their opinions and attitudes, openness to change and trying new methods of doing things, and willingness to learning and expanding knowledge. Candidates should avoid stating what they have always done in their previous jobs. However, they can use their previous experiences in subtle ways in supporting their flexibility as practitioners and confirming to the interviewers that they possess the skills and qualities they seek in the potential case managers.

Questions That may be Asked by Candidates

It is appropriate for candidates to ask questions during the interview process. However, they should be asked when opportunities exist. For example, interviewers may ask candidates at some point during the interview process if they have any questions. If this does not happen, then candidates may ask their questions toward the end of the interview. Questions that are considered appropriate may include the following:

- Patient population(s)
- Area of responsibility (e.g., inpatient unit, outpatient clinic, both areas)
- Expectations regarding performance
- Expected hours of work (e.g., days, evenings, weekends, rotation)
- Reporting mechanism (i.e., the case manager's position in the table of organization)
- Current status in relation to case management and institutional goals
- Support systems
- Orientation process to the work environment and the role

The salary should not be discussed during the interview unless it is brought up by the interviewer. It is always better to negotiate the salary at the time the job is offered.

Candidates may also ask the interviewer about the time frame for filling the job, or how long it will be before they are notified if they are accepted. Candidates may contact the recruiter and inquire if a decision has been made if the indicated time frame has passed. It is acceptable to ask about the reasons for not being hired. Interviewing is a demanding skill and one cannot improve unless made aware of deficient areas.

CHARACTERISTICS LOOKED FOR IN POTENTIAL CANDIDATES FOR THE CASE MANAGER'S ROLE

The role of the case manager is integral to the success of the case management model. Candidates for this job should reflect potential for success in the role during the interview process. There are several significant skills (Box 6-2) case management leaders look for in candidates for the case manager's role. These skills are based on the job description of the case manager and are affected by the environment of work (i.e., the operations/systems of the organization, policies, procedures, standards of care and practice, and status and power embedded in the job as compared with other health care professionals). The most important skills are those that make the potential candidate able to collaborate effectively with other health care providers within and outside the organization.

In this position the case manager is expected to work with minimum direction or supervision. Because case managers are integral members of interdisciplinary teams, they are expected to demonstrate excellent

---

box 6-2
Case Manager's Skills

1. Clinical
2. Leadership
3. Teamwork
4. Time management
5. Decision making/problem solving
6. Critical thinking
7. Organization
8. Delegation
9. Communication/open-mindedness/assertiveness
10. Diplomacy/politics
11. Tolerance
12. Commitment
13. Education/teaching
14. Role modeling
15. Change agent
16. Conflict resolution
17. Power
18. Cultural sensitivity

decision-making and problem-solving skills. In addition, they should exhibit willingness to work with others (i.e., teamwork). Because of their varied responsibilities, case managers should have superior organizational and time-management skills. This is important for increased productivity and efficiency in the role. They work daily with physicians, nurses, patients and families, and other health care providers to ensure that high-quality and cost-effective care and outcomes are achieved. These expectations make assertiveness, ability to communicate well verbally and in writing, diplomacy, and open-mindedness among the many skills required for success in the role.

Case managers spend much of their time in facilitating and coordinating patient care activities and resolving **variances.** In this role function, they are expected to demonstrate skills in leadership, clinical care activities, tolerance, delegation, and negotiation. When they hold patient and family teaching sessions, they apply the adult learning theory into their practice and follow the strategies derived from the health-belief model, which means that they should be knowledgeable in the available theories on patient and family teaching. However, when they are asked for help by a member of the health care team, they are looked at as role models and resource people. They are expected to be able to find answers to challenging situations.

Interviewer's Role

During the interview process, interviewers should evaluate whether potential candidates possess the skills required for the role. If found to be lacking in any of the skills, interviewers should evaluate candidates for potential success in learning these skills. The questions to be asked in an interview should cover the affective, cognitive, and behavioral aspects of the role.

The best questions to be asked are the open-ended ones (Table 6-1). Potential candidates should also be asked to provide practical examples that support their abilities and help demonstrate competence in their skills. Examples are particularly important because they provide concrete evidence related to the candidates' performance in real work situations. Examples usually validate the candidates' answers because they add an objective flavor to the subjective answers. When candidates are found to be struggling with giving examples, the interviewer may use hypothetical situations to help potential candidates express their opinion.

The interviewer must be careful not to ask questions that are considered against the law, as determined by the Americans with Disabilities Act, Equal Employment Opportunity Act, and Age Discrimination in Employ-

ment Act. For example, avoid questions such as the following:

- How old are you?
- How many children do you have?
- How old are your children?
- Are you married?
- What religious holidays do you observe?
- What language do you speak when not at work?
- What is your ethnic background?
- What are your political beliefs?

Interviewers should take their time in conducting the interview. They should avoid making candidates feel rushed. A reasonable interview is one that lasts an average of 1 hour. Similar to the candidates, interviewers are required to be poised, clear, direct, articulate, and skillful in the interview process. It is imperative for the interviewers not to bore the candidates with talking too much about the institution and the job. They should avoid unnecessary rambling.

Interviewers should prepare the interview questions in advance. As much as possible, they should use the same set of questions for interviewing all potential candidates. This pattern makes it easier to compare candidates and select the best one for the job. Most institutions have a standardized interviewing process in place and a predetermined set of questions that can be adapted to each specific job. If this is not the case in your institution, it is helpful to prepare interview questions beforehand.

At the end of the interview, interviewers may summarize the interview by explaining the next step(s) to candidates. This may include whether follow-up interviews are necessary and if so, with whom, when, and where. It is also important that candidates be informed of the time frame for filling the position and the method of notifying the selected candidate. This eliminates any confusion candidates may face while waiting to hear from the interviewer/potential employer.

Follow-Up Interviews

Candidates for the case manager's role are usually interviewed more than once. They are interviewed by the recruiter and the administrator of the case management program. Some institutions also require them to be interviewed by a panel of interviewers as well (i.e., representative from the interdisciplinary team). Depending on the job description and roles and responsibilities, potential candidates may be required to interview with physicians or chairmen of departments. Candidates should prepare themselves well for impressive and successful interviews in all the steps of the process an institution may have in place.

TABLE 6-1
Sample Questions That may be Asked in the Case Manager's Interview

Questions	Behaviors/skills evaluated
Give me an example when you had too many things to do at once, and tell me how you went about accomplishing the tasks.	Time management Organizational skills Prioritization Creating a plan Getting tasks accomplished
Tell me about a problem you have faced in the past with a patient/family member, a co-worker, a physician, or superior. How did you handle the situation?	Conflict resolution Problem solving Dealing with stress Affection/temperament Team work/independence Effectiveness Assertiveness Comfort level with confrontation
Explain to me what makes you the best candidate for the job.	Motivation Self-confidence Esteem Ability to discuss strengths and weaknesses Experience Assertiveness
From your past experience, tell me about a time when you had to promote change. How were you able to do it? What role did you play in it?	Perseverance Change agent Adaptability and flexibility Openness to change and new ideas Creativity Ability to influence others Assertiveness Risk taking
In your opinion, what does a case manager do?	Knowledge and understanding Potentials Keeping up-to-date with changes in health care
Tell me about a time when you were able to influence the behavior of others in a positive way	Encouragement to others Teamwork/team player Provide feedback Interpersonal skills Creativity and paradigm shift Willingness to try new ideas
Describe a situation when you were able to impact on the cost of patient care/resource utilization.	Awareness of health care cost Cost-containment strategies Allocation/management of resources
Tell me about a time when you were faced with a problem and needed to collect some information for solving the problem. Describe to me how you analyzed the information to come to your decision.	Problem solving Critical thinking Use of data and evidence Response to stressful situations/affection Willingness to complete a project/task Commitment
Describe to me a situation when you had to work with little or no supervision. What did you do?	Independence Motivation Commitment Productivity Leadership
What is it that you can bring to this role/institution that will make a difference?	Previous experience Ability to identify one's strengths Confidence/self-esteem Visionary

---

When interviewed by physicians or chairmen of departments, it is important for the candidates to convey a message of openness, collegiality, collaboration and partnership, and clinical knowledge. It is also important that they convey excellence in teamwork, negotiation, leadership, mentorship, and coaching skills when interviewed by a panel.

Candidates are first interviewed by a recruiter, who screens the candidates and selects those who expressed strong potential for success in the case manager's role.

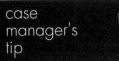

case manager's tip **6-1**

Suggestions for the Interviewer

1. Ask open-ended questions.
2. Establish rapport at the beginning of the interview.
3. Begin with "ice-breaking" questions (e.g., It is a lovely day today; how was your trip coming here?).
4. Allow silence; the candidate may need to collect his or her thoughts before answering the question.
5. Ask behavioral questions.
6. Control the interview; you may need to redirect the conversation if the candidate starts to ramble around.
7. If you want to take notes, explain why.
8. Prepare the questions in advance. Questions should be based on the related job description and/or the resume of the candidate.
9. Ask questions that are based on past job experiences of the candidate. This allows for envisioning the future and investigating the candidate's potential.
10. Ask for contrary evidence, especially when identifying an undesired or a negative skill. Contrary evidence prevents the interviewer from making a one-sided/subjective picture.
11. Validate responses using reflective statements as needed.
12. Avoid judgment, and be objective. Do not allow intuition or "gut feelings" to interfere in your decision.
13. Familiarize self with the skills required for the job (e.g., performance, organizational, interactional).

case manager's tip **6-2**

Suggestions for the Candidate

1. Ask for the job description and the organization's mission and philosophy statements in advance. Study them well.
2. Arrive for the interview on time.
3. Dress for success.
4. Bring your portfolio to the interview. Be prepared to share concrete evidence of your accomplishments when appropriate.
5. Watch for your body language/nonverbal communication. It is a part of the interview too.
6. Do not interrupt the interviewer.
7. Avoid rambling around in your answers. Be poised, concise, clear, and direct.
8. Support your answers with evidence (i.e., examples from previous experiences).
9. Be prepared to discuss what it is that you can provide to the organization.
10. Convey your self-confidence, professionalism, and self-esteem through your answers.
11. Do not hesitate to explain your silence at times. The interviewer is aware that you may need a moment of silence to collect your thoughts before answering a question.
12. Avoid speaking fast or stuttering. Be articulate.
13. Be clear in your career goals.
14. Rehearse your interview if that helps you prepare better.

Next they are interviewed by the administrator of the case management program. Those who are found to be impressive and show strong potential are then called for follow-up interviews. The follow-up interviews, depending on the institution, may include an interview with a physician or the chairman of the department where the case manager will be working and another with a panel of interviewers, including representatives from the interdisciplinary health care team and fellow case managers.

It is important to limit the follow-up interviews only to the candidates who express promising success in the role. The recruiter and the administrator of the case management program may collaborate in selecting these candidates, which are usually limited to two or three in number. Unnecessary interviews waste time and cost money. Candidates should be informed by the interviewer of the next steps, whether follow-up interviews will be conducted, and when they will be informed of such decisions.

Candidates should not forget about the interviewer after the interview is over. It is advisable to send a note or a card thanking the interviewer for the opportunity and the consideration. It is also appropriate for candidates to indicate in the note their continued interest in the job.

Conducting interviews and interviewing are great challenges. One should learn how to meet these challenges. It is beneficial to read about the interview process or attend seminars to polish your interviewing skills. Sometimes it is necessary to practice role playing before your interview. This practice may help you get the job you desire. Case Manager's Tips 6-1 and 6-2 present some tips for the interviewer and the candidate. These tips should help both the interviewer to be better prepared in evaluating and screening the appropriate candidates for the job and the potential candidates to overcome their fear of being interviewed. The skills of interviewing well are important for everyone, because you never know when they may be necessary in your career. You should always remember that the written words (i.e., the resume and cover letter) are the candidate's ambassador to the interviewer. They should be thought of as a glorified list of one's qualities, which when read leaves a lasting impression.

KEY POINTS

1. The interview process is not an easy task. It requires careful and thorough preparation by the candidate and the interviewer. Practice, role play, or rehearsal before the interview could be helpful.
2. Candidates for case management jobs should always send a resume with a cover letter to potential employers explaining their intent for applying for an advertised job.
3. The resume is a compelling source of information for the prospective employer. An impressive resume is one that summarizes the candidate's attributes and skills.
4. The cover letter should delineate the candidate's acquired qualities and skills that are anticipated to meet the requirements of the job applied for.
5. Avoid being rigid, indifferent, or inflexible during an interview (this is applicable for both the candidate and the interviewer).
6. If interviewing several candidates for a job, use a standardized set of questions that could be prepared based on the job description and should reflect the skills and qualities demanded by the job. This makes selecting the best candidate for the job easier.

CHAPTER 7

CURRICULA AND CERTIFICATION IN NURSE CASE MANAGEMENT

Recently, **case management** has become the most desired approach to patient care delivery. Case management had originally been a nursing care delivery model. Today, however, most health care institutions have adopted case management as their patient care delivery system. Nurses who assumed the case manager's role in the 1980s were basically prepared for the role in health care organizations (i.e., hospitals). Training sessions for these nurses were conducted on the premises of the institution itself, particularly at the patient's bedside. Since the beginning of the 1990s, however, nurse case managers have opportunities for training in a variety of settings. In addition to the institution-based case management training programs, today there are several programs that are college based or university based.

The case management programs that exist today can be classified into three types depending on the length of the program and the place where it is provided. These are (1) a certificate program; (2) a noncertificate program; and (3) a graduate degree program. Nurse case managers can choose any of these programs for training. Requirements for entry into the case management role may vary from institution to institution.

Case management is defined by the Commission for Case Manager Certification (1996) as "a collaborative process which assesses, plans, implements, coordinates, monitors, and evaluates the options and services required to meet an individual's health needs, using communication and available resources to promote quality, cost-effective outcomes." Case management programs are designed to train nurse case managers in the case management process. The content of these programs is a detailed discussion of the Commission's definition of case management.

CASE MANAGEMENT CERTIFICATE PROGRAMS

Case management certificate programs are of two types. One is provided by an independent agency or a health care institution in the form of a multiday conference. The other type is provided by a college or university in the form of multiple credits, usually 12 credits. Enrollment in the independent agency program is open to all nurses regardless of educational background or speciality. However, the college-based certificate program is limited to those who hold college degrees. Some colleges offer a postbaccalaureate certificate program. Others offer a postmaster's. Both types of programs include theory, as well as clinical courses. Participants in either type of program are provided with a *Certificate in Case Management* when they complete all the requirements. New England Healthcare Assembly's certificate program is an example of a non–college-based program, whereas Seton Hall University's program is an example of a college/university-based program.

New England Healthcare Assembly's Case Management Certificate Program

The New England Healthcare Assembly's Case Management Certificate Program (New England Healthcare Assembly, 1996) is designed as an integrated program of three modules. Each module is a stand-alone seminar. However, it is an integral part of the overall program and the scope of case management. Each module is given separately over 3 days of coursework. The whole program requires 9 days of coursework for completion. A participant could complete the coursework within 4 months if registering for the three modules consecutively. A comprehensive examination is required after completing the three modules, after which a certificate of completion can be provided.

The program is offered for clinicians, administrators, and support staff who are involved in designing, implementing, and evaluating case management systems. Health care professionals such as nurses, social workers, discharge planners, utilization reviewers, and quality and risk management professionals are eligible for enrollment in this program.

This certificate program includes discussions regarding case management systems in various health care settings and managed care organizations. Organizational development, health care reimbursement systems, and financial analysis processes are also discussed. The skills learned in this program include strategies for successful design, implementation, and evaluation of case management systems and case management plans; management of **variances;** and integration of interdepartmental processes for continuous quality improvement efforts.

The first module includes topics such as the following:

1. Assessment of the external health care environment
2. Managed care and its financial underpinnings
3. Key elements of case management
4. Role of the case manager across the health care continuum
5. Management information systems
6. Utilization review and case management

The key concepts discussed in this module include health care policy, integration of patient care delivery, **managed care, capitation,** reimbursement systems, cost/benefit analysis, case management models, case management plans, roles of case managers in various models and care settings, critical functions of case managers, variance data collection and analysis, financial and administrative information systems, automation in case management, and utilization review procedures and protocols.

The second module includes the following topics:

1. Patient care across the health care continuum
2. Financial reimbursement systems
3. Patient care quality
4. Patient care outcomes
5. Evaluation indicators for case management systems

Participants in this module will learn how to coordinate patient care outside the hospital walls. They become astute in identifying and coordinating community resources and in collaborating with patients and their families, primary physicians, managed care organizations, and community-based case managers. They also learn how to ensure and monitor the quality of patient care in the community. Reimbursement issues are discussed pertaining to **Medicare, Medicaid,** managed care organizations, and other **third-party payors.** How to evaluate a case management model is the last topic learned in this module. Patient care quality, **outcome measures** and indicators, patient's satisfaction, continuous quality improvement and participation in improvement teams, **length of stay,** and cost containment are among the subjects discussed in this module.

The third and last module provided in this certificate program includes topics such as the following:

1. Role of case managers
2. Interdisciplinary teams
3. Customer relations
4. Competency of case managers
5. Organizational change

Case managers are given the opportunity in this module to learn the skills required to be an active and efficient participant in an interdisciplinary team. They learn how to effect positive change, how to manage conflict, and how to promote case management as an integral part of the organizational culture, values, and philosophy. They also learn the ins and outs of their role and responsibilities, priority setting, and how to respond effectively to multiple needs.

Seton Hall University's Certificate Program

The Seton Hall University's Certificate Program (Seton Hall University, 1996) was established in 1996. It is a 12-credit postbaccalaureate program in nurse case management that is offered only to nurses. This program combines theory and practice and may fit into any organizational setting. Admission to this program is restricted to those nurses who meet the following criteria:

1. Baccalaureate degree in nursing from a National League for Nursing (NLN) accredited program
2. Cumulative B average
3. B average in nursing courses
4. Current licensure as a registered professional nurse
5. Minimum of 1 year of clinical nursing experience

Preference for participation in this program is given to applicants who are certified in a clinical nursing specialty and those who are working in the capacity of nurse case managers. The program consists of 6 credits in nurse case management theory, 3 credits of clinical experience/practicum, and 3 credits in nursing resource management.

The Nurse Case Management Theory Course I is designed to teach participants about the role of nurse case managers in a managed care environment and across various health care settings. The exploration of community resources for client support and the concepts of health care insurance (Medicare, Medicaid, managed care organizations, and other third-party payors), **utilization management,** legal and ethical issues, discharge planning, and total quality management are the selected topics of discussion.

The Nurse Case Management Theory Course II is an extension to Course I. It examines the case management process. Participants are developed in patient's screening and selection for case management services, assessment of patient's and family's needs, development of the treatment plan (i.e., the case management plan), ongoing case management, evaluation of patient's responses to treatment, patient and family teaching, and care of the patient after discharge. Health care marketing strategies; financial management and health care cost accounting, particularly reimbursement systems; standards of care and practice; and public policy legislation are discussed. In addition, research as a vehicle for advancing the role of the nurse case manager is also examined.

The Nurse Case Management Practicum Course provides the students with the opportunity to explore, test, and expand the nurse case management theory(ies) in the organizational setting. During this course, enrollees are expected to rotate through clinical areas and be exposed to first-hand experience with case management. They are precepted by seasoned nurse case managers. Socialization with experienced case managers permits the students the opportunity to analyze, synthesize, integrate their learning, and evaluate their effectiveness as potential/future nurse case managers. Students are given control over their clinical experience through designing their own objectives and planning, controlling, and evaluating their learning experiences to achieve these objectives.

The Nursing Resource Management Course emphasizes the health care organizations as "corporate entities." Business perspective of managing nursing services is a major part of this course. Complex management issues are shared and explored as they relate to managing single departments, as well as the health care organization as a whole.

The Seton Hall University's Certificate Program is a four-semester program, in which one or two courses may be taken in each semester. At the successful completion of the program, students are provided with a "certificate of completion" in nurse case management.

CASE MANAGEMENT NONCERTIFICATE PROGRAMS

Case management noncertificate programs are those offered by health care institutions as part of training, orientation, and education of nursing and nonnursing personnel in preparation for the implementation of case management systems. These programs are usually designed by individual institutions based on their policies and procedures and on the job description, roles, and responsibilities of nurse case managers. The design of these programs is affected by who will assume the case manager's role. In addition, the length of these programs varies from one institution to another—2 to 4 weeks depending on the intensity of the program. Some

institutions have been able to obtain approval for offering continuing education units (CEUs) to the participants in these programs. This is a result of successfully completing an application for CEUs submitted to nursing continuing education boards such as the American Nurses Association's Board of Continuing Education.

Health care institution–based noncertificate programs are generally taught by the nursing continuing education department or the institution's training and development department. The staff of these departments are the instructors of the program, in collaboration with the administrator of the case management service/department. Sometimes these programs are taught by a consultant or consulting agency that is charged with overseeing the implementation of case management systems. Topics discussed are similar to those addressed in the certificate programs. The difference, however, is that the noncertificate, institution-based program is individualized to fit the institution's policies, procedures, operations, standards of care, standards of practice, and extent of responsibilities of those to assume the case manager roles (see Case Manager's Tip 7-1 for strategies for developing a solid case management orientation program).

Other noncertificate case management programs are those offered in schools of nursing as one or two courses, earning 3 to 6 credits, in baccalaureate or master's degree programs. The topical outline of these courses varies from one school to another. However, the basics of case management and managed care, financial reimbursement systems, roles of case managers, case management plans, variance data collection and analysis, outcomes management, and quality improvement are common to all schools and programs. The content of these courses is usually approved by the state education department and/or accrediting agencies such as the NLN. Most schools that include case management courses in their programs offer such course(s) as a mandatory part of the curriculum rather than as elective courses.

Students who are enrolled in the school-based programs and nurses who attend the health care institution–based programs are eligible for participation in the certified case manager exam (see the following section). After completion of these training programs nurses are deemed knowledgeable in case management systems and ready for practice.

CASE MANAGEMENT DEGREE PROGRAMS

Case management degree programs are full graduate-level programs offered in a college or university setting. They generally are a combination of traditional master's level and newly developed case management systems–

case manager's tip **7-1**

Strategies for Developing a Solid Case Management Orientation Program

1. Involve a case management expert or consultant.
2. Develop a program that is reflective of the nurse case manager's job description.
3. Include subject matter experts from your institution on the planning team.
4. Have the subject matter experts teach in the program.
5. Refer to what has been published in this area; limit the topics to what nurse case managers will be involved in.
6. Hold classes, as well as on-the-job training.
7. Make sure that topics taught include finance, reimbursement, leadership skills, conflict resolution, problem solving, communication and teamwork, and negotiation skills.
8. Include teaching strategies such as role play, case studies, and discussions.
9. Maximize the use of mentoring.

related courses. At the successful completion of these programs, students earn a master's degree. The case management program established by the College of Nursing, Graduate Program, at Villanova University, Villanova, Pa, is a good example of such programs. Enrollment in this program is limited to students with a baccalaureate degree in nursing from an NLN-accredited school of nursing, a 3.0 grade point average, a minimum of 1 year clinical experience, and satisfactory performance on the Miller Analogies Test or the verbal portion of the Graduate Record Exam.

In July of 1993 the College of Nursing at Villanova University received a 3-year grant from the Division of Nursing of the U.S. Public Health Service to develop a graduate degree program in clinical case management. It is a 45-credit program designed to prepare case managers for acute care settings, community-based organizations, insurance and disability management companies, and other managed care systems. In addition, it prepares case managers in the provision, management, and coordination of the total care of groups of clients. At the completion of this program, graduates are able to apply the theory and advanced knowledge of case management systems in clinical practice (Villanova University, 1996).

Students in the clinical case manager program take courses in budgeting, organizational systems, case management models, case manager role development, community resources, clinical outcomes, and marketing. In addition, they are required to take some core courses in health care delivery systems, nursing science, and nursing research, as well as a theory course and a practicum in a particular specialty. The core courses add up to 15 credits. In addition, there are two elective courses.

Description of the Clinical Case Management Courses

The following description of the courses in the Clinical Case Manager Program at Villanova University is based on the information presented in the 1996-1997 catalog of the university's College of Nursing Graduate Program.

In the *Health Care Organizations and Nursing Care Systems* course, clinical case managers learn about the dynamics, culture, and politics of health care organizations and particularly nursing care systems. They analyze the impact of internal and external forces affecting such delivery systems, with a closer look at the impact of these forces on nursing care delivery. In this course, students are exposed to some of the skills required for success in the clinical case manager role, such as negotiation, conflict resolution, change, and motivation.

Budgeting Concepts for Clinical Case Managers is another required course. It prepares case managers in the budgetary process, types of budgets, and budget development and analysis. This course is important because it provides future case managers with better understanding of health care budgeting and the need for cost-containment strategies.

The *Role of the Clinical Case Manager* course prepares case managers for a thorough understanding of their roles and responsibilities toward the organization, patient and family, and physicians, social workers, physical therapists, and so forth. It puts the various roles assumed by case managers into perspective. This course also analyzes the impact of organizational structures and reference groups on the role of clinical case managers.

Another required course is *Marketing in Health Care,* which includes an analysis of concepts related to creating competitive market planning strategies. Assessment and analysis of the market place, demographics, and health care needs are also addressed.

Examination of the various models of case management, the impact of legislation and health care financing on such models, grant writing, funding sources, and

case
manager's
tip

7-2   **Eligibility Criteria**

All applicants for the Commission for Case Manager Certification examination must meet the following two eligibility criteria:
1. Licensure/certification: completion of a postsecondary program in human and health services
2. Employment/experience in the area of specialty indicated by the license or certificate

ethical considerations in health care are all discussed in the *Models for Case Management* course. In this course, students learn about case management models across the health care continuum and their logistics, similarities, and differences.

Community resources and strategies for accessing federal, state, and voluntary agencies, as well as regional resources, are the focus of the *Community Resources* course. This course is important to case managers because of the role they play in discharge planning and patient care coordination. It provides them with an understanding of the regulations regarding community resources and the different entitlements of patients in relation to their health care insurance coverage.

Clinical case managers enrolled in this program learn how to assess, evaluate, and analyze patient care outcomes in the *Clinical Outcomes* course. They also learn about the development, implementation, and evaluation of case management plans/critical pathways. Care mapping as a quality improvement mechanism and evaluating case management plans through variance analysis are also discussed.

Patient Education: Principles and Strategies is another important course that prepares case managers in their role as patient and family educators. Patient teaching across the life span; teaching/learning process; identifying the learner needs, barriers, and readiness to learning; and motivational factors are some of the topics discussed. Case managers also learn how to incorporate patient and family teaching into the case management plan. The effective utilization of teaching strategies and tools is explored.

In the *Practicum in Clinical Case Management* course, students get the opportunity to apply the theory, knowledge, and skills they learned in class to practice settings. With the help of a clinical case manager as a preceptor, students select a practicum site in which they operationalize their future role in case management into a particular care setting. During this practicum, they practice the clinical case manager role, test their skills and knowledge, and refine them as needed.

This degree program in case management provides case managers with a wide understanding of case management models and systems and prepares them for success in the role of case manager in a variety of settings.

CERTIFICATION IN NURSE CASE MANAGEMENT

Certification in nurse case management is important because it affirms that the nurse case manager possesses the knowledge and skills required to render appropriate and safe case management services to potential clients. There exists only one certification in nurse case management. It has been sponsored by the Commission for Case Manager Certification (CCMC) since July 1, 1995. Before then, it was sponsored by the Certification of Insurance Rehabilitation Specialists Commission (CIRSC).

The CCMC (1996) advocates for case management as a specialized area of practice rather than a profession. Case management experts who developed the eligibility criteria for the certification agree that case management services can be provided by a variety of professionals from different health and human services and professions (e.g., nursing, social work, physical therapy). As a result, these professionals, when certified as case managers, use the credential "certified case manager" (CCM) in conjunction with their professional licensure (e.g., registered professional nurses use the credentials RN, CCM; certified social workers use the credentials CSW, CCM).

The certification examination is offered twice every year, during the months of June and December. The initial certification is valid for 5 years. Renewal of the case manager certification is required every 5 years. It can be achieved through reexamination or if the CCM demonstrates professional development, which entails participation in approved continuing education programs. In addition, the certified case managers applying for certification renewal should also provide evidence that they continue to hold the same license or certification they held at the time of the initial certification (e.g., registered professional nurse, certified social worker, certified physical therapist).

Eligibility Criteria for Case Manager Certification

The CCMC has established two eligibility criteria that have to be met by all applicants at the time applications for the examination are submitted (Case Manager's Tip 7-2). The first criteria is licensure/certification, and the other is employment/experience. In addition, all applicants "must be of good moral character, reputation, and fitness for the practice of case management" (Commission for Case Manager Certification, 1996).

The licensure/certification criteria requires the applicant to have completed a minimum education of a postsecondary program in the field of human and health services. For example, registered professional nurses on all levels of education (diploma, bachelor's, master's, or doctorate degrees) are eligible for participation in this

certification. The Commission only honors the educational programs that provide a license/certificate that permits the holder to legally practice without the supervision of another professional (e.g., registered professional nursing programs).

In addition to meeting the licensure/certification criteria, the applicant for the case manager certification examination must provide verification of employment and experience in the area of specialty as indicated on the license or certificate. To be eligible, one must provide evidence of either (1) 12 months of full-time employment under the supervision of a certified case manager; (2) 24 months of full-time employment without supervision of any professional; or (3) 12 months of full-time employment as a supervisor of case management

---

case manager's tip | **7-3**
Topics to Review for the Certification Examination

1. Patient's bill of rights
2. Legal and ethical issues
3. Patient's privacy and confidentiality
4. Continuum of care
5. Clinical information systems and communication of information
6. Medical terminology
7. Patient's assessment and data-gathering procedures
8. Disease processes and treatment modalities
9. Psychosocial assessment of patients and families
10. Assessment of support systems
11. Coping with and adaptation to illness
12. Evaluation of patient's responses to treatments and quality of care
13. Advocacy
14. Negotiation of services
15. Managed care
16. Insurance policy coverage; inclusions/exclusions
17. Cost/benefit analysis
18. Cost-containment strategies
19. Precertification for services
20. Health care delivery systems
21. Screening and intake of patients for case management services
22. Coordination and facilitation of care activities
23. Patient and family education
24. Discharge planning
25. Case management plans
26. Community resources and services
27. Documentation of case management services
28. Role of the case manager
29. Consultation
30. Legislation and public policy related to case management
31. Liability issues/concerns of case management
32. Outcomes management; variances and variance analysis
33. Utilization review
34. Americans with Disabilities Act
35. Durable medical equipment
36. Evaluating the effectiveness of case management services

services and/or case managers. Applicants should demonstrate that their employment experience entails the components of case management services as defined by the Commission for Case Manager Certification, which are assessment, planning, implementation, coordination, monitoring, and evaluation.

Examination Content Topics

The certification examination consists of 300 multiple-choice questions that address five different broad areas related to the job description and roles and responsibilities of case managers and the case management process. These include the following, as they appear in the CCM Certification Guide (Commission for Case Manager Certification, 1996):

1. Coordination and service delivery
2. Physical and psychosocial factors
3. Benefit systems and cost/benefit analysis
4. Case management concepts
5. Community resources

Case Manager's Tip 7-3 presents a suggested list of topics that may aid case managers in their preparation for the certification examination.

KEY POINTS

1. Case management programs are of different types. They are either college/university-based, institution-based, or independent agency–based.
2. Case management programs could be certificate or degree programs.
3. Regardless of their preparation or background in case management, nurse case managers are eligible to sit for the case manager certification examination.
4. Certification in nurse case management is important because it affirms that nurse case managers possess the knowledge and skills required for rendering case management services to their clients.

References

Commission for Case Manager Certification: *CCM certification guide,* Rolling Meadows, Ill, 1996, Commission for Case Manager Certification.

New England Healthcare Assembly: *New England healthcare assembly's case management certificate program, marketing brochure,* Boston, 1996, New England Healthcare Assembly.

Seton Hall University, College of Nursing: *Seton Hall University's nurse case management certificate program, marketing brochure,* South Orange, NJ, 1996, Seton Hall University.

Villanova University, College of Nursing Graduate Program: *1996-1997's graduate nursing catalog,* Villanova, Pa, 1996, Villanova University.

CHAPTER 8

NURSE CASE MANAGER'S DOCUMENTATION

Over the past decade, greater emphasis has been given to the role nurses play in the provision of patient care as a result of redesigning, reengineering, or restructuring of health care delivery systems. This change has increased the level of importance of nursing documentation. Nursing documentation has become even more important in institutions that developed and implemented new patient care delivery models such as **case management,** care management, integrated care, and collaborative care. The main reason behind the increased importance of nursing documentation is related to the changes that have occurred in the role of the registered professional nurse, particularly the introduction of the role of nurse **case managers.**

The creation of the nurse case manager's role has pressured health care providers other than nurses to rely more on some of the important functions nurses play in the delivery of patient care, which have historically been ignored. These functions include but are not limited to the following:

- Coordination of discharge planning activities
- Facilitation and expedition of patient care activities
- Psychosocial assessment of needs of patients and families
- Emphasis not only on actual patient/family problems but also on potential ones
- Evaluation of patient care outcomes and responses to treatment
- Counseling of patient/family regarding knowledge of health needs and preventive measures
- Service monitoring

These functions have been emphasized greatly in the job descriptions and the roles and responsibilities of nurse case managers in a variety of institutions and patient care settings.

IMPORTANCE OF DOCUMENTATION

Nurse case managers view documentation as an important aspect of their role (Case Manager's Tip 8-1). Docu-

mentation reflects their professional responsibility and accountability toward patient care. In its *Standards of Clinical Nursing Practice,* the American Nurses Association (1991) identifies documentation as an integral part of its six standards of care (Table 8-1). Bower (1992), Cohen and Cesta (1997), and Tahan (1993) also identified documentation as an important role function of nurse case managers. There are several factors that increase the importance of documentation of nurse case managers, including the following:

1. Professional responsibility and accountability to patient care
2. Communication of the nurse case manager's judgments and evaluations
3. Evidence of nurse case managers' plans of care, interventions, and outcomes
4. Legal protection; valuable evidence
5. Standards of regulatory agencies (e.g., the U.S. Department of Health and the Joint Commission on Accreditation of Healthcare Organizations [JCAHO])
6. Health care reimbursement (e.g., the **diagnosis-related group [DRG]** system, managed care organizations, and **third-party payors**)
7. Supportive evidence of quality of patient care

ROLE OF NURSE CASE MANAGERS IN DOCUMENTATION

Documentation by nurse case managers is extremely important, because it is the only concrete evidence of their role in the provision of patient care. Nurse case managers' documentation in the medical record should reflect the case management steps discussed in Chapter 4. It should include documentation related to the following areas:

1. Method of patient referral for case management
2. Patient screening for appropriateness for case management services
3. Assessment of needs
4. Identification of the actual and potential problems
5. Establishing and implementing the plan of care
6. Facilitation and coordination of care activities

The Importance of Documentation

The case manager's documentation is crucial because it is the only evidence of the case manager's role in the provision of patient care.

TABLE 8-1
Evidence of Documentation in the Standards of Care of the American Nurses Association

Standards	Measurement criteria
Assessment	Relevant data are documented in a retrievable form
Diagnosis	Diagnoses are documented in a manner that facilitates the determination of expected outcomes and plan of care
Outcome identification	Outcomes are documented as measurable goals
Planning	The plan is documented
Implementation	Interventions are documented
Evaluation	Revisions in diagnoses, outcomes, and the plan of care are documented

Modified from American Nurses Association: *Standards of clinical nursing practice,* Kansas City, Mo, 1991, American Nurses Association.

7. Patient and family teaching
8. Patient's discharge and disposition
9. Evaluation of patient care outcomes

Appendix 8-1 at the end of this chapter presents an example of a nurse case manager's documentation record.

Method of Patient Referral for Case Management Services

Patient referrals for case management services may take place in three different ways. The first one is through a direct referral by a health care provider such as the primary nurse, private physician, consulting physician, house staff, nurse practitioner, physician assistant, social worker, or physical therapist. The patient could also be referred by personnel in the emergency department or the admitting office. The second method of referral for case management services is done by the patient/family themselves, particularly if they were familiar with the case management process from previous encounters. The third method of patient referrals is not exactly a true referral. However, the nurse case manager may elect to screen all the new admissions and identify those who could benefit from case manage-

ment. In home care settings and insurance companies, nurse case managers may follow all patients regardless of the seriousness of the episode of illness.

In most institutions the case management referral process is preidentified by health care administrators and nursing executives in a policy, procedure, or protocol and made clear to all health care providers through education and training.

The nurse case manager's documentation (Case Manager's Tip 8-2) should include how the patient has been referred for case management services, who made the referral, the reason(s) for the referral, and the date and time the referral is made. If no referral is made and the patient has been identified by the nurse case manager when screening the new admissions, then the nurse case manager's documentation should indicate so.

Patient Screening for Appropriateness for Case Management Services

However the referral process is made, the nurse case manager has to conduct a patient/family screening to determine appropriateness for case management activities. A decision regarding the patient's need for case management is made based on the "criteria for patient selection into the case management process" discussed in Chapter 4 (see Box 4-1, p. 40). Some of these criteria are patient's acuity, age, complexity of diagnosis, teaching needs, discharge planning, noncompliance with treatment regimen, insurance coverage, and financial status.

When patient screening is completed and case management services are deemed appropriate, the nurse case manager then writes an intake note in the patient's record explaining that the patient is accepted into the case management process (Case Manager's Tip 8-3).

Assessment of Needs

Screening of the patient/family for case management services and the initial assessment of needs are usually done concurrently by the nurse case manager because they are interrelated. The assessment of patient/family needs is made during the nurse case manager's first encounter with the patient/family. Careful assessment and

| case manager's tip | 8-2 | Elements to Include in Documentation |

The nurse case manager's documentation should include the following items:
1. How the patient was referred for case management services
2. Who made the referral
3. Reasons for the referral
4. Date and time of the referral

| case manager's tip | 8-3 | Elements of the Intake Note |

The intake note should focus on the following issues:
1. Reason for patient's hospitalization, need for medical attention, need for home care services
2. Indications for case management services (i.e., which criteria for selection of patients for case management are met?) (e.g., age, acuity, complexity of diagnosis, noncompliance)
3. Method of referral (e.g., health care provider, patient/family, nurse case manager screening)
4. The date and time patient's screening took place and the time the intake note was written
5. Method of screening (e.g., patient/family interview, discussion with other health care providers, review of medical record)
6. Certification/approval of current patient's hospitalization or medical services by the managed care organization

| case manager's tip | 8-4 | Elements of the Initial Assessment Note |

In addition to the criteria mentioned in the patient's screening section, the initial assessment note should include the following:
1. Chief complaint
2. Risk for injury
3. Discharge planning needs
4. Social support system
5. Health education needs
6. Justification for the need of medical services/attention

documentation of the patient's/family's needs can enhance the effectiveness of case management. Documentation of the initial assessment of needs by the nurse case manager is a more detailed extension of the intake note (Case Manager's Tip 8-4). Both notes are usually completed consecutively. In most cases one note is written combining both intake and assessment.

The nurse case manager's documentation should not include a thorough health history or a physical examination. A statement indicating that the medical record, including the patient's history and physical assessment (assessments that are completed and documented by other health care professionals, including the primary nurse and the physician), has been reviewed by the nurse case manager is of equal value and importance. The initial assessment note, however, should reflect any significant abnormalities identified by the nurse case manager that would dictate the plan of care, the interventions/treatments, and management of the patient's needs.

Identification of Patient's Actual and Potential Problems

Identification of the patient's actual and potential problems is the starting point for establishing the patient's plan of care. Accurate and comprehensive identification of these problems has a significant effect on patient care **outcomes.** A thorough examination of the patient's medical record, in addition to interviewing the patient and family, makes it easier for the nurse case manager to prioritize the patient's needs that should be stated in the patient's record as actual or potential problems. Regardless of the patient's condition, needs, and chief complaint, the nurse case manager's documentation of the patient's actual and potential problems almost always include problems related to the following:

1. Patient/family teaching
2. Discharge planning and disposition
3. Social support systems
4. Clinical condition (i.e., signs and symptoms)

The problems, identified by nurse case managers, regarding the complexity of patient/family teaching needs, discharge planning, and the absence of a social support system should be clearly and thoroughly documented in the patient's medical record.

For example, an elderly insulin-dependent diabetic patient who is legally blind and unable to self-administer insulin and who is admitted for uncontrolled diabetes cannot be discharged from the hospital before ensuring that he has a safe mechanism in place for administration of insulin injections. Another example is a businessman who is newly diagnosed with myocardial infarction and who is going to be started on cardiac medications for the first time. This patient may not be discharged unless patient teaching is completed and the patient discharge is deemed safe. Nurse case managers are well trained in how to be proactive planners, particularly in how to meet the discharge planning and teaching needs of their patients before discharge.

The documentation of the nurse case manager's assessment of the needs of these two patients on admission should include the potential problems regarding discharge planning and complexity of patient teaching. The plans of care developed should be reflected in the documentation, particularly how the identified needs will be met before the patients' readiness for discharge. Problems similar to the ones discussed in these examples may delay the patient's discharge. Careful documentation of these problems by nurse case managers helps justify the delay for administrators, insurance companies, and so on. This kind of documentation also justifies the patients' needs for services after discharge (i.e., home care). Managed care organizations usually look for such documentation in the medical record, which justifies the need for intensive services, when conducting medical record reviews.

Establishing and Implementing the Plan of Care

Planning patient care is a key element in the role of nurse case managers. Accurate and careful planning based on the data collected during the initial screening

and assessment of patients, as well as the appropriateness of the identified actual and potential problems, enables nurse case managers to provide individualized, efficient, and high-quality care. The plan of care is extremely important, because it serves as a communication tool for everyone involved in patient care. Articulating the plan of care in writing and making it clear to all those involved in the provision of care promotes continuity and consistency of care.

Nurse case managers are responsible for making sure that the written plan of care includes the patient's actual and potential problems/nursing diagnoses, the expected/desired outcomes of care, and the interventions/treatments needed to meet the expected outcomes (Table 8-2). It is important for nurse case managers to document in the patient's record the patient/family agreement to the plan of care as discussed on admission and at the time the initial assessment of patient's needs is completed. Documenting that the goals of treatment are collaboratively set with the patient/family, the nurse case manager, the attending physician,

---

TABLE 8-2

Example of a Patient Problem as Written by a Nurse Case Manager in the Plan of Care of a Patient With Fluid Retention Related to Congestive Heart Failure

Patient problem/nursing diagnosis	Expected outcomes of care (patient/family goals)	Nursing interventions
Fluid balance: excess	Stabilized fluid balance	
	Downward trend in patient's weight; no sudden increase	Weigh patient daily before breakfast
	Balanced intake and output	Monitor accurate intake and output
	Adherence to fluid restriction	Restrict fluids intake to 1000 ml per day
	Electrolytes within normal; no changes in potassium level	Monitor serum electrolytes, notify physician of any abnormal results
	Increased urine output	Give diuretics as ordered and monitor patient's response
	Reduction in severity of peripheral edema	Assess peripheral edema daily

case manager's tip   **8-5**   # Characteristics of Outcomes

Outcomes should be:
1. Patient and family oriented
2. Realistic and practical
3. Clear and concise
4. Measurable and observable
5. Concrete and doable
6. Time/interval specific

---

box 8-1

Examples of Patient Care Outcomes for a Diabetic Patient With a Nursing Diagnosis of Knowledge Deficit

The patient/family will be able to:
1. Describe the signs and symptoms of hypoglycemia
2. Describe the signs and symptoms of hyperglycemia
3. Demonstrate correct insulin injection technique
4. State the appropriate sites for insulin injections
5. Demonstrate appropriate syringe filling technique
6. Describe the preventive measures of diabetes foot care

---

box 8-2

Issues to be Addressed by Nurse Case Managers in the Reassessment Note

1. Assessment of new needs
2. Follow-up on treatments/interventions
3. Patient and family teaching efforts and progress
4. Facilitation and coordination of tests and procedures
5. Patient/family and interdisciplinary team conferences
6. Referrals to and consults with ancillary or specialized services
7. Discharge planning issues and status of discharge plans
8. Evaluation of patient responses/outcomes
9. Necessary revisions in the plan of care

---

and others involved in the care is essential. This improves compliance with the JCAHO's standard of patient's rights.

The nurse case manager should document the goals of care to be met both before and at the time of discharge. These goals are the expected outcomes of care agreed on with the patient and family and the interdisciplinary team. The expected outcomes of care should be documented following a specific format (Box 8-1) and focusing on specific elements (Case Manager's Tip 8-5).

Nurse case managers individualize the nursing interventions based on the signs and symptoms evidenced in the patient's condition. In addition, they include interventions that prevent any undesired symptoms or untoward outcomes. Nurse case managers formulate nursing interventions that are specific, realistic, individualized and patient/family oriented, and based on the signs and symptoms of the disease.

Documentation in the plan of care should reflect the nurse case manager's ongoing evaluation of the patient responses to treatment and the required revisions in the plan of care as necessitated by the patient's responses.

Nurse case managers are also required to reassess the patient and family on a continuing basis, evaluate the patient's condition for any improvements or changes, follow up on the appropriateness of the nursing interventions, and identify any new problems that may have arisen and ensure their inclusion in the plan of care. When the patient reassessment is completed, the nurse case manager is expected to write a reassessment note in the patient's record (Box 8-2). It is recommended that nurse case managers who work in acute or subacute care settings write a minimum of three reassessment notes for every patient each week of hospitalization. In long-term care settings, one reassessment note every week is considered appropriate. However, in ambulatory care settings such as clinics and home visits a note is recommended for every encounter with the patient. In addition, a reassessment note is suggested as necessitated by the patient's condition.

Facilitation and Coordination of Care Activities

Because nurse case managers are held responsible for coordinating and facilitating the provision of care on a day-to-day basis, their documentation in the patient's record should reflect these functions. Such progress

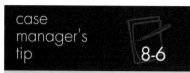

8-6   Documentation of Patient and Family Teaching

The nurse case manager's documentation of patient and family teaching, based on the patient's condition and needs, should include the following:

1. Assessment of health care teaching needs
2. Review of the disease process, signs and symptoms, risk factors, possible complications, and preventive measures
3. Review of the medical/surgical regimen, compliance with the treatment, and the importance of continuous medical follow-up
4. Instructions regarding medications intake, dosage, actions, side effects, route, and special observations
5. Preoperative and postoperative teaching
6. Wound care
7. Pain management
8. Instructions regarding the required use of medical equipment (e.g., glucometer)
9. Ongoing review of the plan of care and the discharge plan
10. Availability of and the need for support from community resources after discharge
11. The level of understanding of the teachings held, and whether there is a need for further reinforcement of the information shared and discussed

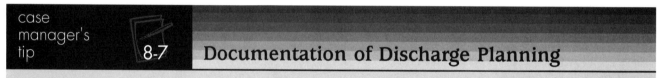

8-7   Documentation of Discharge Planning

The nurse case manager documents discharge planning in the following manner:

1. Assessment of discharge needs in the initial assessment of the patient (i.e., at the time of screening of the patient for case management services) (Box 8-3)
2. Ongoing assessment of discharge needs, because they may change based on changes in the patient's condition
3. Actual patient's disposition at the time of discharge in the form of discharge note (Box 8-4)

notes usually include facilitation and coordination of care activities such as the following:

1. Scheduling and expediting of tests and procedures, and prevention of any delays
2. Patient care–related conferences with the family and the interdisciplinary team
3. Coordination of complex discharge plans
4. Preparation of patients and families for operative procedures
5. Transition of patients from acute to subacute or long-term care settings
6. Consulting with other health care providers
7. Ongoing communication with managed care organizations

Patient and Family Teaching

Nurse case managers are responsible for supervising the patient and family teaching activities. This role responsibility should be evidenced in their documentation. Nurse case managers make sure that patient/family teaching is included in the plan of care and appropri-

ately documented in the patient's record. They document all the patient/family teaching activities they conduct (Case Manager's Tip 8-6).

Patient's Discharge and Disposition

Patient's discharge and disposition are important responsibilities of nurse case managers (Case Manager's Tip 8-7). Assessment of the patient's discharge needs starts at the time of admission and continues throughout the hospitalization, until the patient is ready for discharge.

Documentation of discharge planning to support safe discharge is important, because it may be scrutinized by peer review organizations (PROs) if the patient is readmitted with the same problem shortly after discharge. Such situations may increase the institution's financial risk. If the patient is to receive home care services after discharge, the discharge note should then include the reasons for such services and what is expected to take place at home regarding the care of the patient. Because nurse case managers discuss home

---

box 8-3

Areas of Documentation Related to the Assessment of Discharge Planning Needs of Patients

1. Services used before hospital admission
2. Projected needs of services after discharge (e.g., home care, physical therapy)
3. Availability of good social support system
4. Need for referrals to specialized personnel/services (e.g., social work, home care intake coordinator)
5. Patient's condition (e.g., mental stability, functional abilities)
6. Financial status and insurance coverage
7. Necessary paperwork when requesting community services after discharge (e.g., medical request for home care services) or nursing home placement (e.g., patient review instrument)

---

box 8-4

Areas of Documentation Related to Patient's Discharge

1. Disposition (e.g., home, nursing home, group home, rehabilitation facility, hospice)
2. Mode of discharge; transportation provided, if any
3. Person who accompanied the patient on discharge
4. Communication with appropriate people regarding confirmation of discharge (e.g., home care agency, managed care organization, patient's family)
5. Confirmation of availability of any equipment needed (e.g., wheelchair, crutches, glucometer, walker)
6. Completion of necessary paperwork related to discharge (e.g., medical request for home care, patient review instrument [for patient's placement in a nursing home])
7. Confirmation of services needed by the patient after discharge (e.g., hemodialysis center, special doctor's clinic)
8. Condition of patient at the time of discharge
9. Discharge instructions

---

care needs with home care planners, it is suggested that such discussions be included in the discharge documentation.

Evaluation of Patient Care Outcomes

Evaluation of the patient's responses to treatments is essential for better decision making regarding patient's progress and discharge. Progress notes of nurse case managers should reflect documentation of the patient's status in relation to the desired outcomes established at the time of admission and proactively identified in the plan of care. The frequency with which nurse case managers document patients' progress and responses to treatments depends on the institutional policies and procedures regarding documentation, the charting system, the type of treatments and nursing interventions needed by the patient, and the standards of care.

Nurse case managers are also required to track **variances** of care and delays in achieving patient care outcomes (see Chapter 11 for a detailed discussion on variance). They are cautioned not to document any subjective judgments or system and practitioner variances, because they increase the institutional liabilities.

CASE PRESENTATION

Documentation by nurse case managers is essential to patient care, because it eliminates confusion and uncertainty from the plan of care and promotes its understanding by all the health care providers involved in the provision of care of the particular patient. Documentation reflects the professional responsibility and accountability of nurse case managers toward patient care and provides concrete evidence of their role in the provision of care. To better understand the nurse case managers' role in documentation, the rest of the chapter will be a discussion around a case presentation of an elderly patient with exacerbation of heart failure who needed acute care. Although this case presentation focuses on acute care, the concepts and skills discussed may be applied in any care settings.

Documentation of patient's care in the medical record is an important means of communication between health care professionals. It eliminates misunderstanding and improves awareness of the patient's condition, plan of care, and responses to treatments. Nurse case managers' documentation is necessary to the understanding of their role in patient care. The case study and excerpts on documentation shared in this chapter are only examples of nurse case manager's documentation. Nurse case managers are advised to review the policies and procedures related to documentation that are available in the institutions where they work and make every effort to comply with those policies and procedures.

KEY POINTS

1. Documentation by nurse case managers is important, because it is the only concrete evidence of their role in the provision of patient care.

Elderly Patient With Exacerbation of Heart Failure

In this case study, an 86-year-old male was admitted to the coronary care unit (CCU) of a major academic medical center through the emergency department (ED). Mr. D lives by himself in an apartment building on the fourth floor. He has been admitted to the hospital four times in the past 2 months. Each time he spent 3 to 4 days, of which 2 days were in the CCU. This time, he presented to the ED with chest pain and shortness of breath even when resting. On physical exam, he was found to have bilateral audible crackles and 3+ edema in the lower extremities, which was worse around the ankles (pedal). No new changes were identified on the electrocardiogram when compared to the ones taken on the previous hospitalizations. According to the results of his blood tests, he was found to have a potassium serum level of 3.3 mEq, a creatinine of 2.8, and a blood urea nitrogen of 22.

When Mr. D was asked about the home care services arranged before discharge during his last hospitalization, he claimed he did not get along well with the visiting nurse and the home health aide so he asked them not to visit him again. Mr. D also informed his nurse case manager that he has no relatives or friends, no money, no insurance, and that he has not been taking his medications (diuretics, digoxin, potassium, and ACE inhibitor). He has not been compliant with his restrictive diet and has been eating whatever he could find. Mr. D was referred to the heart failure nurse case manager by the ED physician and later on by the primary nurse in the CCU.

The heart failure nurse case manager, after meeting with Mr. D and reviewing his medical history and record, wrote a screening/intake note. She assessed Mr. D for appropriateness for case management services and wrote an acceptance note while the patient is still in the ED. The following is an excerpt from the heart failure case manager's note.

Case management screening and intake note, Tuesday, August 13, 1996, 10:00 AM

Called to see patient by Dr. Jones from the ED. An 86-year-old male with frequent hospitalizations (four times in 2 months) with same complaints of exacerbation of heart failure and noncompliance with medical regimen (medications, activity, diet, and community services). Mr. D has no insurance coverage and no primary physician. Patient is accepted into the case management services program. Will follow up for full assessment and establishment of the plan of care in the CCU.

Jane Doe, MSN, RN, Heart Failure Case Manager

The screening and intake note written by the heart failure nurse case manager is concise and to the point. It includes the source of referral, the reasons for acceptance for case management services, and the necessary follow-up to be made. On arrival of Mr. D to the CCU, the case manager conducted a thorough assessment of the patient, reviewed the medical record (current and previous hospitalizations), and contacted the cardiologist/heart failure team taking care of Mr. D to discuss the plan of care. The heart failure nurse case manager then explained to Mr. D the reason(s) for his hospitalization, the goals of his treatment, and his plan of care (as discussed with the heart failure team). The nurse case manager also involved Mr. D's primary nurse in the discussion and in the decisions made regarding his care. The heart failure case manager then proceeded to write an assessment and plan of care note in Mr. D's medical record. The note read as follows.

Case management services follow-up note, Tuesday, August 13, 1996, 12 noon

A thorough assessment and interview of Mr. D regarding his past medical history and hospitalizations, medications intake, compliance with medical regimen, insurance coverage, and community services before hospitalization were completed. Medical record was reviewed, and case was discussed with the heart failure team and Mr. D's primary nurse.

Assessment of needs

Mr. D's complex condition is related to his noncompliance with the medical regimen and the prescribed community services. His needs are summarized as the following:

1. Health care insurance coverage and accessibility to a primary care provider
2. Teaching regarding medical regimen and importance of compliance with the regimen
3. Discharge from the hospital into a safe environment in the community

Plan

1. Verify Mr. D's health insurance coverage, and contact outpatient heart failure service for follow-up on Mr. D after discharge.
2. Teach/ensure patient teaching is done regarding medical regimen and self-care expectations after discharge.
3. Refer patient to home care services. Contact the home care intake coordinator (HCIC). Also refer patient to the nutritionist for dietary counseling.

Jane Doe, MSN, RN, Heart Failure Case Manager

During Mr. D's hospitalization, the heart failure nurse case manager continued to work with him, the heart failure team, the primary nurse, and the HCIC to facilitate Mr. D's care and expedite his discharge back into the community. She worked on meeting the goals of his hospitalization and the needs that were identified on admission. Every time she was able to confirm the successful completion of Mr. D's required care activities, she wrote a note in his medical record. The following are some examples of follow-up notes written by the heart failure case manager during Mr. D's stay at the hospital.

Case management services follow-up note, Wednesday, August 14, 1996, 9:00 AM

Contacted noninvasive cardiology laboratory to expedite Mr. D's echocardiogram. Was able to successfully schedule the echo for today, to be done at 1:00 PM.

12:00 noon

Discussed discharge planning with Mr. D. Reinforced his need for visiting nurse services and home health aide. He states, "I have been very dissatisfied with the agency, the nurse does not answer all my questions . . . always in a rush" . . . "the home health aide does not spend the 4 hours with me every day, she frequently tells me that she likes to leave early, because she's got something to do. Could you do something about this?" Reassured Mr. D of the follow-up.

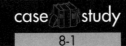
case study
8-1

Elderly Patient With Exacerbation of Heart Failure—cont'd

2:00 PM

Called for results of echo. Preliminary report to be sent to the CCU. Discussed the report with the heart failure team. No significant changes from previous echo that was done 9 months ago. Patient is stable enough to be transferred to a telemetry bed. Arranged for telemetry bed, and primary nurse will transfer Mr. D out of the CCU by 3:00 PM. Discussed the plan with Mr. D; he understands the plan and is in agreement. Reassured him of case management follow-up while in the telemetry unit.

Jane Doe, MSN, RN, Heart Failure Case Manager

Case management services follow-up note, Thursday, August 15, 1996, 10:00 AM

Home care agency was called; discussed Mr. D's concerns, and negotiated a change in the assignment of home care services. The agency agreed to send a different nurse and home health aide. Informed Mr. D of the change in services; he was pleased. Also discussed the importance of compliance with the medical regimen and the home care services. Mr. D promised to try his best.

Contacted the social security and welfare offices and checked on Mr. D's insurance. Found out that he has Medicare and Medicaid coverage. Reactivated his coverage and requested new cards, because Mr. D could not locate the originals.

Called the outpatient heart failure services, and scheduled Mr. D's follow-up appointments for the next 3 months. Arranged for an ambulette for transportation to the hospital for each follow-up appointment.

Jane Doe, MSN, RN, Heart Failure Case Manager

As all nurse case managers do, the heart failure nurse case manager reviewed Mr. D's medical record, particularly regarding patient teaching activities, to ensure positive patient care outcomes and to identify any variances in the care of Mr. D that might require the nurse case manager's interventions. It was noted that Mr. D has good understanding of his disease process, diet restrictions, and the dosages and actions of his cardiac medications. However, he seemed to experience some problems understanding the importance of fluid restrictions, the side effects of medications, and the necessity of monitoring his weight. The heart failure nurse case manager interviewed Mr. D regarding teaching and reinforced the areas that still required continued teaching. The nurse case manager then wrote the following note in the medical record.

Case management services follow-up note, Thursday, August 15, 1996, 2:00 PM

Mr. D's medical record was reviewed. Mr. D seems to still be experiencing some problems understanding the significance of fluid restrictions and daily weights, as well as the side effects of his medications.

Action

1. Provided Mr. D with written instructions regarding his medications; reviewed with him the importance of his medications, dosage, schedule, and side effects. Assessed what he was familiar with and reinforced the areas lacking. Reinforced information regarding sided effects, particularly the importance and reasons of the need for potassium supplements while on diuretics. Mr. D was still unable to verbalize complete understanding of the side effects of medications. He was reassured that this issue will be shared with the visiting nurse for further follow-up at home after discharge.
2. Fluid restriction was also discussed with Mr. D and corrected his impression that restrictions are related to water only. He was provided with instructions on how to control his fluid intake. He was able to verbalize the instructions successfully.
3. When discussed further, it was identified that Mr. D had no problem understanding the importance of monitoring his weight. The real issue was that he did not have a scale at home. A scale was ordered for him, to be delivered to his house on discharge. He was provided with a daily log to record his weights and instructed to bring it with him every time he is back for a follow-up visit with the outpatient heart failure service.

Jane Doe, MSN, RN, Heart Failure Case Manager

It is as important for the nurse case manager to write a discharge/disposition note in the medical record as it is to write a screening and intake note on admission. Disposition notes usually summarize the patient's progress toward recovery and whether the goals of treatment, identified on admission, are met at the time of discharge. The heart failure nurse case manager summarized Mr. D's discharge as follows.

Case management services discharge/disposition note, Friday, August 16, 1996, 3:00 PM

Mr. D is scheduled for discharge on August 17, 1996. The needs identified on admission have been met. His clinical status has improved significantly: no shortness of breath while at rest; able to ambulate around the unit comfortably and without oxygen. He lost 15 pounds with the diuretics. Home care services have been reinstated with new personnel. He has better understanding of his disease and medical regimen. Mr. D's health care insurance cards will be mailed to him by social services. A scale and oxygen for emergency use at home will be delivered to his house by Saturday morning. Ambulette has been arranged for transportation back and forth on the day of his follow-up appointment. Ambulette service has also been arranged for discharge by 11:00 AM tomorrow. Telephone numbers of the heart failure nurse case manager and outpatient services were provided.

Jane Doe, MSN, RN, Heart Failure Case Manager

2. Documentation acts as a means of communication among the health care professionals.
3. Documentation improves awareness of the patient's condition, plan of care, and responses to treatments.
4. Documentation of nurse case managers should follow the case management process. For each step in the process, a note is expected.

References

American Nurses Association: *Standards of clinical nursing practice*, Kansas City, Mo, 1991, American Nurses Association.

Bower KA: *Case management by nurses*, ed 2, Kansas City, Mo, 1992, American Nurses Association.

Cohen EL, Cesta TG: *Nursing case management: from concept to evaluation*, ed 2, St Louis, 1997, Mosby.

Tahan HA: The nurse case manager in acute care settings: job description and function, *J Nurs Admin* 23(10):53-61, 1993.

NURSE CASE MANAGER'S DOCUMENTATION RECORD

This appendix presents an example of a nurse case manager's documentation record. The use of a standardized record streamlines and improves documentation. The record acts as a trigger for better documentation. It also reduces the amount of time required for thorough documentation. Such records can be made flexible to fit the needs of nurse case managers in any patient care setting.

IMPORTANT ASPECTS OF DOCUMENTATION

Effective documentation provides a written record of the following items:
- Patient and family needs
- Actual and potential problems
- Patient and family interview on admission
- Goals of treatment
- Case conference
- Assessment and reassessment
- Patient and family teaching
- Discharge planning
- Referrals to other services (e.g., home care)
- Completion of patient care–related paperwork (e.g., applying for nursing home placement)
- Facilitation and coordination of patient care activities
- Ongoing involvement in patient care activities
- Resolving variances and delays in care activities
- Discharge summary

APPENDIX 8-1—cont'd

BETH ISRAEL MEDICAL CENTER

**PATIENT CARE MANAGER/CASE MANAGER
DOCUMENTATION RECORD**

DIAGNOSIS: _____

PCM/CM: _____

2200

A. **INITIAL ASSESSMENT**

DATE: _____ / _____ / _____

☐ Consulted with: _____
☐ Review of medical records
☐ Goals mutually set with:
  ☐ Patient ☐ Significant Other: _____

_____
_____
_____

B. **NEEDS AS IDENTIFIED BY PCM/CM OR PATIENT/SIGNIFICANT OTHER**

☐ parenting/bonding
☐ acceptance of illness
☐ emotional support
☐ grieving process
☐ support systems
☐ nutrition
☐ social work
☐ PT/OT
☐ respiratory therapy
☐ psychiatry
☐ medical/surgical
☐ patient representative
☐ other

C. **MEETINGS/ROUNDS**

_____
_____

MAP 066 (Rev 12/94)

PATIENT CARE MANAGER/CASE MANAGER DOCUMENTATION RECORD

DATE INITIATED	D. REQUIRED FACILITATION/COORDINATION AND OUTCOMES TO INTERVENTIONS	DATE REVIEWED/ COMPLETED

A P P E N D I X 8-1—cont'd

PATIENT CARE MANAGER/CASE MANAGER DOCUMENTATION RECORD

DIAGNOSIS: _____

PCM/CM: _____

‖‖‖‖‖‖‖‖‖‖‖‖‖‖‖‖‖‖‖‖
2200

E. TEACHING NEEDS AS IDENTIFIED BY PCM/CM OR PATIENT/SIGNIFICANT OTHER

☐ signs and symptoms of disease

☐ potential complications

☐ disease process

☐ medications

☐ tests/treatments/procedures

☐ equipment

☐ Reviewed MAP for completion of patient teaching

Patient/Significant Other Teaching

Key: U = Verbalized understanding   D = Able to demonstrate   R = Needs reinforcement

TOPICS TAUGHT	OUTCOME	DATE REVIEWED	FOLLOW UP/COMMENTS

APPENDIX 8-1—cont'd

PATIENT CARE MANAGER/CASE MANAGER DOCUMENTATION RECORD

F. DISCHARGE PLANNING

Anticipated needs upon discharge:

☐ equipment

☐ home care evaluation

☐ long term care/facility

☐ short term residence

☐ hospice care

☐ transportation

☐ home, no needs

☐ home with ☐ HHA ☐ RN
                    ☐ LPN ☐ Homemaker

☐ special services

☐ other

Forms Required for Completion

☐ M11Q

☐ PRI

☐ VNS

Comments:

CHAPTER 9

DEVELOPING CASE MANAGEMENT PLANS*

There is no doubt that the current health care delivery system is experiencing massive and revolutionary changes. With the increased infiltration of **managed care** and managed competition, health care administrators, nursing executives in particular, are pressured to seek intelligent changes to the way care is delivered. Most health care institutions, whether acute, ambulatory, long term, or home care, have undergone some sort of reengineering and redesign. Regardless of the setting, **case management** continues to be the best way to deliver high-quality, efficient, and cost-effective care.

Case management delivery systems have been proven successful in various care settings (Cohen and Cesta, 1997; Guiliano and Poirier, 1991; Hampton, 1993; Tahan and Cesta, 1995; Zander, 1991; Zander, 1992). They rely heavily on **case management plans** (CMPs) that delineate the best/ideal practice. In this chapter a 10-step process for developing such plans is discussed. The process provides a template for health care professionals who are interested in implementing CMPs and a step-by-step guide to developing these plans, with practical examples to simplify the process.

Although CMPs are not new to many organizations, the lack of a deliberate and systematic process to develop these plans holds these organizations back from creating timely and efficient results. This chapter is highly beneficial for health care providers, case managers in particular, who are involved in the development of CMPs. They may acquire new knowledge and strategies to simplify the task of developing CMPs, or they may even choose to implement the proposed process if they currently do not have a formal one in place.

DEFINITION OF CASE MANAGEMENT PLANS

Since their inception, CMPs have been used as tools to define practice and as guides for patient care activities.

Whatever they are called, the format is either an abbreviated, one-page version or a comprehensive, detailed booklet (Cohen and Cesta, 1997; Tahan and Cesta, 1995). They are available in paper or computer formats. However, their purposes, the way they are used, and the process in which they are developed are approximately the same (Bozzuto and Farrell, 1995; Esler et al, 1994; Ferguson, 1993; Hydo, 1995; Ignatavicius, 1995; Ignatavicius and Hausman, 1995; Katterhagen and Patton, 1993; Meister et al, 1995; Thompson et al, 1991).

Case management plans are labeled differently in different institutions. Some are copyrighted, such as care maps; some are not, such as multidisciplinary action plans (MAPs). Examples of CMPs include critical path, anticipated recovery path, clinical pathway, care guide, collaborative plan, coordinated plan, integrated plan of care, or action plan. Throughout this chapter, these plans will be referred to by using the generic term *case management plan*. Case Manager's Tip 9-1 lists the characteristics of CMPs.

The use of CMPs has created a multitude of advantages. Among the most important ones are cost effectiveness and reduction in **lengths of stay,** readmissions to acute care settings, or home care visits; improved quality of care and customer satisfaction; better allocation of resources and coordination of services that result in eliminating redundancy, fragmentation, and duplication of care activities; clearly defined plans of care and delineation of responsibilities; and improved communication systems among the various disciplines (Cohen and Cesta, 1997; Giuliano and Poirier, 1991; Ignatavicius, 1995; Ignatavicius and Hausman, 1995; Tahan and Cesta, 1995; Zander, 1991).

PROCESS OF DEVELOPING CASE MANAGEMENT PLANS

Case management plans are developed best through an interdisciplinary team that is granted the authority and responsibility by a higher administrative team, usually a steering committee charged with implementing case management systems, to develop a specific plan for a particular diagnosis or procedure. The interdisciplinary

*Part of this material first appeared in *Nursing Case Management* 1(3):112-121, 1996, Lippincott-Raven, Philadelphia, PA.

case
manager's
tip
9-1

Characteristics of Case Management Plans

1. Each plan addresses a specific diagnosis, surgical procedure, or a phase in the care needed.
2. They represent a time line of patient care activities based on the clinical service. This could be minutes or hours in the emergency department, days in the acute care setting, weeks in the neonatal intensive care unit, months in long-term facilities, or number of visits in ambulatory or home care settings.
3. They include well-defined milestones or trigger points that aid in expediting care and indicate an impending change in care activities (e.g., switching from intravenous to oral antibiotics when temperature is within normal range for 48 hours) or readiness of patients for different care setting (e.g., criteria for transferring a patient from an acute to a subacute or nursing home care setting).
4. The length of each plan depends on a predetermined length of stay based on the diagnosis/procedure and reimbursement rules, guidelines, and mechanisms.
5. They clearly delineate the responsibilities of the various health care team members as they relate to each particular department.
6. The plans identify the outcome indicators or quality measures used to evaluate the appropriateness and effectiveness of care.
7. Each plan may include a specific variance tracking section to evaluate any delays in care activities/processes.
8. The plans may be used as one strategy for ensuring compliance with the standards of care of regulatory and accreditation agencies.
9. The plans are interdisciplinary in nature—a mechanism that reinforces a seamless approach to the delivery of care.
10. The plans can be used as an educational tool for house staff, student nurses or nurses in training, and newly hired employees.
11. The plans help improve performance in the areas of patient and family teaching, coordination of services, collaboration and communication among the health care team members, and discharge planning.
12. The plans may also be developed as a "patient version," which can be given to the patient and family at the time of admission into the hospital or community care setting. This plan helps the patient understand what is projected to take place during the course of treatment.

team is given the responsibility of developing the actual content of the plan. The steering committee, however, provides the team with ongoing expert and administrative support throughout the process.

Team members meet numerous times to discuss and develop the CMP. Sometimes they work individually in between meetings. The length of time needed for the development and completion of one CMP usually depends on the complexity of the diagnosis or procedure; the number of physicians or practitioners that will use the plan; the extent of disagreements among physicians regarding the content of the plan that may arise while attempting to build **consensus;** the number of disciplines involved; the experience of the team members involved in the process; the availability of team members, their commitment, their productivity, and how well they can work together (i.e., group dynamics); and the presence or absence of a support person or an expert in CMP development. One CMP may take as long as 6 to 9 months for completion, particularly if the team is developing a CMP for the first time, or as little as a few weeks if team members are well experienced in the process.

Steering Committee

The steering committee is composed of professionals who hold executive-level positions in the institution. The

departments represented on the steering committee may include, depending on the sophistication of the institution, operations, finance/cost accounting, marketing, nursing/patient care services, information systems, medical records, legal and risk management, quality improvement and **utilization** review, **managed care** and **case management,** data management, research, and others as deemed necessary. Members of the steering committee may be the high-ranking officers of each of these departments or their designee. Some institutions may choose not to create a new, stand-alone committee for this purpose. Responsibilities of a steering committee, in this case, may be added to a preexisting committee such as a quality council or a **length-of-stay** or cost-reduction task force.

The major role of the steering committee is to put together a strategic plan for the implementation of case management systems, training and educating those involved in the process, selecting and prioritizing the diagnoses and procedures for which CMPs are to be developed, and providing support for the teams charged with developing CMPs. Members of the steering committee provide leadership and direction of the development, implementation, and evaluation of the case management system.

Most institutions have established a standardized process for the development of CMPs. The steering com-

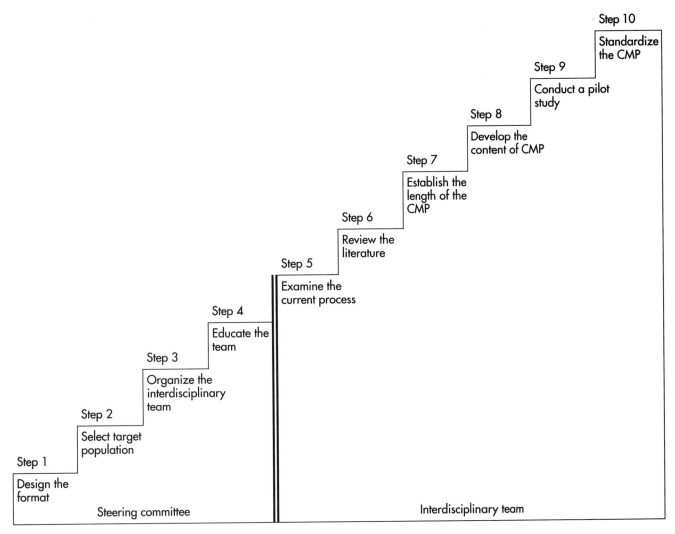

Fig. 9-1   The process of developing case management plans (CMPs).

mittee is responsible for the development of this process. Having established a formal process is very important, because it provides the interdisciplinary team with the foundation for successful development and implementation of CMPs. An ideal process is a simple one that clearly identifies the steps in a systematic way and makes it easier for the team to follow.

This chapter includes an example of such processes (Figure 9-1) for health care administrators to adapt into their organizations and adjust as needed. This example follows a 10-step process that differentiates between the work and responsibilities of the steering committee and the interdisciplinary team.

The steering committee is responsible for the first four steps, because they require higher administrative authority in decision making. They are related to the logistics of case management systems and plans and are part of the overall case management implementation plan put together by the steering committee and approved by key executive personnel in the institution.

The remaining six steps are the responsibility of the interdisciplinary team. They address the actual work of the team and the creation of the plan.

Step 1: Design the format of the plan. Deciding on the format is crucial, because it guides the development of the content of the plan (Case Manager's Tip 9-2). The format should be made easy for all health care professionals to follow and use. This step is integral to the establishment of case management systems, because it affects clinical practice and other care activities and processes (e.g., documentation, performance improvement processes, coding of the medical record, presentation of the standards of care and practice).

The CMP should be designed in such a way that includes the various elements of patient care (Box 9-1) (Ferguson, 1993; Ignatavicius and Hausman, 1995). Some of these elements are related to the medical/surgical care of the patient, whereas others are nursing in nature. In addition, there may be elements related to support or administrative services. Specific sections of

case
manager's
tip

9-2

Factors That Affect Choosing a Particular CMP Format

1. Whether the CMP will be used for documentation
2. The number of disciplines that need to be represented in the plan
3. Complexity of the diagnosis/procedure
4. The clinical area or service or care setting
5. Whether the plan will replace any existing preprinted physician orders or protocols
6. The appropriate time line
7. Forms that must be eliminated from the patient's record on implementation of the plan
8. Related risk management and legal issues
9. Whether the plan will be a permanent part of the medical record
10. Existing standards of regulatory bodies and accreditation agencies
11. Plans for automation of the medical record

---

box 9-1

Elements of Patient Care as They Appear on the Plan

1. Assessment of patient monitoring
2. Tests and procedures
3. Care facilitation and coordination, including care milestones
4. Consultations and referrals
5. Medications
6. Intravenous therapy
7. Activity
8. Nutrition
9. Patient and family teaching
10. Treatments—medical, surgical, and nursing interventions
11. Wound care
12. Physical therapy and occupational therapy
13. Pain management
14. Outcome indicators and projected/desired responses to treatments
15. Safety
16. Discharge planning
17. Psychosocial assessment

---

the CMP should be allotted to quality indicators, **outcome** measures of care, **variances** tracking, and data collection. The number of the different care elements for each CMP depends on the diagnosis or surgical procedure addressed. For example, a plan for chest pain evaluation may include a pain management section but not physical or occupational therapy sections. Speech pathology and physical and occupational therapy are important when addressing a stroke CMP. A CMP to be used in a subacute care facility designated for ventilator-dependent patients should always include a respiratory care section that stresses the institution's protocol for weaning patients off mechanical ventilation.

The final format of the CMP (see Appendix 9-1 for an example) should be presented to the institutional medical records committee, legal department, and medical board for review and approval before it is made official. A decision regarding the format should be in place before authorizing any interdisciplinary team to start working on a CMP. The approved format becomes the desired CMP's template that is followed by all interdisciplinary teams to maintain consistency and uniformity of plans. The format also provides the framework based on which the team can construct the content details of the CMP. The steering committee then develops guidelines for the use of the template/final format of the CMP. The guidelines explain in detail how the template should be followed or used, the definitions of each of the care elements, and examples of the various patient care activities that could be listed under each care element (Box 9-2). This is important because it maintains continuity and consistency of CMPs across the various interdisciplinary teams. When a team is established, a copy of the template/format and a copy of the guidelines should be presented to and discussed with the team members.

Step 2: Identify/select target population. The mechanism for selecting target populations can be done at any time during the design phase of CMP format. The steering committee studies the patient populations/groups served by the institution. It then selects the groups that need improvement regarding cost and quality, that present a risk for financial loss, or that are a potential for revenue.

There are several criteria that must be considered when selecting target populations for which to develop CMPs. These include volume of the patient group, cost of care, complexity of care needed, institutional length of stay compared with other benchmarks, variations in practice patterns, the need for multiple services/care

box 9-2

Guidelines for the Placement of Patient Care Activities in the Case Management Plan

Each patient care activity should be indicated in the appropriate "care element" category. The following is a master list that should be used as a guide by interdisciplinary teams during the process of developing a case management plan.

ASSESSMENT AND MONITORING

1. Physiological assessment measures (e.g., blood pressure, temperature, pulse[s], respirations, hemodynamic monitoring)
2. System assessment (e.g., cardiac, pulmonary, gastrointestinal)
3. Intake and output
4. Drainage of bodily fluids
5. Weights

TESTS AND PROCEDURES

1. Laboratory tests (e.g., blood work, urine, sputum, pathology)
2. Unit tests (e.g., glucose fingerstick, guaiac, urine dipstick)
3. Routine diagnostic tests (e.g., electrocardiogram, chest x-ray, ultrasound)
4. Diagnostic/therapeutic procedures (operations, cardiac catheterization, angiogram, angioplasty, gastrostomy tube placement)

TREATMENTS (PREVENTIVE AND THERAPEUTIC)

1. Dressing change and wound care
2. Intermittent compression device
3. Chest physiotherapy
4. Oxygen therapy and ventilator-related care
5. Central line site care
6. Tracheostomy care

MEDICATIONS

1. Routine medications necessary for the particular case type (standing, p.r.n., and single dosages; premedication needs when preparing a patient for a particular procedure)

PAIN MANAGEMENT

1. Pain management protocol
2. Frequency of evaluating pain status and response to medications
3. Indications/recommendations for nonpharmacological actions
4. Medications for pain management

INTRAVENOUS THERAPY

1. Intravenous fluids (e.g., D_5W, D_5NSS)
2. Blood and blood products

NUTRITION

1. Type of diet/meal
2. Instructions for diet progression
3. Fluid restrictions
4. Tube feedings
5. Parenteral nutrition

ACTIVITY

1. Activity limitations/ambulation
2. Safety instructions
3. Physical and occupational therapy
4. Fall risk assessment
5. Skin integrity risk assessment
6. Functional measures

CONSULTS

1. Routine consults (e.g., infectious disease, anesthesiology)
2. Specific consults (e.g., speech pathology for a stroke patient)

PSYCHOSOCIAL ASSESSMENT

1. Coping and adjustment to illness and hospitalization
2. Support system
3. Anxiety level

PATIENT/FAMILY TEACHING

1. Assessment for readiness to learn
2. Assessment of limitations/barriers to learning
3. Assessment of learning needs
4. Education plan, including areas of teaching (e.g., medications, disease process, activity/exercise, dietary limitations, specific medical/surgical regimen after discharge)
5. Need for particular equipment (e.g., glucometer for diabetic patients)

DISCHARGE PLANNING

1. Assessment of discharge needs
2. Referrals of high-risk patients to home care, social work, nutrition
3. Completion of any necessary paperwork for nursing home placement

OUTCOME INDICATORS (EXPECTED OUTCOMES OF CARE)

1. Intermediate outcomes
2. Discharge outcomes

VARIANCE TRACKING

1. Instructions on the use of variance section of the case management plan
2. Classifications/coding
3. Action plan
4. Date and time

PATIENT PROBLEMS

1. Delineate how patient problems should be stated (i.e., medical/nursing language)
2. Actual and potential problems

TABLE 9-1
Different Procedures in DRG 112

Percutaneous cardiovascular procedures	ICD-9 codes
Angioplasty, coronary, PTCA, multiple vessel with or without thrombo-lytic agent	36.05
Angioplasty, coronary, PTCA, single vessel with thrombolytic agent	36.02
Angioplasty, coronary, PTCA, single vessel with-out thrombolytic agent	36.01
Catheterization, heart, le-sion or tissue	37.34
Mapping, cardiac	37.27
Removal, obstruction, coro-nary artery, other speci-fied	36.09
Valvuloplasty, percutaneous	35.96
Simulation, cardiac, electro-physiological	37.26

PTCA, percutaneous transluminal coronary angioplasty.

TABLE 9-2
Different ICD-9 Codes in DRG 96

Bronchitis and asthma, age greater than 17 with complications and comorbidities	ICD-9 codes
Bronchitis, chronic, muco-purulent	491.1
Bronchitis, chronic, obstruc-tive	491.2
Bronchitis, chronic, simple	491.0
Asthma, extrinsic	493.01
Asthma, intrinsic	493.11
Asthma, chronic obstruc-tive, with status asth-maticus	493.21
Asthma, chronic obstruc-tive, without status asth-maticus	493.20

settings, feasibility of developing the plan, potential revenue (i.e., control of resources, fragmentation and duplication of care), opportunity for improvement in quality of care, reports from payor groups, problem-prone/high-risk diagnoses or procedures, and results of internal and external quality management monitoring (Cohen and Cesta, 1997; Ignatavicius and Hausman, 1995; Tahan and Cesta, 1995).

It is important to evaluate the number of patients seen in a particular **diagnosis-related group (DRG)** when selecting a target population. The decision of which DRG should be targeted is made based on the number of patients seen in a particular DRG during a whole year. The larger the number of patients seen, the better the opportunities for improvement. The established CMP will then be applied to a larger population, which maximizes the benefit.

Because a DRG is too broad and may include several procedures that require different resources, whereas International Classification of Diseases, version 9 Conversion Manual **(ICD-9-CM)** is very specific, evaluation and analysis of patient populations should be made at the ICD-9 code level. Consider DRG 112 (percutaneous cardiovascular procedures) as an example. It includes several different procedures, with each designated a separate ICD-9 code (Table 9-1) (St Anthony Publishing, 1992). The treatment plans for each of these procedures are different—cardiac catheterization is a diagnostic procedure, whereas angioplasty is a therapeutic procedure, and electrophysiological cardiac stimulation is a

diagnostic procedure but very different than catheterization, which makes developing a CMP for DRG 112 more difficult. However, developing a separate CMP for each procedure/ICD-9 code is more feasible. As a result, it is better to consider developing a separate CMP for each ICD-9 code than for the DRG.

Another example is DRG 96: bronchitis and asthma, age greater than 17 with complications and comorbidities (Table 9-2). There are major differences between treating these two disease entities. It is best to deal with this DRG based on ICD-9 codes (St Anthony Publishing, 1992). Sometimes it is appropriate to combine two or more ICD-9 codes in one CMP. For example, combining asthma ICD-9 codes 493.20, 493.21, 493.01, and 493.11 in one CMP that delineates the standard of care of adult asthma is relevant, because there exist minimal to no variations in the treatment of asthma in the different ICD-9 codes. However, combining ICD-9 codes 493.20, 493.21 and 491.1, and 491.2 is not appropriate, because treating asthma is different than treating bronchitis, and the standard of care for both diagnoses cannot be combined into one standard.

The volume of patients seen in one DRG should not be considered in isolation from other measures, such as cost per case, cost per day, consumption of resources (e.g., the number of x-rays, blood tests, or electrocardiograms in one hospitalization), average length of stay, and profit and loss ratios. Patient populations that exert financial loss on the institution are considered the best target for CMP development.

Table 9-3 is an example of one administrative report that can be used to identify a target population. Examining the data presented, one can see that DRGs 88 and 127 have longer lengths of stay and at the same time have profit losses. Thus considering the development of

TABLE 9-3
Example of Administrative Report Used to Identify Target Populations

DRG	Description	Total cases*	Average length of stay	Excess days†	Profit (Loss)‡
88	Chronic obstructive pulmonary disease	150	6	2	($1145.43)
89	Simple pneumonia and pleurisy, age greater than 17 with complications and comorbidities	165	7	2	($989.56)
90	Simple pneumonia and pleurisy, age greater than 17 without complications and co-morbidities	100	3	(1)	$1120.56
127	Heart failure and shock	200	7	3	($1895.62)
143	Chest pain	116	3	(1)	$460.75

*Total number of patients seen annually in each DRG.
†Total number of days above or below average length of stay at comparable institutions.
‡Amount per case.
NOTE: The figures in this table are hypothetical and are presented for clarification purposes only.

CMPs for these two DRGs is worthwhile, because the opportunities for improvement and profit are high. To address these two DRGs requires the establishment of two different teams for CMP development, because the DRGs are related to two different services—pulmonary and cardiology.

Conversely, DRGs 90 and 143 are not a high priority for CMP development, because the length of stay is lower than that in comparable institutions and they are financially profitable. The institution may decide to develop CMPs for these diagnoses based on other factors and improvement efforts, such as quality of care, practice patterns, and allocation and use of resources.

Step 3: Organize an interdisciplinary team. Members of the interdisciplinary team are selected by the steering committee. Recommendations from department heads are usually considered when organizing the team. The selection of members is based on their communication skills and ability to work in a team, their clinical competence and past experiences, and their commitment to their work. Becoming a member of an interdisciplinary team and contributing to the development of processes that improve patient care can be a rewarding experience for staff members.

Based on the type of the CMP to be developed, members from the various disciplines involved in patient care are selected to serve on the team. It is important to include all disciplines so that the completed plan is thorough and well written. Every team should include representatives from various departments or disciplines such as medicine (including house staff), nursing, case management, quality improvement and utilization management, social services, home care, and nutrition. Members from other departments may participate on a consultation basis. These departments may include pharmacy, medical records and coding, finance, patient representative, materials management, laboratory, and radiology. Some departments may be represented as needed based on the diagnosis being worked on. For example, representation from rehabilitation and occupational therapy and speech pathology is essential for a team working on a stroke CMP, respiratory therapy for asthma, chronic obstructive pulmonary disease, or pneumonia plans.

The interdisciplinary team should be moderate in size (i.e., 6 to 10 members). A larger team reduces its productivity, increases the risk for disagreements, and delays the process. The team is empowered by the steering committee to make independent decisions. The steering committee may designate one of its members to act as a sponsor for the team. The sponsor's role (Case Manager's Tip 9-3) includes coaching the team through the process, removing obstacles and answering unresolved questions, acting as a liaison between the team and the steering committee, and overseeing the administrative activities that keep the team functioning. In addition, it is important that the steering committee appoint two members of the interdisciplinary team to

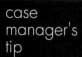

case
manager's
tip
9-3

Roles and Responsibilities of the Team Sponsor

1. Provides the team with administrative support and power
2. Acts as a resource
3. Answers any unanswered questions or, when unable, facilitates obtaining the answer
4. Acts as the team's liaison with the steering committee
5. Ensures that work is on track
6. Helps the team in problem solving
7. Alerts the team not to make decisions regarding issues that are beyond their realm of responsibilities or power
8. Brings feedback about the team to the steering committee

case
manager's
tip
9-4

Roles and Responsibilities of the Team Leader and Team Facilitator

Team Leader

1. Chairs the meeting
2. Prepares the agenda
3. Introduces team members, and explains the charge and goals of the team
4. Guides team members through the process of developing CMPs
5. Keeps the team focused on its goals
6. Stimulates discussion regarding treatment modalities and patient care activities, and seeks different opinions
7. Encourages active participation of members
8. Helps members reach common understanding and resolutions on disagreements
9. Builds consensus of members regarding ideal/best practice to be included in the CMP
10. Guides members through problem-solving process when necessary
11. Elicits information, ideas, opinions, comments, and recommendations
12. Ensures that every member gets the opportunity to contribute
13. Obtains commitments for actions
14. Follows up on unresolved/unconcluded issues
15. Clarifies and summarizes conclusions and decisions
16. Collaborates with the facilitator of the team
17. Collaborates with the sponsor of the team

Team facilitator

1. Coaches the team leader and the members
2. Serves as a role model
3. Ensures participation of every member
4. Monitors group processes, and relieves tension when it arises
5. Interjects as needed
6. Keeps the team focused
7. Maintains a positive and collegial atmosphere during meetings: openness, acceptance, trust, respect, support, cooperation, collaboration, listening, cohesiveness, and teamwork
8. Makes suggestions to keep the team moving forward
9. Confronts interpersonal or process problems
10. Serves as a liaison with team members between meetings
11. Offers support and training sessions as necessary
12. Clarifies ideas and decisions and makes recommendations during meetings
13. Collaborates with the team leader and the sponsor

case manager's tip	9-5 **Roles and Responsibilities of the Team Member**

1. Participates actively in meetings
2. Attends meetings
3. Provides relevant information
4. Collects data
5. Supports the team's charge and goals
6. Cooperates in achieving consensus when needed
7. Completes assignments
8. Maintains a positive and collegial atmosphere during meetings
9. Respects the team's ground rules
10. Represents co-workers
11. Seeks guidance when needed
12. Acts as a recorder
13. Collaborates and cooperates in the team process

act as the team leader and the facilitator (Case Manager's Tip 9-4). These two members play an important role in keeping the work of the team progressing and ensuring that the goals and objectives of the team are met within the established time frame. Some institutions may require the team to present its recommended CMP before the steering committee when it is completed and ready for implementation.

Direct care providers should be well represented on the team as team members (Case Manager's Tip 9-5), because they are instrumental in sharing their firsthand experiences with the day-to-day patient care activities. To prevent physician's resistance to the use of CMPs, it is recommended that they be involved in the process from the beginning and given the leader or co-leader role on the interdisciplinary team (Cohen and Cesta, 1997; Tahan and Cesta, 1995). Past experiences show that physicians who participate on a team become promoters of case management systems and CMPs in their institutions and continue to be the best supporters and sellers.

Step 4: Educate/train the team in the process. Before the team launches the development process for a CMP, members should be trained in the process. Formal training must include topics such as general overview of case management systems and plans; the process of developing CMPs; the responsibilities of the team leader, facilitator, and members; and tools and strategies for success. Examples of the work of other teams, if they exist, should be shared (Cohen and Cesta, 1997; Ignatavicius and Hausman, 1995; Tahan and Cesta, 1995). It is in this forum that the expectations from the team, the administrative support available to the team, and the role of the sponsor and the steering committee as they relate to the role of the interdisciplinary team should be dis-

cussed. The team should be given the opportunity to ask any questions or raise any concerns. It should also be informed of the ongoing support of the steering committee throughout the process. After completing the required training, the team starts its work on the plan.

One may ask who prepares the steering committee regarding case management systems and how members of the steering committee acquire their related knowledge. Most institutions hire an outside consultant (an expert in case management systems) to help and guide them through the process. The consultant plays an important role in helping the steering committee develop the best case management system for the institution. The consultant also develops an education packet specific to the institution's policies, procedures, and operations to train members of the steering committee and the interdisciplinary teams that will be starting to develop CMPs. Sometimes institutions may prefer to hire a full-time employee (instead of a consultant) who is an expert in the area of case management to assume full responsibility for the program. The employee is usually responsible for coordinating all the activities of the program; educating committee members, interdisciplinary team members, and staff; and acting in place of the consultant.

Developing the Plan's Content

Step 5: Examine the current practice. This step represents the start of the work on the actual content of the plan. The team members usually begin with brainstorming regarding the care of a patient. Members are asked to concentrate on the routine rather than the exception (i.e., the normal recovering patient and not exceptions or extraneous situations), because exceptional patients usually represent a small number of cases. During brainstorming, members attempt to list any quality barriers regarding patient care and any experienced delays in the past. Discussing the quality barriers helps members better understand the current situation and identify the improvement efforts the CMP will address.

After brainstorming is exhausted, team members move on to developing a flow diagram for the current process. A flow diagram that highlights the most important steps in the process of caring for a patient is recommended to prevent the team from getting bogged down with the unnecessary details. The flow diagram (see Figure 1-1, p. 11, for an example of a flow diagram) should reflect the projected care of the patient from admission until discharge and in some cases until after discharge.

There are several ways to examine current practice patterns. The two most important ways are review of medical records and interviews of care providers. In medical record reviews, members are asked to concentrate on the critical elements of care discussed earlier and presented in Box 9-1, such as assessment, tests and procedures, treatments, consultation and referrals, care facilitation and coordination, medications, intravenous therapy, activity level, nutrition, patient and family teaching, wound care, physical and occupational therapy, pain management, outcome indicators and projected desired responses to treatment, and discharge planning. Data collection regarding the critical elements and the attached time frames of delivery of patient care activities is essential in the development of CMPs. Mostly, tools to simplify and standardize the process of collecting data are developed by the team members before starting the data collection process.

Particular attention is given to the care activities considered as critical milestones of care or trigger points for a change in the treatment plan. For example, it is important to collect data about when an intravenous antibiotic is switched to its oral form during the hospitalization of a patient with pneumonia or when an intravenous corticosteroid is switched to an oral form while caring for a patient with asthma. These milestones are important because they affect the length of stay and are considered outcome measures or quality indicators. It is recommended that a thorough chart review be done regarding the most significant care activities that are required for a case type, with particular evaluation of their time frames for completion. For example, caring for a patient hospitalized for a coronary intervention procedure may require health care professionals (physicians, nurses, and others) to ensure the successful completion of several different care activities (Box 9-3) preprocedure, intraprocedure, and postprocedure, and at the time of discharge. These activities, as specified in Box

TABLE 9-4
Example of Physicians' Practice Patterns for DRG 89: Simple Pneumonia and Pleurisy, Age Greater Than 17 With Complications and Comorbidities

Physician	Number of patients	Average length of stay	Cost per case
A	55	6.5	$9280.56
B	50	4.5	$6985.44
C	34	7.0	$9986.53
D	30	7.0	$9895.32
E	25	6.9	$9643.50
F	18	5.8	$7856.64

NOTE: The above data are presented for clarification purposes only.

9-3, should be the center of medical record reviews when developing a CMP for coronary interventions.

Practice patterns of individual physicians should be assessed for variables such as length of stay and cost per case (Table 9-4) by examining the effect of starting time of antibiotic therapy on length of stay (Figure 9-2) or by reviewing the use of resources per case (e.g., counting the number of electrocardiograms, x-rays, scans, blood tests). In the example seen in Table 9-4, physician B has the lowest average length of stay and the least cost per case. This physician appears to be providing care differ-

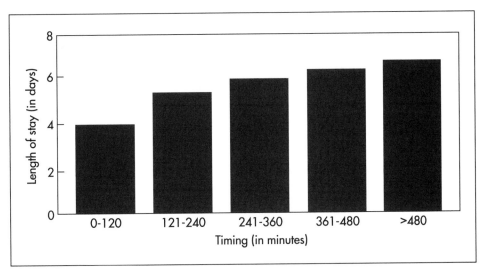

Fig. 9-2 Example of physician's practice pattern. Timing of first antibiotic dose and length of stay for patients in DRG 89. (NOTE: The data in this figure are presented for clarification purposes only.)

ently from the others. Medical records for this physician's patients must be reviewed and compared with other physicians' records to identify differences and determine appropriate practice patterns for the CMP.

Using the example in Figure 9-2, one can see that the earlier the first dose of antibiotic is started in a pneumonia patient, the shorter the average length of stay will be. Based on this conclusion, the interdisciplinary team might recommend that the antibiotic to be used to treat pneumonia should be started as early as the time of admission. This recommendation should be reflected in the time line of the CMP for pneumonia.

After completing the medical record reviews, team members interview representatives of the health care team who provide care for the patient population in question. This includes physicians, house staff, nurses who provide direct patient care, and ancillary and professional staff. Similar to the medical records review, the interviews concentrate on the critical elements of care and their attached time frames.

Other important documents available in the organization are also reviewed by the team and are studied carefully for their relation to and impact on the delivery of care. These may include any data reports on file in the institution (e.g., utilization, financial, quality assurance and improvement, and medical record reviews), the standards of care and practice, the preprinted physician orders, protocols, and guidelines (Cohen and Cesta, 1997; Ignatavicius and Hausman, 1995; Tahan and Cesta, 1995).

Step 6: Review the available literature. A thorough review of the literature is essential, because it raises awareness of team members to the latest trends and technology in patient care. The available research should be studied carefully and used to validate the recommendations made in the CMP. This creates an opportunity to provide patient care that is research based.

Review of the literature should also include an examination of any published related quality improvement efforts, CMPs, and existing standards of care that are developed by professional organizations such as the Joint Commission on Accreditation of Healthcare Organizations (JCAHO), physician groups and societies, nursing organizations, or governmental agencies such as the Agency for Health Care Policy and Research (AHCPR).

Step 7: Determine the length of the plan. The length of the CMP is determined based on several factors. These factors include institutional administrative reports regarding the average length of stay and reports of length of stay per physician, DRG's length of stay for Medicare and non-Medicare populations, managed care contracts and their respective organizations, variations in practice patterns as they relate to the length of stay, physician preference, reimbursement reports, and improvement targets (Bozzuto and Farrell, 1995; Cohen and Cesta, 1997; Esler et al, 1994; Ferguson, 1993; Ignatavicius, 1995; Ignatavicius and Hausman, 1995; Tahan and Cesta, 1995).

The team should study the length of stay issue very carefully. It should seek the steering committee's support and guidance as needed. The length of the CMP, as decided by the team, should be within the reimbursable range and lower than the institution's current average length of stay for that particular diagnosis or DRG. Also, it is crucial that improvement targets regarding length of stay, mostly decided by the steering committee, are made known to the interdisciplinary team before launching the development process of the CMP.

Step 8: Write the content of the plan. This step involves compiling together all the data collected in the previous steps. Representatives from each department are asked to write a draft of their respective part in the provision of care following the approved format of the plan and based on the results of the data collected from chart reviews, interviews, and review of the literature. All the drafts are then put together on one form to be discussed and finalized by the team members.

The content of the plan should reflect the ideal/best practice that was agreed on by the team, in realistic time frames. For example, expecting to complete an echocardiography by day 2 of hospitalization of a chest pain patient, knowing that the system requires a turnaround time of 72 hours from ordering to completion, is not realistic. Such unrealistic expectation will result in delays in care, compared with the plan, every time a patient with chest pain is admitted for treatment. However, the team may make a recommendation to the steering committee that the process for completing an echocardiogram in 72 hours should be evaluated so that a 2-day turnaround is possible. It then becomes the responsibility of the steering committee to make a final decision regarding the time frame.

When the team finishes the plan, it should be circulated for review by a group of physicians, nursing leaders, ancillary department heads, and support services involved in the care of the specific patient population. The CMP also must be sent to the pharmacy department to review whether the medications selected are cost effective and sent to the coding division of the medical records department for a review of word choices that may enhance coding and improve reimbursement. This review must be done before concluding the content of the plan, and it could be done earlier in the process.

The CMP will then undergo a final review by the team regarding the recommendations of the reviewers. The final draft of the plan is then presented to the steering committee for approval. The team clarifies any questions asked and presents the reasons why a particular practice pattern was recommended. Finally, the CMP is put into practice.

Step 9: Conduct a pilot study of the plan. In this step, the team implements the use of the CMP. Training and education regarding the CMP for all health care providers involved in the particular specialty or diagnosis should be completed before implementation of the plan. The CMP is then evaluated for quality, feasibility of use, appropriateness of time line, length of stay, any delays or variations in care, practice patterns of physicians and other care providers, and compliance.

The CMP is piloted on a group of patients. The results of the pilot are then analyzed and discussed by the interdisciplinary team, and revisions are made accordingly. The plan is then printed in the final version for official use.

Step 10: Standardize/normalize the plan. After completing the pilot study of the CMP and making the required changes, the interdisciplinary team meets to develop policies and procedures regarding the use of the plan. It should be made clear to all involved health care professionals that the CMP represents the standard of care for that particular population and should be followed when caring for the patient. It should also be made clear that some patients might not fit the CMP, and it is appropriate not to use the CMP in these situations. The final plan is then added to the master manual of CMPs and circulated in the final format to key people in the institution. The plan can be shared with various health care providers in different forums such as grand rounds, newsletters, and administrative and departmental meetings.

Policies and procedures on the use of CMPs, particularly documentation of patient progress and variances, what to do when a patient does not fit the CMP, and why it is important to individualize the CMP, are extremely important and should be in place before implementing the use of CMPs. Such policies and procedures serve as a guide and reference for any health care practitioner required to use the CMPs.

STRATEGIES FOR PHYSICIAN PARTICIPATION AND BUY-IN

Physicians play a key role in the success of the team charged with developing a CMP for a particular diagnosis or procedure. Physician participation in developing the plan is integral to improving consistency (i.e., eliminating variations in physician practice patterns) in the care of patients with similar diagnoses who are cared for by different physicians. Obtaining physician support is a prerequisite to achieving the identified goals of the team. Physician buy-in to the use of CMPs before their development and implementation is a key to compliance in their use afterward. Case Manager's Tip 9-6 lists some strategies that can be employed to obtain physicians and increase their participation in the interdisciplinary teams for CMP development.

ORGANIZING THE WORK OF THE INTERDISCIPLINARY TEAM

The steering committee may provide the interdisciplinary team members with guidelines that define what is expected from the team and how the work should progress in each meeting. These guidelines are used to facilitate, simplify, and expedite the process of develop-

case manager's tip 9-6 Gaining Physicians' Support of CMPs

Some strategies and benefits that can be communicated to physicians to gain their buy-in and increase their participation in the interdisciplinary teams to develop CMPs include the following:

1. Involve physicians in the process of developing CMPs from the beginning.
2. Approach influential physicians who are interested in improving the quality of care and reducing the related cost for participation.
3. Demonstrate the benefits of CMPs to physicians' personal practice.
4. Share related published materials (e.g., evaluative research, description of case management systems, physician's opinions from other similar institutions) with all physicians.
5. Emphasize that CMPs are recommendations for treatment rather than rigid guidelines or standing orders. Make clear to all physicians that the CMP should be individualized for each patient on initiation and that changes are possible.
6. Delineate how CMPs enhance quality of care:
    a. Clearly and proactively defined care expectations and physicians' preferences
    b. Improved continuity of patient care, especially if a patient requires care across different patient care units within same institution
    c. Detailed patient/family education requirements
    d. Open communication patterns among various disciplines involved in the care
    e. Care-related variance data tracking; the use of variance data for continuous quality improvement efforts
7. Delineate how CMPs enhance cost of patient care:
    a. Predetermined patient care activities that are sequenced in a timely manner to achieve appropriate length of stay and expected outcomes
    b. Modifications of physicians' practice pattern
    c. Consistency in patient care across physicians
    d. Improvement in patient care as a result of variance tracking
    e. Benefits of the CMP in reducing risk management issues
8. Communicate how CMPs improve compliance with the standards of regulatory agencies.
9. Explain how the plan could be used as an education/training tool for residents, house staff, nurses, and students.
10. Emphasize that the plans may be used as marketing tools to attract more participation from managed care organizations.
11. Stress opportunities for research and creativity in patient care delivery.
12. Emphasize that data from tracking variances facilitate changes in hospital systems to eliminate inefficiencies in patient care.
13. Share individual physician's performance data/practice pattern and how it compares to that of other physicians in the hospital and in comparable institutions.

---

ing CMPs. The steering committee assigns the team's leader and facilitator before the team's first meeting. These two members are specially trained to assume these roles. Interdisciplinary team members are also trained regarding the roles they play. Preparing all members of the team, including the facilitator and leader, is important because training improves the team's productivity and increases members' skills in teamwork and CMP development. Interdisciplinary teams need an average of six to eight meetings, 1 hour each, to complete a CMP. The following sections outline an example of how the work of the team should be planned.

Preparation Meeting

The steering committee assigns the team leader and facilitator based on the specific case type/CMP to be developed. A meeting is then held between representative(s) from the steering committee and the leader and facilitator, during which the goals and expectations of

the interdisciplinary team are discussed. During this meeting, the following issues are finalized:

- Membership of the team, including physicians
- Length of stay of the CMP
- Training and education of the team members
- Date, time, and place of the team's first meeting
- Finalizing the agenda of the first meeting
- Notifying team members of their participation on the team
- Establishing a time line for the team's work and a target date for completion of the CMP
- Sharing of the available data (previous administrative, length of stay, and utilization review reports) related to the CMP type

Interdisciplinary Team's First Meeting

During the first meeting, the interdisciplinary team leader discusses the team's goals and expectations and the time line for completion of the expected work. A list of all team members and their phone numbers is distributed. This meeting is geared toward educating the team members. The issues discussed include the following:

- The process of developing a CMP
- Goals for improvement
- Specific discussion regarding the responsibilities of each member in the development of the CMP
- The template of the CMP as provided by the steering committee
- The available data related to the particular case type, and examples of CMPs from other institutions
- Assignments for next meeting (plan of care related to each discipline)
- Finalizing the meetings schedule (date, time, location, and frequency)

Second Meeting

During the second meeting, team members conduct medical records review and discuss the following:

- The preliminary plan of care prepared by each member of the team as it relates to the discipline he or she represents
- The time line placement of the recommended interventions
- The assignment for next meeting (finalize the plan of care of each discipline)

Third and Fourth Meetings

During the third and fourth meetings, the team finalizes the recommended plan of care, compares the ideal/best practice with the review of literature available, and makes changes as needed. The team starts to discuss the expected outcomes of care. The team does the following:

- Finalizes the interventions and the treatment plan
- Starts discussing the intermediate and discharge outcomes of care
- Begins looking at preprinted physician order set
- Ensures that the patient's actual and potential problems are included in the plan

Fifth Meeting

In the fifth meeting, members of the interdisciplinary team present the intermediate and discharge outcomes of care related to their portion of the CMP. A discussion on whether these outcomes are feasible within the time line recommended takes place. If any problems are identified, adjustments are made. The preprinted physician order set and the list of patient's problems are also confirmed. At this point the CMP is near completion. The team starts to discuss vari-

ance tracking and what type of data are to be collected.

Sixth Meeting

The sixth meeting is spent by the team finalizing the significant data for variance tracking. The team also prepares the final CMP to be shared with the chief of the department where the CMP will be implemented. It is important to also obtain the steering committee's feedback on the recommended CMP before it is finalized. In addition, the team starts planning for pilot testing of the CMP.

Seventh Meeting

During the seventh meeting, the interdisciplinary team discusses the recommendations made by the chief of the department and the steering committee. The CMP is revised accordingly. The pilot-testing plan is finalized, and the CMP is confirmed in its final version that is ready for testing.

Eighth Meeting

The last meeting is spent on reviewing the pilot data. Data are analyzed, and a decision of whether the CMP is ready for wide implementation is made. Based on the data collected during the pilot period, the CMP is revised and finalized. At this point the CMP is ready to become the standard of practice. It is usually submitted to the steering committee in its final version with recommendations for implementation. The report generated by the interdisciplinary team, which is based on the pilot of the CMP, is also given to the steering committee. In this meeting the work of the interdisciplinary team is completed. The team may also decide on follow-up dates for meetings to evaluate the use of the CMP and the variance data collected to determine if any changes should be made in the CMP.

The interdisciplinary team members work on their assignments in between meetings. The actual meeting time is used for follow-up on work progress and for discussions around identified concerns or issues. Case Manager's Tip 9-7 presents strategies for holding effective meetings. These strategies can be applied by nurse case managers when being involved in running meetings, whether related to developing CMPs or not.

SUMMARY AND CONCLUSION

The use of CMPs has become more popular in virtually all patient care settings. The standardization of the process of developing these plans is extremely important. The previous discussion provides health care and nursing administrators and case managers with a practical,

case
manager's
tip

9-7

Strategies for Running Effective Meetings

1. Identify the purpose of the meeting.
2. Prepare an agenda before the meeting, distribute it to the members, and allow them to add items/issues to it.
3. Be sure that all agenda items are necessary and appropriate.
4. Allocate in advance the time needed for discussing each agenda item.
5. Start and finish the meeting on time.
6. Stay on schedule during the meeting. Adhere to the allotted time for the item. If discussion is not concluded within the allotted time, follow up on the item in the next meeting.
7. Assign subgroups to work on certain issues in between meetings to maximize the utility of the meeting time. Ask these subgroups to report back with the outcomes/decisions during the next meeting.
8. Allow and encourage participation of all members.
9. Clarify and summarize discussions/decisions before an issue is concluded.
10. Ensure that the environment is conducive to the meeting: room, ventilation, temperature, seating.
11. Keep interruptions to a minimum.
12. Record minutes.
13. Maximize the use of visual aids (e.g., handouts).
14. Prevent disagreements. Use consensus building when issues arise.
15. Generate a sense of team spirit.
16. Ensure normal group dynamics as they are essential to accomplish the purpose.
17. Limit participation in the meeting to the necessary players.
18. Schedule the meeting on a date and at a time when all necessary people are available.
19. Be sensitive to organizational politics.
20. Avoid mixing business with pleasure.
21. Keep conversations relevant and discussions balanced.
22. Avoid editorializing.
23. Promote active listening.
24. Recognize individual expertise and talent.
25. Do not dominate the discussion.
26. Avoid value judgment statements.
27. Allow for difference of opinions.
28. Negotiate win-win resolutions.
29. Conclude the meeting with a summary of accomplishments.
30. Express appreciation.

step-by-step approach to developing CMPs. It can be used as a tool to train members of interdisciplinary teams involved in developing CMPs. The method presented is flexible and can be tailored to any organization or care setting. It can be used to develop CMPs for the care of patients in acute, ambulatory, long-term, or home care settings. The process to be followed in these settings is the same, but the content and format of the plans may vary.

The use of CMPs has successfully contained health care costs, reduced lengths of stay, improved quality of care, streamlined use of resources, and opened communication lines among the health care team members. Formalizing the process of developing CMPs is the first step toward ensuring that these benefits will be met. The proposed process is beneficial to all health care providers in any care setting, particularly case managers, whether they are involved in developing CMPs or are planning to get started. It can be used by members of

the interdisciplinary teams as a blueprint to develop CMPs. It serves as a guide or safety mechanism to ensure that all bases are covered during the developmental process and before the plan is concluded.

KEY POINTS

1. It is necessary for each institution to have a steering committee to oversee the development, implementation, and evaluation of case management plans.
2. It is more effective to have a formal process and structure for developing case management plans.
3. Case management plans should be developed based on the literature, particularly research, expert opinion, and recommendations of professional organizations and societies.
4. It is important to seek the input of all health care providers involved in the care of a particular patient when developing a case management plan.
5. The case management plan, after it is piloted and approved, should become the institution's standard of care and applied by all practitioners.

6. The interdisciplinary team charged with developing a particular case management plan should be given enough guidance by the steering committee and provided with appropriate training and education regarding the process.

References

Bozzuto B, Farrell E: A collaborative approach to nursing care of the open heart surgical patient, *Case Manage* 6(3):47-53, 1995.

Cohen EL, Cesta TG: *Nursing case management: from concept to evaluation,* ed 2, St Louis, 1997, Mosby.

Esler R et al: A case management success story, *Am J Nurs* 94(11):34-38, 1994.

Ferguson LE: Steps to developing a clinical pathway, *Nurs Admin Q* 17(3):58-62, 1993.

Guiliano HH, Poirer CE: Nursing case management: critical pathways to desirable outcomes, *Nurs Manage* 22(3):52-55, 1991.

Hampton DC: Implementing a managed care framework through care maps, *J Nurs Admin* 23(5):21-27, 1993.

Hydo B: Designing an effective clinical pathway for stroke, *Am J Nurs* 95(3): 44-50, 1995.

Ignatavicius D: Clinical pathways: the wave of the future, *Healthcare Travel* 2(5):23-25, 46-47, 1995.

Ignatavicius DD, Hausman KA: *Clinical pathways for collaborative practice,* Philadelphia, 1995, WB Saunders.

Katterhagen JG, Patton M: Critical pathways in oncology: balancing the interests of hospitals and the physician, *J Oncol Manage* 2(4):20-26, 1993.

Meister S et al: Home care steps protocols, *J Nurs Admin* 25(6):33-42, 1995.

St Anthony Publishing: *DRG: working guide,* Alexandria, Va, 1992, St Anthony Publishing.

Tahan HA, Cesta TG: Developing case management plans using a quality improvement model, *J Nurs Admin* 24(12):49-58, 1995.

Thompson KS et al: Building a critical pathway for ventilator dependency, *Am J Nurs* 91(7):28-31, 1991.

Zander K: Care maps: the core of cost and quality care, *New Definition* 6(3):1-3, 1991.

Zander K: Physicians, care maps, and collaboration, *New Definition* 7(1):1-4, 1992.

CASE MANAGEMENT PLAN

This appendix presents a template for case management plans. Case management plans usually delineate the standards of care; identify patients' actual and potential problems, the goals of treatment, and the necessary patient care activities; and establish the projected outcomes of care.

THINGS TO REMEMBER ABOUT DEVELOPING CASE MANAGEMENT PLANS

- Establish an interdisciplinary team.
- Identify team members based on the diagnosis or surgical procedure in question. Members should be chosen based on their clinical experiences, leadership skills, communication skills, tolerance to hard work, and commitment to the institution and the project.
- Identify a team leader and a facilitator.
- Provide the team with administrative and clerical support.
- Establish a project work plan (time line of activities) before the team's first meeting.
- Train team members in the process of developing CMPs.
- Team members should prepare their work in between meetings. Meetings should be held to review the work and determine the next steps.
- Regardless of the format of the CMP, it should always include the patient care elements as identified by the organization, the patient problems, projected length of stay and outcomes of care, a variance tracking form, and patient care activities and interventions.
- Time line the CMP as indicated by the care setting. For example, minutes to hours in emergency departments, number of visits in clinics and home care, days in acute care, weeks in areas of longer length of stay such as neonatal intensive care area, and

months in nursing homes and group homes. The time line of CMPs in subacute care and rehabilitation centers can be established based on the length of stay, goals of treatment, and intensity of activities. For the most part, it is daily or weekly.

- Preestablish the expected (acceptable) length of stay.
- Determine the mechanism for tracking variances and define the variance categories to be evaluated.
- Ensure that the CMP is the standard of care applied by all health care providers, including physicians.
- Include patient and family teaching and discharge planning activities in all CMPs.
- Determine whether CMPs are a permanent part of the medical record.
- Maximize documentation on the CMP. Require all patient care services to use the CMP for documentation.
- Develop CMPs based on the latest recommendations of research and professional societies.
- Avoid being rigid in recommending treatments. For example, use words like "consider" when including treatments, medications, or interventions that may not be applicable to every patient, completion may not always be possible within the indicated time frame, or progress may be dependent on patient's condition.
- Identify the intermediate and discharge outcomes of care in each CMP.
- Delineate the ICD-9 code or the DRG number of the CMP on the cover page.
- Include all disciplines involved in the care of patients as indicated by the diagnosis or surgical procedure considered.
- Stress the importance of patient care activities that historically were identified as problem areas or requiring improvement.
- Establish a time frame for reviewing and revising the CMP.

TEMPLATE OF A CASE MANAGEMENT PLAN

Diagnosis: _____

Admit Date: ___ / ___ / ___

Attending MD: _____

Date: ___ / ___ / ___

DRG#: _____ Expected LOS: _____

Discharge Date: ___ / ___ / ___ Actual LOS: _____

Primary Nurse: _____

Day _____ of _____

CARE ELEMENTS	RESPONS. PARTY*	INITIALS	EXPECTED OUTCOMES	COMMENTS / NOTES
Assessment/ Monitoring				
Lab Work				
Tests / Procedures				
Treatments				
Medications				
Consults				
Activity				
Nutrition				

APPENDIX **9-1**—cont'd

CARE ELEMENTS	RESPONS. PARTY*	INITIALS	EXPECTED OUTCOMES	COMMENTS / NOTES
IV Therapy				
Respiratory Therapy				
Physical Therapy/ Occupational Therapy				
Wound Care				
Pain Management				
Patient/Family Education				
Psychosocial Assessment				
Discharge Planning:				

Initial	Signature	Initial	Signature

* Responsible Party: Registered Nurse (RN), Attending Physician/House Staff (MD), Nurse Practitioner (NP), Social Worker (SW), Home Care Intake Coordinator (HCIC), Physical Therapist (PT), Occupational Therapist (OT), Nutritionist (NUT)

CHAPTER 10

QUALITY PATIENT CARE

Perhaps the most important topic in health care today is quality. Although health care organizations have always had quality at the top of their priority list, especially when the prospective payment systems (PPSs) began, only recently has it been recognized that continuously improving quality can make a difference. The difference can be as vital as survival or providing the health care organization with a competitive advantage in the marketplace.

IMPORTANCE OF QUALITY

Today's competitive health care environment demands constant attention to improvements in quality. Consumers are demanding that they receive full value for their health care dollar. The goal of any health care provider is to have customers desire to return if necessary for their health care needs. If health care organizations fail to strive for quality, they will fall behind in the highly competitive marketplace.

Meaning of Quality

Probably the most difficult hurdle is to agree on what quality means. What are the properties, characteristics, and attributes of care that lead us to a judgment of good or bad quality? Quality may include, but not be limited to, available health care services, standards of providers, comprehensive assessment and documentation, collaborative and informed relationships with patient and family, minimal injuries or complications for hospitalized patients, evaluation of new technology and resources, and effective management of health care resources (McCarthy, 1987).

The patient's view of what is important in his or her care may be seen as one aspect of quality, along with patient satisfaction, when defining indicators of quality. The overall quality of health care will be judged on the entire package, including health outcomes, accessibility, timeliness and efficiency of services, interdisciplinary communication, and the direct and indirect costs of illness and care (Case Manager's Tip 10-1).

From the customer's point of view, there are three types of quality characteristics: "take-it-for-granted" quality, expected quality, and exciting quality. Take-it-for granted quality is what a health care setting must offer to be acceptable (e.g., staff competency). Expected quality includes those things that are necessary and expected (e.g., food quality). Exciting quality pertains to those items that are nice to have but are not necessary (e.g., environmental features) (Nelson and Larson, 1993).

Effective case management must work within a framework that demonstrates quality improvements while taking the patient's perceptions and expectations into account.

Another approach to defining quality includes the following attributes Donabedian (1980) outlines when assessing for quality:

1. *Effectiveness:* The ability to attain the greatest improvements in health now achievable by the best care
2. *Efficiency:* The ability to lower cost of care without diminishing attainable improvements in health
3. *Balance:* The balancing of costs against the effect of care on health so as to attain the most advantageous balance
4. *Acceptability:* Conforming to the wishes, desires, and expectations of patients and their families
5. *Legitimacy:* Conformity to social preferences as expressed in ethical principles, values, norms, laws, and regulations
6. *Equity:* Conformity to a principle that determines what is just or fair in the distribution of health care and its benefits among the members of the population

Health care providers historically have been concerned with the maintenance and improvement of quality of care for hospitalized patients (Dash et al, 1996). Most health care organizations today have a mission statement that tends to incorporate the institution's culture or values and beliefs. Phrases usually include honesty, commitment to patient/customer satisfaction, and

case
manager's
tip   10-1   **Perception of Quality**

A patient's perception of quality is only as good as the last encounter.

case
manager's
tip   10-2   **The Role of Customer Service in Quality**

Customer service will be what defines quality in the future and will more than likely play a major role in a hospital's survival as we become more deeply involved in a managed care environment.

commitment to employee satisfaction in an environment that is conducive to performing the best work. The values are what the organization regards as important. They are the principles that the organization will uphold and defend, the fabric that holds the organizational structure together, and the foundation on which it rests.

Quality Categories of Organizational Values

Commonly, organizational values can be divided into five categories of quality: patient/customer focus, total involvement of taking responsibility for quality, measurement or monitoring of quality, systems support, and continuous quality improvement (Organizational Dynamics, Inc, 1991). It is necessary to define each more fully and give examples of a strong organizational commitment vs. a weak organizational commitment to quality.

Patient/customer focus. Patient/customer focus is related to service, products available, and sharing of information to both an institution's internal and external customers (Case Manager's Tip 10-2). Customer service has become a common buzzword. Determining whether your external customers received the quality they valued is a powerful tool for an organization to use. In the past, most facilities believed that if they tracked the number of problems or occurrences and they remained within an acceptable level, then the organization was providing quality customer service. More recently, the technique of asking the consumers about their expectations of quality care was found to be much more telling and accurate rather than a hospital making random assumptions as to what the customer needed or considered as quality care. Patient care surveys are now widely used in all types of settings as successful tools toward quality care assessment and improvement.

An example of one patient care survey is produced by Press Ganey Associates, Inc. (1996). On average, the customer is asked to reply to 40 or more questions covering the hospitalization from admission to discharge. These surveys can be tailored to any organization's specificities that will help benchmark it with the surrounding hospitals. This system has moved quality from a vague, subjective process to an objective, measurable tool serving many purposes. This tool is able to grade the entire hospital and break down the results to specific areas, patient units, or departments. The survey can then place the organization in a ranking order with its competitors and benchmark its success or reveal areas for improvement.

As **case management** programs become more and more visible, patient satisfaction surveys may need to be altered so that they capture not only environmental amenities of things such as food and room comfort but also include professional care received. Case management should be added to patient care surveys in the future.

It is appropriate to consider an example of an organization's commitment to quality customer service: patients are called after discharge to hear if their expectations were met. Their suggestions and complaints are taken seriously, addressed, and responded to. The organization that does not incorporate customer service into its quality program, does not respond to patient complaints, and ignores suggestions made by its customers is jeopardizing its reputation, market share, and financial status.

Total involvement. The total involvement of taking responsibility for quality relates to the fact that management personnel or quality assurance personnel cannot be the sole people involved in quality assurance efforts. It is everyone's responsibility to be involved in the achievement of quality. Quality is the direct result of positive employee behavior (Williams, 1994). Positive employee behavior is usually the result of staff job satisfaction. Employees tend to feel ownership of their organization's values when they have been involved in the selection of those values. Productive behavior will be evident when an organization's goals are clear and understood by its employees, their role in the organization is defined, and the policies and procedures governing their role are well communicated. For example, the hospital that supports a strong case management team and empowers its members with the permission to solve problems is an organization with a commitment to quality. The hospital showing weakness in this area of quality commitment will not address the need for a case management program and will wait for some divine intervention to solve its problems.

Measurement or monitoring of quality. Measurement or monitoring quality must be done to meet goals. Improvement is impossible without measurement (Organizational Dynamics, Inc, 1991). The case manager's role is to ensure that the patient is moving along in the acute level of care, subacute, or even home care stay in a timely fashion. If any **outcomes** are not achieved or are delayed, it is the case manager in these settings who is responsible for determining why and for facilitating a corrective action plan. These untoward occurrences are called **variances** (see Chapter 11). By reviewing a patient's progress regularly and anticipating the plan, patient variances will be kept to a minimum and **length of stay** issues avoided. Health care provider variances are related to omission or error made by a practitioner. Regulations and policies govern this area. If a health care provider omits a medication, this is a variance that could affect the treatment plan. Operational variances are those that happen within the health care setting, such as a patient waiting for a rehabilitation bed that is not available and delays discharge or equipment failures or scheduling delays. Retrospective analysis and trending of variances result in identification of frequently occurring variances. This analysis will help monitor quality and identify areas for improvement. Outcomes are paramount criteria of good quality either by themselves or as related to costs if efficiency and optimality are to be determined (Donabedian, 1991).

Systems support. Systems support includes planning, budgeting, scheduling, and performance management needed to support the quality effort. If systems are well coordinated, the time it takes to accomplish the work will be reduced. Everyone should be invested in providing quality work. A team effort should be fostered to accomplish unified goals. A good example of this is a health care delivery system called *patient-focused care* that is being adopted in many acute care settings. This

---

box 10-1

Quality Improvement Plan: a 14-Step Approach

1. Management commitment
2. Quality improvement plan
3. Measurement
4. Cost of quality
5. Quality awareness
6. Corrective action
7. Zero defects planning
8. Employee education
9. Zero defects
10. Goal setting
11. Error cause removal
12. Recognition
13. Quality councils
14. Do it all over again

From Crosby-Philip B: *Quality is free: the art of making quality certain*, New York, 1979, McGraw-Hill.

---

system is based on the philosophy that the patient is the center core of focus and that all disciplines involved with the patient must be able to access that patient easily. Patients should not have to seek out the area needed for their treatment; it should come to them. The patient requiring physical therapy should not have to be transported to the physical rehabilitation department; the department's physical therapist should be available in the unit in which the patient resides. This decreases the nonproductive time of transport and can ultimately have the effect of shortening the hospitalization.

Continuous quality improvement. Through continuous quality improvement, organizations foster creativity to do things better tomorrow than they did yesterday. It is a way of correcting flaws and making improvements. Well over a decade ago, the industrial leaders of the world realized that to remain competitive and survive in our economy today, quality improvement techniques were needed. There are three individuals who stand out as pioneers in the development of quality improvement techniques: Philip B. Crosby, W. Edwards Demming, and Joseph M. Juran. Crosby (1979) designed a 14-step approach for his quality improvement process (QIP) (Box 10-1).

Demming and Juran's work dates back to the 1920s and 1950s and was responsible for enormous improvements in Japanese manufacturing. In 1986 Demming's approach to quality improvement came to America. He is best known for involving the employee in the quality improvement effort. This approach involved groups of employees coming together to discuss problem identification and problem solving. When this process is applied to health care it involves strategies not only to improve quality but also to reduce costs.

In the United States, the concept of quality has matured first from the early quality control or inspection and testing effort to the middle ground of quality assurance, in which selected specialists monitored quality, identified errors or incidents, and kept report cards on each individual blamed for the problem. The quality assurance specialists tend to lack the authority or clout necessary to change the way work is performed. Moreover, quality assurance and its inspection techniques never catch the real issues affecting patient care. The fully mature quality effort is known as *continuous quality improvement* or *total quality management*. The organizations that embrace this concept are those advanced in the ability to empower their employees to be responsible for quality. The Joint Commission on Accreditation of Healthcare Organizations (JCAHO, 1996) has set forth the charge to integrate quality improvement endeavors that focus on actual performance and outcomes.

The JCAHO has designed the quality cube (Figure 10-1) to depict a model for assessing quality. It illustrates the relationship of performance and important func-

tions to a range of patient populations and services provided. The cube is a tool that stimulates thought related to improvement priorities.

Over the past few years health professionals have shifted their efforts from quality assurance (QA) to quality improvement (QI) and most recently advancing to such terms as continuous quality improvement (CQI), total quality management (TQM), and JCAHO's latest term—process improvement (PI). QA, as stated earlier, tends to focus on reduction of errors, meeting standards set up by regulatory agencies, and measuring defined outcome. This model functions in response to problems and has a retrospective view of tracking occurrences after they have happened. QI, on the other hand, focuses on improving a process, meeting customer needs, and measuring customer-identified outcomes. It is a continuous proactive process involving all employees at all levels. The QI approach is one in which the advantage is clear, and it assumes that most people want to do the right thing well. According to the Health Outcomes In-

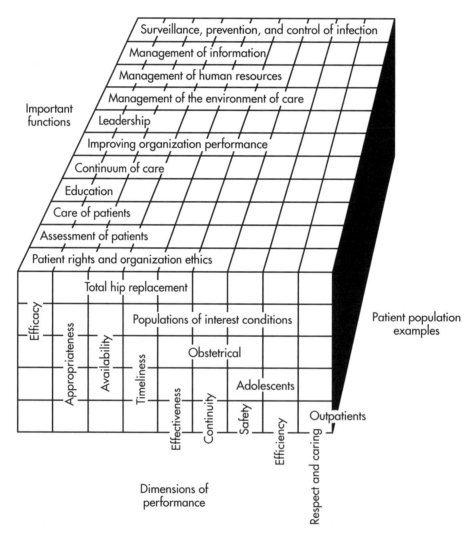

Fig. 10-1 The quality cube: a model for assessing the quality of health care. (Redrawn from JCAHO: *The 1996 accreditation manual for hospitals,* Oakbrook Terrace, Ill, 1995, JCAHO.)

stitute (1994), quality in health care is achieved by "doing the right thing right," where "the right thing" is outcome management and one does it "right" by controlling the process.

We have moved from the paradigm of QA, where provider-defined outcomes (such as morbidity, mortality, and clinical endpoints) rule, to QI, which relies on user- and customer-defined outcomes (such as cost of care, health-related quality, and patient satisfaction). QI focuses on the continued improvement of all processes rather than just those identified as a problem. This type of an approach can improve quality of care of the majority of patients and also decrease statistical outliers. **Outlier thresholds** are set by the Health Care Finance Administration (HCFA). This is the range of days a patient may stay hospitalized at the maximum reimbursement rate. Outliers are those who exceed the set range of days. In contrast, QA governs itself by the 80/20 rule (or "Pareto Principle"), which states that 80% of costs are generated by 20% of the patients. Therefore, those who abide by this principle will only address a small percentage of issues. Table 10-1 provides a snapshot summary of QA vs. QI activities.

CASE MANAGEMENT AND CQI

How does the QI approach to health care fit in with a case management model? Case managers' skills and role characteristics, as discussed in previous chapters, exemplify many of the descriptive elements of QI: problem solving, negotiation, mentoring, quality monitoring, and outcome analysis. Usually the first task for a case manager is to select those patients who would benefit from case management. The next task is to facilitate patient treatment goals and discharge plans. In a successful case management program all patients should be monitored for quality, use of resources, and length of

TABLE 10-1
Summary of QA vs. QI

Topic	Quality assurance	Quality improvement
Focus	Licensure satisfaction	Strategic planning
Approach	Top-down	Top-down/bottom-up
Goals	Reduce errors	Satisfy the customer
Actions	Track outliers	Improve processes
Type of change	Incremental	Incremental
Employees	Not invested	Participation in QI teams

Modified from Newell M: *Using nurse case management to improve health outcomes,* Gaithersburg, Md, 1996, Aspen.

stay. Once a patient is identified as one who would benefit from case management, a management plan is designed. The management care plan is developed to optimize the treatment plan, streamline the care to avoid delays or road blocks, and avoid any compromise in quality. By following these guidelines quality issues are easily tracked. Two tools that are commonly used to track issues of quality are indicator reports and variance reports. Indicator reports are usually geared more to physician practice patterns and untoward occurrences as sequelae to their practice (e.g., an unplanned return to the operating room during the same hospitalization, postoperative complications, or abnormal laboratory results not addressed)—simply put, identifying anything that does not happen when it should. Variance reporting will be discussed in much more detail in Chapter 11.

In general, the case manager is the driving force behind the success of quality patient care through the case management. The case manager who checks on quality indicators and variances not only identifies problems but also must find remedies for the patient's care to continue to successfully move through the hospital system.

A case management program has a major importance to any quality effort. Case managers have the potential to reduce readmissions and the ability to evaluate the possibility of meeting a patient's health care needs in an alternative and probably less-costly setting. The case manager must ensure that a patient receives adequate and appropriate care while acute and must provide adequate quality follow-up care. By doing this efficiently case managers reduce premature discharges at health care facilities and help to guarantee that patients' discharge plans are adequate to meet their needs, with the ultimate goal of quality care, patient satisfaction, and avoiding unnecessary readmissions.

You can quickly conclude after reviewing Case Study 10-1 that had all the health care disciplines involved in the discharge plan of Mrs. Lopez been consulted, the outcome could have been avoided. By simply reviewing with the home care agency the equipment that the patient was using in the hospital vs. the equipment being used at home, the undue anxiety of the patient's family would not have occurred. Had the home health nurse and case manager assessed the ventilator and related supplies that would be used in the home, the patient's well-being could have been maintained by altering the education of the caregivers in the home.

CONSUMER/PATIENT SATISFACTION

An important outcome of any case management program is customer satisfaction. Patient and family satis-

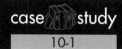

case study
10-1

Example of Unnecessary Readmission to Hospital

Mrs. Lopez is a 68-year-old woman who was admitted with a diagnosis of congestive heart failure. She developed acute respiratory problems and was placed on a ventilator. Her family was very involved in her care and met with the case manager regularly to organize a quality-of-life discharge plan. The case manager worked diligently to provide this patient and her family with all the necessary tools and provisions to meet their needs of going home. The plan was to go home even if Mrs. Lopez remained on the ventilator. A respiratory company was closely involved and worked with the case manager and family to teach the necessary skills to the family and prepare the home for a ventilator. The case manager worked with Mrs. Lopez's daughter to teach her basic respiratory care and Ambu-bagging techniques and to improve her confidence when dealing with her mother's ventilator. After many weeks of preparation, the doctor, case manager, patient, family, and respiratory therapy company all believed they provided a high-quality dis-

charge plan. Within 3 days of discharge Mrs. Lopez was readmitted in respiratory distress. The family was devastated and complained that the visiting nurse from home care was very delayed and did not provide the same information taught to the family in the hospital. The Ambu bag that they were using in the hospital did not work like the one provided at home; the daughter became distraught and called an ambulance.

- What went wrong with the quality of this care plan?
- Was this the most effective discharge plan?
- Did the case manager include all caregivers in this plan, including those involved in follow-up care?
- If the case manager included the skilled home care agency in the discharge plan, could this outcome and readmission have been avoided?
- Were costs, patient satisfaction, and caregiver needs affected by this incomplete plan?

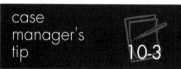

case manager's tip
10-3
Customer Service Rule of Thumb

A customer service rule of thumb says that a satisfied customer will tell 3 people, but a dissatisfied customer will tell 20.

---

faction are essential outcomes to measure; physician, team members, and other involved agencies, as in the previous example, are also important customers. Case managers must work closely with all members of the health care team to assess, monitor, and analyze the delivery of care, the case management plan, and the patient/family response to the care to continuously improve the organization's quality of performance (Flarey and Smith-Blanchett, 1996).

A **case management plan** is designed typically through a multidisciplinary process; when executed correctly, the team's collaboration designs the single best treatment plan for a specific patient case. The plan also provides for a collection and ongoing evaluation of potential quality issues. These issues are usually identified through variances or complications. The entire process enables a focus on quality by continually assessing and identifying opportunities for improvement (Flarey and Smith-Blanchett, 1996).

Case management's efforts for improvement must be accomplished case by case. Case management plays a crucial role in evaluating and monitoring a patient's case management plan and discharge goals. Case managers are the professionals most aware of the patient's functional, physical, and cognitive abilities and know

best how these abilities will affect and determine a patient's level of functioning after discharge from an acute care setting. Offering the best-possible discharge plan is vitally important because of the potential for reducing readmissions and providing alternative care methods for less cost—and thus the ultimate outcome of heightened patient, family, physician, and payor satisfaction.

Being able to exceed your customers' expectations for quality service must be the driving force; this central concern is a primary reason a registered nurse becomes a nurse case manager. Quality service should be a way of life for any case manager's day-to-day functions, and it is one of the standards necessary for health care today to prosper and survive (Case Manager's Tip 10-3).

Cost/Quality/Case Management

As health care costs increasingly become a public issue and managed care organizations spend more and more time examining documentation of health care expenses and charges, it is more apparent that quality monitoring must also include elements of not only practice patterns and patient satisfaction but also cost-containment strategies.

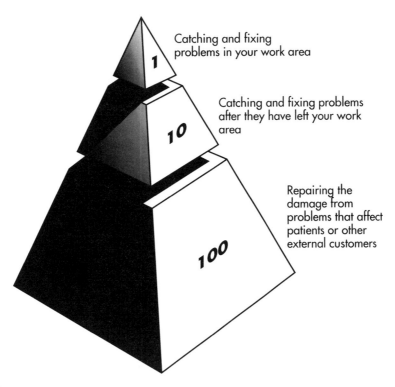

Catching and fixing problems in your work area

Catching and fixing problems after they have left your work area

Repairing the damage from problems that affect patients or other external customers

Fig. 10-2   The 1-10-100 rule. It makes a difference *when* a problem is fixed. The 1-10-100 rule states that if a problem is not fixed when it occurs, it will only become more costly to fix later in terms of both time and money. (Redrawn from Organizational Dynamics, Inc: *The quality advantage,* Burlington, Mass, 1991, Organizational Dynamics, Inc.)

In health care organizations problems that go undetected can have devastating effects that involve wasted time and money. When a problem is not fixed at the time it occurs, it will only become more costly to fix later in terms of time and money (Organizational Dynamics, Inc, 1991) (Figure 10-2).

Costs usually involve the necessary expenditures and those that are avoidable. A *necessary cost* is one that is needed to sustain a certain standard. *Avoidable costs* are those that occur whenever things are done wrong or the wrong things are done right. Necessary and avoidable costs can be further defined by prevention, inspection, and failure costs. *Prevention costs* are those intended to ensure that things will not go wrong. *Inspection costs* are the costs of finding an error and fixing that error. *Failure costs* are those incurred when patient or customer satisfaction is negatively affected. Any institution will pay a big price for a marred reputation, rework, waste, legal penalties, extra charges, or loss of business.

Poor quality is very costly. To help reduce the potential costs poor quality incurs, it becomes imperative that case managers facilitate QI by making sure they get involved and have the confidence and skills required to do their job well. This does not mean that case managers are solely responsible for the cost of quality. They must work in concert with all of the members of the interdisciplinary team. For example, a physician writes

an order for a medication that the patient has an allergy to. If the nurse notices this error as the order is picked up, it would involve a simple solution of ordering another medication that is more appropriate for the patient. If, however, the order goes to the pharmacy and the allergy is not noted, the pharmacist fills the order, and the nurse administers the drug; the result could end in terrible tragedy. The cost of the incorrect drug is only the tip of the iceberg for this error. The dollars alone cannot fully measure the impact of this error on the patient and the hospital. The real cost of this undetected problem shows the heightened damage as illustrated in the 1-10-100 rule. Not only has a medication occurrence added increased cost, but patient satisfaction is at stake as well.

The obvious key to reducing costs and maintaining quality is prevention. The case manager, in the daily review of patient care, works toward preventing errors, problems, and bottlenecks to care. The next-best strategy after prevention is early detection and treatment of the problem. Again consider the scenario of the drug error. If the immediate physician order error is not detected, then the first level of prevention does not occur. However, if the nurse detects the problem before administration of the drug, then early detection prevents the potential full impact of the error. If the nurse, on the other hand, administers the incorrect drug, then early detection is not employed. To compound this error, perhaps the patient is aware that a mistake has taken place. Now the confidence in the physician and hospital staff has been marred. The case manager is now involved in identifying this quality issue and must now get the physician and perhaps a hospital representative in to speak with the patient and attempt to make amends. It now becomes clearer that the cost of quality in this example could have the worst effect of all—a dissatisfied patient who will never return to that health care facility.

A second area where cost and quality intertwine is the cost associated with misuse of personnel or equipment resources. For example, a case manager specializing in cardiac care began to notice a strange occurrence on the unit. Many of the cardiac patients were being monitored simultaneously on both the telemetry units and physician-ordered Holter monitors. The case manager began to ask the obvious question, "Why?" The Holter monitors were an added expense for the hospital not only due to the fact that the equipment was costly but also because of the misuse of personnel required to read the Holter monitor data and file a report. The same data were available on the telemetry monitors. The case manager decided to investigate the problem by analyzing the cost of the Holter monitoring. In addition, the case manager met with various physicians and the medical director to troubleshoot the rationale behind ordering the Holters on telemetry patients. What was discovered by the case manager was the fact that new telemetry technicians had been hired by the hospital and the physicians did not have the confidence that their patients' monitors were being read with the same caliber as the previous telemetry team. The case manager then set out to reassure the physicians of the qualifications, training, and orientation of the new telemetry technicians and personally reviewed a number of cases in which the Holter and telemetry were used, comparing the diagnostics of both to show the physicians that the quality of their patients' care had not been compromised. Due to the perseverance of this case manager, the additional use of Holter monitors with telemetry units was diminished. By analyzing this problem the case manager identified an opportunity for QI through the most cost-effective method available to the patients.

The last area is the cost of delays. There is much at stake when quality is affected by a delayed service. All of the issues mentioned thus far come into play here. The cost associated with delays, the impact on patient satisfaction, and the misappropriation of resources and personnel will significantly affect the cost of outcomes. Delays are very costly to hospitals and can negatively influence how they are judged by managed care companies, other physicians, customers, and patients.

The example of the ventilator-dependent patient is useful here as well. Suppose that the patient appears to have the potential to be weaned from the ventilator. Weaning can be an arduous task, but the ultimate payoff is so exciting and cost effective that if done successfully it can save the hospital many costly dollars. The challenge of weaning a patient from a ventilator lies with an experienced team who follows the patient very closely. This involves the efforts of case management, as well as social work, dietary, respiratory therapy, speech therapy, physician, nursing staff, patient, and family. The multidisciplinary approach to this complex patient's care management plan is essential to its success.

First the case manager and social worker must work with the family to help them adjust to the idea that weaning their loved one may take some time and may or may not be successful. This alone is difficult and at times frustrating and disappointing for a family. Once the case manager has established that the patient and family are emotionally prepared, the next step is for the other disciplines to educate the family on the care required at home. The timing and availability of the other departments can make or break the length of time it takes to wean a patient. It becomes crucial for the case manager to stay on top of the whole process from start to finish so that everything is in place at the right time. The social worker must work on applications for personal care attendants or any financial arrangements that need to be finalized before discharge. The dietitian must be closely involved with the patient, watching all food intake. The right balance of protein, fat, and carbohydrates must be monitored, because weaning cannot take place without the proper caloric intake. A negative nitrogen balance from inappropriate intake can significantly delay the weaning process. The speech therapist has the vital role of training the patient in different speech and swallowing techniques. If this is attempted with a dedicated positive approach toward the patient's progress, the odds of success are greater. Not all patients are able to meet the criteria for successful speech therapy. It is the case manager who will discuss the potential with the speech therapist and physician to see if the patient is a good candidate. Successful speech and swallow training can make the difference between a patient who will require tube feedings and the patient who can go home on oral food intake. Imagine the delays that can occur in this area alone if no one takes an aggressive risk in attempting to train the patient. Should this area not be explored or attempted with strong expertise, the patient will require tube feedings, which will surely cause a delay because of the added teaching required. The family will need to learn the tube feeding procedures, and the patient will have an additional psy-

case manager's tip	10-4	The Importance of Keeping the Physician Informed

An informed physician is better equipped to intervene appropriately and not react to inconclusive data.

case manager's tip	10-5	Key Elements to Help Avoid Delays in Patient Care Planning

1. Make sure that family/patient education is begun early.
2. Maintain open physician communication.
3. Include all disciplines on the team.
4. Use case management to guide progress.
5. Use patient teaching tools to assist disciplines in tracking progress.
6. Include outside agencies such as home care or respiratory therapy companies early.
7. Be persistent, persevere, and have patience to achieve your goals.

chological hurdle to get over. This is an area in which the case manager can again be involved. A patient-teaching checklist can assist all disciplines in tracking the progress of the family and their ability to learn various tasks such as tube feedings. Without the use of such a tool an additional delay can occur, because there will be no record of the progress or lack of progress a family is making in learning the necessary skills required. Another discipline that must coordinate its intervention when weaning a patient is the respiratory therapy department. They must monitor all the oxygen saturation data and be willing to try the patient on and off the ventilator for periods of time knowing that this is a tedious task that requires patience and perseverence. Any missed opportunities to try the patient off the ventilator could delay the ultimate weaning process and may even cause a failed weaning of the patient. Obviously if the attempts are failed the medical costs of this patient's care increase dramatically.

All interdisciplinary efforts should be to work toward keeping the cost of this patient's care as low as possible. It is very important for the physician to have a trusting relationship with all the involved disciplines in the patient's discharge plan. If the physician becomes discouraged with the progress being made, chances are he or she will make the decision that the patient is not weanable. The physician must be kept well informed by the nursing staff whenever progress is being made (Case Manager's Tip 10-4).

The case manager again has the important role of assisting the physician in making educated decisions regarding whether the patient is making significant enough progress to be weaned off of the ventilator. The case manager must also have the expertise to know when to call the skilled nursing agency to begin the preparations for discharge. If the timing is off on this phase of the discharge plan a major delay will be incurred. As in the scenario discussed earlier in this chapter, if the skilled nursing piece is not included in the discharge plan the risk of an unnecessary readmission is significant. Similarly, if the outpatient home respiratory therapy company is not brought into the loop at the right time, the home may not be properly prepared for a ventilator if this patient cannot be weaned. It behooves the company to check the home electricity to accommodate the ventilator. Thus if the patient does not come off the ventilator, the potential delay of wiring the home for appropriate electricity can be avoided.

There are other tools that can assist the case manager's efforts toward a successful weaning and cost-effective quality discharge plan. The use of a clinical pathway or multidisciplinary action plan that is specific to weaning a patient off the ventilator will serve as an excellent guideline for all disciplines involved in the case to help track areas of strengths and weaknesses. It will help to standardize the process and yet individualize it to specific patient needs. Patient teaching pathways or patient education tools can help to include the patient and family in the plan. The teaching guidelines can assist as a resource for the patient and family at times when the information being taught becomes overwhelming. Anything that can help to reinforce teaching will ultimately be a benefit to the patient/family and ultimately lead to a timely discharge not hindered or delayed by lack of understanding on the patient's or family's part (Case Manager's Tip 10-5).

SUMMARY

Case management and continuous quality improvement are connected very closely in terms of the basic philosophy and process. The asset that case management has is the ability to simultaneously consider quality and cost. The tracking methods used by case management help to measure the cost of good quality vs. inferior quality.

The ongoing goal of any formal case management program is to identify the optimal treatment plan and most cost-effective discharge plan achievable. If such a plan is developed, quality is sure to follow. A case manager's quality effort takes place case by case. It is an organized approach to improving quality and efficiency in patient care and cost.

In the face of today's perceptions and expectations it is an ongoing challenge for case management to significantly impact quality and cost effectiveness; the challenge must be accepted if we are to survive this tidal wave that the health care industry is experiencing.

KEY POINTS

1. Today's competitive health care environment demands constant attention to improvements in quality.
2. There are three types of quality: take-it-for-granted quality, expected quality, and excited quality.
3. Organizational values consist of 5 categories of quality: patient/customer focus, total involvement for taking responsibility for quality, measuring/monitoring quality, systems support, and continuous quality improvement.
4. It is everyone's responsibility to be involved in the achievement of quality.
5. Quality assurance focuses on reduction of errors, whereas quality improvement focuses on improving a process.
6. The key to reducing costs and maintaining quality is prevention.

References

Crosby-Philip B: *Quality is free: the art of making quality certain,* New York, 1979, McGraw-Hill.

Dash K et al: *Discharge planning for the elderly,* New York, 1996, Springer.

Donabedian A: Exploration in quality assessment and monitoring, vol 1, *The definition of quality and approaches to its assessment,* Ann Arbor, Michigan, 1980, Health Administration Press.

Donabedian A: *The role of outcomes in quality assessment and assurance,* Miami, 1991, Excerpts from Annual Conference on Nursing Quality Assurance.

Flarey D, Smith-Blanchett S: *Handbook of nursing case management,* Gaithersburg, Md, 1996, Aspen.

Health Outcomes Institute: *Introduction to outcomes,* Bloomington, Minn, 1994, Health Outcomes Institute.

Joint Commission on Accreditation of Healthcare Organizations: *The 1996 accreditation manual for hospitals,* Oakbrook Terrace, Ill, 1996, JCAHO.

Larson-Nelson C: Patients' good and bad surprises: how do they relate to overall patient satisfaction? *QRB* 19(3):89-94, 1993.

McCarthy C: Quality health care inches closer to precise definition, *Hosp Peer Rev* 12(2):19-20, 1987.

Newell M: *Using nursing case management to improve health outcomes,* Gaithersburg, Md, 1996, Aspen.

Organizational Dynamics, Inc: Excerpts from conference presentation, Burlington, Mass, 1991, Organizational Dynamics, Inc.

Press Ganey Associates, Inc: Weston, Mass, 1996, Press Ganey Associates, Inc.

Williams RL: *Essentials of total quality management,* New York, 1994, American Management Associates.

CHAPTER 11

MEASURING THE EFFECTIVENESS OF A CASE MANAGEMENT MODEL

As a **case manager** in your organization you may be called on to participate in the evaluation of the **case management** model, its effects on the organization, or its effects on patient **outcomes.** You may have direct responsibility for evaluating the model's effectiveness, the success of the case manager's role, or your personal job performance. Some of the evaluation criteria to be discussed in this chapter may require an organizational effort in terms of data collection and/or analysis. Some you may be able to facilitate as part of your own daily job activities.

Whenever possible, it is important to have an evaluation process set up before implementation of the model. This is particularly true for those outcomes that affect the organization. Categories such as **length of stay,** patient and staff satisfaction, and costs of care should have baseline benchmarks against which the hospital can judge success or failure. Additional measurement points will be identified prospectively during the course of the hospital stay or course of treatment or intervention and then at the point of discharge or completion of services, depending on the care setting. Other indices, particularly those related to clinical or patient outcomes, will evolve over time.

OUTCOMES AS INDICES OF QUALITY

Broadly speaking, outcomes can be grouped by those that have an effect on the organization vs. those that have an effect on patients. These indicators may be the best measures of quality, because they provide an understanding of the functioning of the organization and its effects on the product of services and patient care. Outcomes are the results of actions or processes. In patient care they are defined as the goals of the health care process. A good outcome is one that has achieved the desired goal.

Case management, through the use of tools like multidisciplinary action plans (MAPs) and clinical pathways, and through case management team conferencing, al-

lows health care providers to prospectively identify the expected outcomes or goals of care. There are no organizational or clinical processes or tasks that are carried out that do not have an expected outcome attached to them. Therefore, outcomes in their narrowest sense allow us to understand the effects on an individual patient and in their broadest sense provide us with an understanding of the functioning of an organization or the health care system at large. These linkages provide us with an understanding of the structure (the organization), the process (the delivery system), and the expected outcomes (goals of care).

Expected outcomes of care are of different types (Box 11-1). Some are related to the organization's performance but are not directly related to the patient's health. Others are related to the patient's health but are not directly related to the organization's performance. Still others are solely related to the clinical process, meaning they are purely clinical in nature.

Patient Satisfaction

Understanding our patient's satisfaction with the care and services we provide helps us to improve those services over time and to continuously improve patients' level of satisfaction with the care they receive. Patient satisfaction data are either collected toward the end of the hospital stay or soon after discharge. All hospitals and many other health care organizations collect and monitor data on patient satisfaction. Unfortunately there may not always be a mechanism for feeding that information back for the improvement of system processes or expected clinical outcomes.

Patient satisfaction data collection instruments must be carefully analyzed to determine whether the instrument is valid and reliable. Some instruments, if not tested and determined to be valid and reliable, can only be used to monitor trends and not for statistical analysis. Some organizations mail questionnaires to patients after discharge. Some administer them just before discharge while the patient is still on the institution's

Expected Outcomes Not Directly Related to the Patient's Health

1. Increase patient satisfaction
2. Increase staff satisfaction
3. Improve the turn-around time for tests/treatments/procedures
4. Reduce the cost of care
5. Reduce length of stay
6. Improve interdepartmental and interdisciplinary communication

TABLE 11-1

Advantages and Disadvantages of Mailing Vs. On-Site Distribution of Questionnaires

Method	Advantages	Disadvantages
Mailing	Greater reflection of patient's true feelings	More satisfied and dissatisfied patients respond
On-site	Timely, "live" responses; face-to-face interactions	Patient may fear retribution; labor intensive

premises. The advantages and disadvantages of both methods are summarized in Table 11-1.

Whether organizations mail their customer satisfaction surveys to patients after discharge or distribute them on-site with discharge papers or through some other means, there exist some pros and cons with either method. Mailing questionnaires means that patients can respond at home, where they may feel safer to share their true feelings. Unfortunately the majority of responses will reflect those patients who had either a very positive or a very negative experience. Those who had a positive experience will want to share. Those who had a negative one will be lodging a complaint. This skewing of the responses may mean that the sample of people responding does not reflect the experiences of the average patient.

On-site distribution can be accomplished in various ways. Some organizations include the questionnaire as part of the discharge process. Some may include it on the patient's meal tray some time before discharge. These methods also have pros and cons. On-site responses may not reflect the patient's candid and true feelings, because the patient may fear retribution from the hospital staff if responding negatively. On the positive side, the patient's immediate feelings can be captured.

On-site collection is the more labor-intensive process. It requires a distribution and collection process, whereas the return process is built in when the questionnaires are mailed in. One method of collecting on-site responses that may reduce fear of retribution is to manually distribute the questionnaire to the patient at the bedside 24 to 48 hours before discharge. Along with the questionnaire, provide the patient with a pencil and an envelope. Give the patient a short period of time to complete the questionnaire, and ask him or her to seal it in the envelope when finished. Tell the patient that sealing the envelope ensures there will be no association made between patients and their responses, the sealed

envelopes will be retrieved as a later time, and responses will be anonymous. Come back and pick up the envelope later. This technique is effective in getting a more representative sampling of patients, and the responses are then more timely. Unfortunately it is a labor-intensive process that requires a dedicated employee or volunteer. Not all organizations may have such resources at their disposal. In addition, make an effort to randomize the sample of patients chosen to be included in studying customer satisfaction. Randomization may be applied to both procedures that are followed in the distribution of the questionnaires, on-site or mailed.

Whenever possible, use a questionnaire that is scientifically valid and reliable. One such instrument is the Hinshaw and Atwood Patient Satisfaction Instrument (Hinshaw and Atwood, 1982). *Validity* indicates that the instrument is indeed measuring what it is supposed to be measuring; *reliability* is a measure of the instrument's consistency, meaning that the results are consistent from one data collection time to the next.

Staff Satisfaction

Measuring and monitoring staff satisfaction carry many of the same issues in interpretation of the data as those presented by the patient satisfaction data. It is difficult to prove a direct correlation between changes in staff satisfaction scores and case management. There are so many variables at play in an organization at any period in time that only relationships may be concluded from any data. Care must be taken in measuring staff satisfaction by using instruments that are valid and reliable whenever possible. If the results are statistically significant, a stronger and more powerful argument can be made between the implementation of the case management model and the changes in staff satisfaction scores.

Staff to be tested should include all those directly affected, such as registered nurses, physicians, social workers, and physical and occupational therapists. Staff should be questioned before implementation of the model and then consistently thereafter in appropriate time periods that will reflect change over time. Generally a minimum of every 6 months or once annually is sufficient. Unfortunately, during these longer time periods, staff may leave their positions and ones may be added. Matching samples over a long time period will be difficult to maintain due to attrition.

Turn-Around Time for Tests, Treatments, and Procedures

Turn-around time can be used as a measure of the organization's process improvement after the introduction of case management. Facilitating care and managing the patient through the health care system should improve the turn-around time for completion of tests. The turn-around time should be measured from the time the physician places the order until the order is completed and results are recorded in the medical record. Acceptable time frames should be decided in advance. For example, the completion time for CAT scans may be 24 hours from the time the order is written until the results of the CAT scan are placed in the medical record.

Monitoring of these time periods can be done concurrently or retrospectively through the medical record. Concurrent data collection is always preferred, because it is both more accurate and more timely. If any problems or delays are identified, they can be addressed immediately. Retrospective data collection, on the other hand, may be more difficult because of lapses in documentation in the patient's medical record or simply the inability to obtain the necessary information. In addition, when problems are finally identified, it is rather late to try to resolve them.

Finally, relationships should be shown between the reduction in turn-around time and the length of stay. As before, it may be difficult to prove sound relationships between length of stay reductions and turn-around time, because many other factors may have an effect on the length of stay.

Cost of Care

Clinical cost accounting methods are being used more and more as a means of understanding not only hospital charges but also the true costs of care. This information can be used to negotiate realistic and appropriate managed care contracts, because the hospital understands exactly what costs are associated with the care of a specific population of patients. Cost accounting can also be used as a way of measuring the financial impact of case management on the organization. Although understanding that reduction in length of stay of a particular patient population is clearly important, it is also important to determine the amount of resources con-

---

TABLE 11-2

Example of Physicians' Cost-Per-Case Comparisons for DRG 89: Simple Pneumonia and Pleurisy, Age Over 17 With Complications and Comorbidities

Physicians	Number of patients	Average length of stay	Cost per case
A	55	6.5	$9280.56
B	50	4.5	$6985.44
C	34	7.0	$9986.53
D	30	7.0	$9895.32
E	25	6.9	$9643.50
F	18	5.8	$7856.64

---

sumed in the management of that population. Reducing the length of stay but consuming the same amount of resources should be avoided. This will not have the same long-term benefits of shortening the length of stay but also reducing the amount of resources used in the care of that case type of patient (Cohen, 1991).

The two main goals of clinical cost accounting are first to identify the hospital's standard use of materials for a particular **diagnosis-related group (DRG)** and then to define the standard cost of each clinical service. An understanding of these costs allows the organization to assess its costs relative to the normal reimbursements, such as Medicare, Medicaid, and other payors. This information also provides a frame of reference or benchmark against which the hospital can compare itself relative to competitors. This can be particularly useful during managed care contract negotiations when the hospital wants to make the most competitive bid possible (Schriefer et al, 1996).

Internally, clinical cost accounting helps the hospital measure its internal treatment patterns. This information can be linked to the medical staff to determine which physicians are rendering the most cost-effective care. Allowing the physicians to compare their cost per case with that of their colleagues may provide them with information they can use in the creation of their **case management plans** (see Chapter 7).

In the fictitious example in Table 11-2, Physician C has the greatest length of stay and the highest cost per case compared to other physicians caring for the same type of patients. This report reflects the intensity of Physician C's use of resources such as medications, antibiotics, radiology, blood products, and other related supplies. This information might be used by Physician C and his colleagues to develop standard protocols that address the use of product resources and how it can be reduced or controlled.

Clinical cost accounting can be used by physician department heads or chiefs of service as part of staff education programs. The cost information can be used to help them gain a better understanding of the costs of clinical services and their contribution to those costs. Where differing treatment patterns exist, they can review the patient outcomes and relative costs.

On a managerial level, clinical cost accounting can be used as a component of departmental performance reports, providing administrative staff with financial information related to the efficiency of their departments. Medical staff reports such as that shown in Table 11-2 can provide clinically related information to guide physicians in changing their clinical practice patterns and can provide information to the finance department in terms of the cost vs. volume vs. profit to the organization.

Length of Stay

Length of stay is a broad umbrella term that can be interpreted in various ways to indicate the amount of time allotted to the care, treatment, or recuperation of a case. In the inpatient setting it can be measured by the number of bed days, or the number of days the patient remains in the hospital. In the home care setting it is calculated by the number of visits to the home. In the emergency department the length of stay may be measured in hours or parts of an hour (15 minutes). Length of stay statistics are most commonly used in the hospital setting. They are often used as an indicator of the success of case management in conjunction with or in the absence of a cost accounting system.

To determine success or failure of case management and its effect on length of stay, hospitals must have a clear understanding of what their length of stay goals are and compare those with the current length of stay statistics in the organization. Comparisons can be made between the hospital and a variety of benchmarks. The first should be the Medicare and nonMedicare DRG average lengths of stay. Although DRGs are not the primary reimbursement system in every state, they are still used for analytical purposes. It is important to understand the history for the organization so that realistic length of stay reduction goals can be set. The hospital should also benchmark against comparable hospitals. These may or may not be close geographically.

Interdepartmental and Interdisciplinary Communication

Measuring changes in communication may be difficult to do. The best way to capture such changes is through anecdotal comments from the team members affected by implementation of the case management model. Try to capture these comments before implementation and then at designated periods of time after implementa-

tion. It is suggested that this be done in the form of focused groups. Questions asked should focus on the team's ability to communicate in a timely fashion, the level of respect afforded them by other team members, and their sense of team spirit or *esprit-de-corps*. In addition, patient care–related questions should also be asked, such as the staff's perceptions of the effectiveness of case management on patient care delivery and efficiency, cost, quality, and so on. Ask them to identify any barriers to communication, as well as ideas for resolving those barriers.

OUTCOMES RELATED TO PATIENT HEALTH

Each time a clinical intervention is applied in health care, there is an associated expected outcome (Box 11-2). Case management provides the structure for identifying those outcomes prospectively. Clinical outcomes should be interdisciplinary and come as a result of the collective efforts of the entire clinical team.

Avoid Adverse Effects of Care

The hospital environment can be a dangerous place, and one goal of care is always to get the patient in and out of the hospital without doing any harm. Many of the quality indicators traditionally used in health care have focused on errors or problems related with the way care was provided. These have included falls, nosocomial infections, medication errors, returns to the operating room, readmissions, morbidity and mortality reports, and deaths. These indicators are focused on the negative, untoward effects of the care provided to the patient and less on the identification of areas for clinical improvement that appear as patterns. Nevertheless, it is important to continue to track these untoward outcomes after implementation of the case management model.

Improve the Patient's Physiological Status

The next set of indicators is concerned with the patient's clinical response to treatment. A goal of care

---

box 11-2

Expected Outcomes Directly Related to the Patient's Health

1. Avoid adverse effects of care
2. Improve the patient's physiological status
3. Reduce signs and symptoms of illness
4. Improve functional status and well-being

is for the patient to be discharged in a better clinical condition than at the time of admission. One measure of this is the patient's physiological status, which refers to the functioning of the various parts of the patient's organs and other body parts. The physiological status can be measured by such things as vital signs, laboratory values, and physical assessment. It is anticipated that these measures will improve between the time of admission and the time of discharge.

The patient's physical abilities are assessed through a thorough review of the major body systems. These include the cardiovascular, respiratory, gastrointestinal, genitourinary, neurological, musculoskeletal, and integumentary systems.

Improve Signs and Symptoms

Signs and symptoms are the first stage of illness. In this stage three things generally occur: (1) the physical experience of symptoms such as pain, shortness of breath, or fever; (2) a cognitive awareness of the symptoms and a placing of meaning on them; (3) emotional response to this awareness in the form of fear or anxiety (Ignatavicius and Bayne, 1991). At this point the person may self-treat or seek a medical opinion. In either case it is anticipated that the signs and symptoms will be reduced or eliminated. If this occurs, the patient returns to the optimal level of wellness.

It is therefore anticipated that after the clinical interventions of the case management team, the patient's signs and symptoms will be improved.

Improve Functional Status and Well-Being

Functional status and well-being address the patient's ability to perform in a variety of areas. These areas include physical health, quality of self-maintenance, quality of role activity, intellectual status, attitude toward the world and sense of well-being related to self, and emotional status. Functional ability refers to the patient's ability to perform activities of daily living (ADLs). ADLs include an assessment of the patient's ability to perform personal care, ability to communicate, and perception of needs (Ignatavicius and Bayne, 1991).

There are a variety of tools to measure functional status. Among these is the commonly used Functional Independence Measure (FIM), developed by Granger and Gresham (1984). The FIM helps to quantify what the patient actually can do, regardless of the clinical diagnosis. Assessment categories include self-care, sphincter control, mobility and locomotion, communication, and social cognition. The FIM helps care providers measure the level of dependence/independence of their patients in an effort to decide what kind of help they may need after discharge to the community.

CLINICAL OUTCOMES

When developing clinical outcomes, the previously discussed categories should all be considered. Some will be more relevant to the clinical picture than others. One approach for monitoring the expected clinical outcomes is through the identification of intermediate and **discharge outcomes.** These should be specific to the clinical issue at hand. **Intermediate outcomes** are those expected goals that occur during the course of the hospital stay. Achievement of the goal or outcome should be based on the patient's expected response to treatment. These expected outcomes can occur at any point in the hospital stay and usually trigger the move to the next phase of treatment.

Discharge indicators are those expected outcomes that the patient must achieve to be discharged from the hospital. The intermediate and discharge outcomes should be the basis for the case management tools. The expected outcomes must be identified before the clinical course of events can be determined. Determination of the expected outcomes should be based on an assessment of both the appropriateness of the care (a determination of who should receive what care) and the effectiveness of care (how good the outcomes of the care are). This review of the evidence will help to relate the process of care to the expected outcomes. This review should be based on all the available evidence rather than solely on the **consensus** of opinion of the practitioners involved in its development (Crosson, 1995). Physicians, when presented with the factual and scientific evidence behind the case management tool or guideline, will be more likely to favor it and use it to guide their practice.

EXAMPLES OF OUTCOMES

The following examples (Boxes 11-3, 11-4, and 11-5) of expected outcomes are presented to help understand the differences and the relationships between intermediate and discharge clinical outcomes. Each example does not include an exhaustive list of the outcomes related to diagnosis or procedure under which they are listed. The expected clinical outcomes are usually decided on by members of the interdisciplinary team working on developing the particular case management plan. They are finalized after a thorough discussion of their implications on the care of the patient, the length of stay, cost, and quality. They are always

---

box 11-3

Inpatient Management of Mastectomy Patients

INTERMEDIATE OUTCOMES

1. Ambulation: Ambulate when fully awake
2. Encourage ambulation within 2 hours of surgery
3. Encourage regular diet when patient is able to tolerate solids
4. Change/switch pain medication(s) to oral if pain scores are 5 or less for 24 hours

DISCHARGE OUTCOMES

Patient may be discharged as soon as the following criteria have been met:

1. Proper functioning of drains
2. Site is free of signs of hemorrhage and infection
3. Pain is controlled with oral analgesics
4. Patient demonstrates ability to care for drains, or home care is arranged for follow-up
5. Able to ambulate independently

---

box 11-4

Lower GI Surgery

INTERMEDIATE OUTCOMES

1. Ambulation: Out of bed and walking with assistance within 12 hours of surgery
2. Gastric decompression: Nasogastric tubes to be removed 24 to 36 hours postop for drainage under 250 cc or less than 100 cc residual; gastrostomy to be clamped using the same criteria
3. Diet: Begin clear liquids 24 to 36 hours after removal of nasogastric tube or clamping of gastrostomy; advance to full liquid diet the same day; begin with full liquid diet and advance to regular diet on the following day

---

box 11-5

Uncomplicated Myocardial Infarction

INTERMEDIATE OUTCOMES

1. Intravenous nitroglycerin: Taper/convert to oral or topical beginning on second day
2. Supplemental oxygen: Discontinue once patient is hemodynamically stable (usually begins on day 3)
3. Ambulate on day 3 or when free of chest pain and shortness of breath

DISCHARGE OUTCOMES

1. Absence of chest pain and signs of ischemia (should occur within 48 to 72 hours)
2. Resolution of ischemic ECG changes
3. Cardiac enzymes returning to baseline
4. Medications converted to oral/topical
5. Activity progressed to preadmission level
6. Patient/family verbalizes understanding of:
   a. Signs and symptoms of heart attack
   b. Risk factors for heart disease
   c. Medications
   d. Diet restrictions
   e. Cessation of smoking (if indicated)
   f. Activity balanced with rest

---

included as an integral part of the case management plan.

PATIENT CARE VARIANCES

Variance occurs when what is supposed to happen does not take place. It is defined as a deviation from a standard or omission of an activity or a step from a predetermined plan, norm, rate, goal, or threshold (Strassner, 1996). Generally, variances are expectations that are not met. According to *Webster's Third New International Dictionary* (1986), variance is defined as "the fact, quality, or state of being variable or variant, . . . a difference of what has been expected or predetermined and what actually occurs." In relation to patient care, variances are outcomes or health care providers' actions that do not meet the desired expectations. In relation to case management, variances are deviations from the recommended activities in any of the care elements delineated in the case management plan (Cohen and Cesta, 1997; Ignatavicius and Hausman, 1995; Pearson, Goulart-Fisher, and Lee, 1995; Tahan and Cesta, 1995). Variances often result from delays, interruptions, additions, or omissions of patient care activities and processes. They may sometimes be related to expediting patient care (e.g., performing a patient care activity before it is due is considered a variance).

In an era of increased competition in health care, case management plans have emerged as the most desirable tools for improving patient care quality through the elimination and/or prevention of variances, reduction in duplication and fragmentation of care elements, and the standardization of patient care activities. When followed appropriately, case management plans result in consistency in practice patterns of physicians, nurses, and other health care professionals and thus reduce variations in patient care. With this comes the significance of patient care variance data collection and analysis, which are integral elements of case management. Variance data collection cannot occur until the expected outcomes of care, as they relate to the case management plan, have been identified. These expected outcomes become the benchmark against which variation in patient care can be determined.

Variance data collection is important because it pro-

---

box 11-6

Examples of Patient- and Family-Related Variances

PATIENT-RELATED VARIANCES

1. Refuses tests/treatments/procedures
2. Unable to decide on treatment
3. Feels unready for discharge
4. Refuses discharge
5. Noncompliance with medical/surgical regimen, medications, treatments
6. Medical status change/complications
7. Postoperative complications
8. Unable to wean from ventilator
9. Secondary diagnosis with admission (e.g., hospitalized for asthma and diabetes)
10. Language barrier
11. Reaction to medications/allergy
12. Reaction to blood transfusion
13. Poor historian
14. Withholding pertinent information
15. Sign out against medical advice (AMA)
16. Refusing discharge because of religious beliefs, holiday, or inconvenience
17. Noncompliant with diet restrictions
18. Unable to self-administer medication (e.g., insulin)
19. Unable to learn about disease
20. Inability to care for self after discharge
21. No clothes
22. No keys for apartment/left keys at home
23. Lost glasses while in the taxi; can't see well
24. Lost dentures before admission
25. Lost insurance card
26. Pressure ulcer present on admission

FAMILY-RELATED VARIANCES

1. Unavailable to pick up patient at time of discharge
2. Unable to provide support for care after discharge
3. Language barrier
4. Late to pick up patient on discharge
5. Inadequate level of knowledge regarding patient care
6. Difficulty with compliance
7. Unable to learn
8. Want another opinion
9. Unable to bring patient's clothes until after business hours
10. Cannot be reached
11. Cannot afford buying necessary medical equipment or medications

---

box 11-7

Examples of System Variances

HOSPITAL/INSTITUTION-RELATED (INTERNAL) VARIANCES

1. Unavailable rehabilitation therapy program on weekends
2. Weekend medical coverage delays requiring changes in treatment (e.g., cannot switch intravenous antibiotic to an oral form)
3. Operating room overbooking
4. Cancellation of an operative procedure, test, or treatment
5. Unavailable messenger/transport services
6. Machine breakdown
7. Shortage of supplies
8. Laboratory errors/delays
9. Lost requisitions for tests or procedures or treatments
10. Pending infectious disease approval of medications
11. Nonformulary medications
12. Pending results: radiology, pathology
13. Conflict in scheduling tests, treatments, procedures
14. Not enough personnel to perform tests/procedures
15. Prolonged turn-around time for tests/procedures
16. Prolonged turn-around time for referrals, consults
17. Unavailable beds in the intensive care unit
18. Unavailable beds for emergency admissions
19. Specialty patients diverted to nonspecialty beds
20. Hospital-acquired pressure ulcer
21. Hospital-acquired infection (nosocomial)
22. No pneumatic tube/carrier available

COMMUNITY-RELATED (EXTERNAL) VARIANCES

1. No nursing home bed available
2. Transfer to another institution
3. Delayed ambulette transportation
4. No home care available over the weekend
5. Inappropriate transfer from another facility
6. No bed available in a rehabilitation facility
7. Child protective services are late to come
8. Company delivered medical equipment late
9. Managed care company disapproves home care services
10. Managed care company did not certify patient's admission to the hospital
11. Managed care company did not certify an extension in hospitalization (increased days)

---

vides the basis for improvements in patient care activities, processes, outcomes, and quality. The mechanism of variance data collection is usually decided on by the steering committee charged with implementing the case management model and the use of case management plans. Some institutions have delegated this responsibility to a case management department or a quality improvement committee/council. Regardless of who is responsible, the process should be made consistent across the various care settings that exist in the same institution.

There is no standardization in the method of classifying variances. Variances are classified into different categories in different institutions. Traditionally the most common broad categories used to classify variances are patient/family (Box 11-6), system (Box 11-7), and practitioner (Box 11-8). Patient/family variances are the result of the patient's behavior or activity or the behavior/activity of a family member (family is used here

---

box 11-8

Examples of Practitioner Variances

1. Delay in communicating the plan of care
2. Miscommunication between interdisciplinary team members
3. Physician not communicating to the patient
4. Physician not communicating to the family
5. Medication error
6. Wrong test, treatment, procedure ordered
7. Incomplete documentation
8. Incomplete admission assessment/history
9. Omission of an order
10. Delayed request for a consultant
11. Delayed response by a consultant
12. No consent obtained for treatment
13. Delay in processing forms
14. Delay in initiating treatment, plan of care
15. Lack of coordination of discharge plan among the interdisciplinary team members
16. Inappropriate use of medical equipment
17. Patient teaching not done/completed
18. Delay in scheduling tests
19. Inappropriate/early discharge
20. Nurse busy with other patients
21. Failure to or delay in obtaining preapproval for treatments/interventions or community services
22. Physician did not prepare/inform patient of discharge
23. Failure to conduct financial screening

---

in its generic sense to denote a patient's spouse, caregiver, significant other, or family member). Variances may be refusal of treatments, or they may occur as a result of changes in the patient's condition or complications of a medical or surgical procedure (e.g., refusal to sign a consent for an operative procedure, infection, fluid and electrolyte imbalance, or family unavailable to accompany the patient home on discharge). Some institutions separate patient variances from the family-related ones. They may classify changes in the patient's condition as they result from the disease process under a separate category (e.g., physiological). The family-related variances may be classified into a separate category and labeled as "community" variances.

Practitioner variances occur due to behaviors of health care providers. Examples of practitioner variance are omission of a treatment, test, or procedure; giving the wrong medication; incomplete follow-up and documentation of the patient's response to treatments; or a visiting nurse not showing up for a prescheduled home visit. These variances represent the areas that health care providers may have the most control over, and if prevented they can influence positive patient care out-

comes, lead to timely discharge, eliminate unnecessary work, and reduce cost.

System variances are those related to the way an institution operates, and they result in delays in patient care processes. They usually occur because of inefficient operations and systems, and they may be called *operational* variances. Mostly these variances require administrative attention or intervention for resolution. System variances can also be classified as *internal* (i.e., within the walls of the health care facility [institution based]) or *external* (i.e., outside the walls of the health care facility [community based]). Examples of system variances are lost laboratory requisition slips or specimen, failure of an infusion pump, no nursing home bed available, payment denial, or managed care organization not approving certain patient care services.

Variances are also classified as *positive* or *negative* (Bueno and Hwang, 1993; Hampton, 1993; Ignatavicius and Hausman, 1995; Mateo and Newton, 1996; Tahan and Cesta, 1995). A *positive variance* is defined as a desired outcome that occurs before it is expected (i.e., before the time frame that is indicated/projected in the case management plan). It is also a justified type of variance. An example of positive variance is switching a recommended antibiotic to a different one because of a patient's allergy; changing the diet of a cardiac patient, who is admitted for the management of heart failure, from the salt- and fat-restricted diet recommended in the case management plan to include diabetic restrictions because the patient is also diabetic; or a patient's early discharge because all the outcomes are met earlier than expected.

A *negative variance* occurs when a patient care activity is delayed and the patient does not meet the expected/desired outcomes (i.e., the recommended patient care activities in the case management plan are not achieved within the specified time frames). For example, a patient was on anticoagulation therapy and required prothrombin time (PT) testing every 6 hours on the initial day of treatment. He was due for a PT test at 12:00 noon, but the test was not completed until 4:00 PM. The result could not be retrieved from the laboratory information (automated) system until 5:30 PM. The result of the PT was found to be very high, and the patient required an immediate intervention, putting the anticoagulation therapy on hold temporarily. In this example, a delay in performing the prescheduled PT test was identified as a practitioner variance. This variance resulted in a delay in changing the anticoagulation therapy/plan of care, and the patient was required to stay an extra day in the hospital.

Another variance category is an *add-on variance*. It is

defined as an unplanned or extra patient care activity or process. Usually this type of variance occurs as an addition to what is indicated in the case management plan. An example of such variance is added laboratory tests. An add-on patient care activity is considered a variance because it may contribute to an increase in cost or a delay in discharge. Most often this type of variance results in duplication of services or performance of unnecessary patient care activities.

Because there is no standardization in classifying variances, it is difficult to share variances across care settings or institutions for the purpose of benchmarking. It is even more difficult to conduct a joint trending analysis of variance data from several health care institutions located in a particular community, an analysis that could sometimes be important for improving health care in a whole community rather than a particular hospital population. To avoid this, Hoffman (1993) recommends that the standardized critical elements of patient care included in case management plans be used as the classification system for variances (e.g., assessment and monitoring, treatments, medications, patient/family education, discharge planning). If this classification system is followed, then data become transferrable within and across institutions, which is highly beneficial for improving the quality of patient care.

VARIANCE DATA COLLECTION AND ANALYSIS

Designing an effective method for documenting, collecting, and analyzing variances remains a great challenge for most health care institutions. Whether the process of variance data collection is automated or manual, most institutions have made the nurse case manager the one responsible for collecting variances. Variance data could be collected any time during the patient's hospitalization. The best time, however, is at the time it happens or when it is identified. Timely identification and resolution of variances result in the delivery of cost-effective and high-quality care and increase patient/family satisfaction. A variety of sources for variance identification can be used, such as the progress notes of physicians, nurses, and other health care professionals; verbal communication with other members of the interdisciplinary care team during case conference or one-on-one; or communication with other departments.

Deciding the extent to which variance data should be collected is extremely difficult to generalize and varies from institution to institution. How to collect data and what is needed should be prospectively determined. Some institutions collect data at random or as they relate to every single patient care activity without consid-

---

| box 11-9 |

Guiding Questions to Better Decision Making Regarding Variance Data Collection

1. What are the most important patient care elements/ activities that should be monitored?
2. In what format should variance data be collected?
3. Should both intermediate and discharge outcome indicators be monitored?
4. Should any type of variances be collected or only those that affect the quality of care and length of stay?
5. How easy is it to collect the suggested variance data?
6. How accessible are the desired variance data?
7. Where are the variance data located?
8. How can variance data be identified?
9. Who is responsible for variance data collection? Analysis? Reporting?
10. How will the data collected be used?
11. How will the data collected be interphased with the existing quality improvement efforts, if any?
12. What is the benefit of the variance data collected in revising the case management plan?

---

ering their impact on the length of stay and quality of care. In such situations, data might become overwhelming and unmanageable. Because of the volume, collected data can be difficult to analyze, trend, or use to efficiently generate reports that can be used for quality improvement. It is recommended that the interdisciplinary team developing the case management plan spend some time defining the significant patient care activities that need to be evaluated for variance data collection. A decision as to what should be included should be individualized to the specific diagnosis or procedure of the case management plan. In addition, variance data collection should be limited to those that affect the predetermined outcomes of each case management plan. The steering committee overseeing the process of implementing case management systems and developing case management plans is the best group to guide the interdisciplinary teams in this process. A set of questions (Box 11-9) can be used by the interdisciplinary team members as a guiding tool for better decision making when faced with the dilemma of what variance data should be collected.

Variances must be identified and corrected as soon as possible for better-quality patient care outcomes and prevention of unnecessary delays in the patient's discharge or prolongation in the length of stay. Regardless of who is made responsible for variance data collection, there should be the following:

• Concurrent medical record reviews
• Immediate communication of any delays in pa-

tient care to the appropriate people (e.g., physicians, department chiefs, nurse case managers, nurse managers, interdisciplinary team members)

- Immediate attempts to resolve the situation causing the variance
- Prospective plans for what, how, and when variance data should be collected

If the primary nurses are given the responsibility of collecting patient care variances, then they, rather than the nurse case manager, are responsible for responding to the identified variance. However, the ideal way of correcting variances is for the interdisciplinary team member who has identified the variance to immediately begin to try to correct or resolve it. This approach will then result in the most timely results and should help to avoid delays in the length of stay or deterioration of quality. Members of the interdisciplinary health care team should be made aware of their responsibilities toward variance data collection and resolution. Open lines of communication should be established to promote effective and timely communication of variances to the appropriate administrative personnel, particularly when direct care providers such as staff nurses are made responsible for identifying and resolving variances as they occur.

Strategies for Handling Variances

When a patient care variance is identified, certain questions should be answered immediately to resolve the situation and improve outcomes. The answers to these questions will determine the urgency and seriousness of the situation and indicate the corrective action plan. The questions appear in Case Manager's Tip 11-1.

After careful collection of variance data, the data are analyzed. The variance analysis process (Figure 11-1) is a systematic and scientific interpretation of the data collected, through categorization/grouping, trending, and statistical analysis. Variance data are usually compiled and analyzed over time to allow for better opportunities for quality and patient care process improvement. The ideal way of dealing with variance data is to link the process to the quality improvement efforts taking place in the institution. Evaluating variances and constructing and implementing an appropriate action plan for improvement ensure better patient care outcomes and prevent the situation from happening again.

Improvement efforts should be spent on addressing the recurring variances rather than the isolated, random, or single events, because better patient care outcomes are affected by the extent to which the recurring variances are eliminated or prevented. The isolated variances are known to happen due to special causes (i.e., not directly related to the systems, operations, or processes an institution has in place). However, recurring variances are the opposite of isolated variances and take place as a result of common causes. These variances require an evaluation and analysis of the systems and processes of patient care the institution follows, as well as the policies and procedures and in some cases the standards of care and practice. It is suggested that efforts to address the isolated variances be decided based on the individual situation, particularly if these events interfere in the length of stay, patient/family satisfaction, and cost and quality of care.

It is not enough to identify and resolve a variance when it occurs. It is equally important to track variances. The purpose of tracking variance is to conduct a trend-

case manager's tip 11-1

Questions to Help in Handling Variances and Improving Outcomes

1. What is really happening?
2. Is the situation indicative of a variance?
3. How serious is it?
4. What is causing the variance?
5. What is the effect of the variance on the patient's condition?
6. What is the category of the variance?
7. What action must be taken to correct it?
8. Who should be involved in correcting the variance?
9. How urgently should it be corrected?
10. What should be shared with the patient and the family?
11. When should follow-up take place?
12. What should be documented in the medical record?
13. What should be documented on the variance tracking tool?

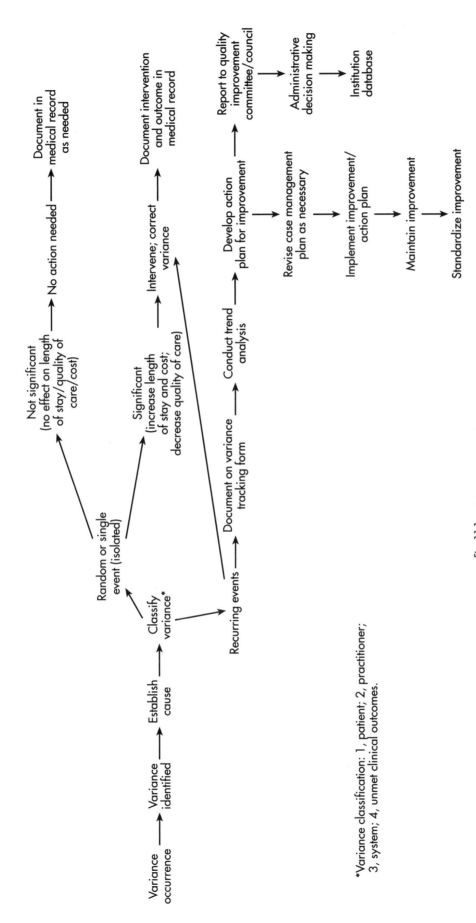

Fig. 11-1   The variance analysis process.

case manager's tip

11-2

Strategies for Making Variance Data Reporting Easy

1. If an institution decides to report variance data by source, it is useful to determine these sources (e.g., patient/family, care provider/practitioner, system), standardize them across the various care settings, and include them in the variance tracking tool. It is also helpful to include subcategories for each source. In addition, designating a code for each source and subcategory makes it easier to track, document, collate, analyze, and trend variances.

2. If an institution decides to report variance data by patient care elements applied in the case management plan (e.g., assessment and monitoring, tests and procedures, activity, medications, treatments, nutrition, patient/family teaching), it is important to determine how variances will be tracked and documented in the variance tracking tool. It is not enough to document variances as they relate to patient care elements only. Based on this method, one will only be able to report the frequency (number of occurrences) of variances in each care element. Another clarifying classification should be used in conjunction with this method. One example is the use of positive and negative classification. This way the data could be analyzed in relation to its impact on patient care processes and outcomes.

3. During the process of variance data analysis, some questions may occur that cannot be answered based solely on the data included in the variance tracking tools. In this situation, a review of medical records is suggested. The review should be conducted carefully and in a way that will answer the questions raised.

4. As much as possible, variance tracking tools should include specific places to identify the type (diagnosis, procedure) of the case management plan and the physician in charge of the care of the patient. This information is important for data analysis. It helps in analyzing the data specific to a case management plan and in identifying the physicians with minimal compliance with the plan.

5. Variance data reports should include data on the effectiveness of the case management plans, practice patterns (i.e., how well and how often the case management plan is followed by care providers), and recommendations for improvement opportunities.

6. Making recommendations for improvement opportunities may be made mandatory in each report. Areas to be addressed when recommending improvements may include the processes of care (e.g., improving the promptness of consults, developing patient education materials to be used in patient/family teaching); revisions in the case management plan (e.g., revising a time frame for an outcome or an intervention, adding a test); and the systems of the institution (e.g., reducing the turn-around time for an echocardiography).

---

ing analysis of each variance category. The results of such analyses are the basis for revising and improving the case management plan, reducing the incidence of variances in the future, and studying the data for necessity of quality improvement efforts, particularly those that are system/operations related.

Variance data collection and analysis allow health care executives to look beyond length of stay and cost of care. They are ongoing processes that are helpful in continuously improving the systems of the institution, case management plans, patient care activities, processes and outcomes, and quality of care. It is through this process that standardization of the best/ideal approach to patient care can be achieved and maintained.

Establishing variance data collection tools and formalizing/standardizing the process are integral to the accuracy and reliability of the data collected (Case Manager's Tip 11-2). Before the initiation of variance data collection, it is imperative to determine what should be measured and how and when assessment and evaluation of care are conducted. It is not uncommon that a variance tracking tool be developed as a part of the case management plan (Figure 11-2). In this case, the tool is made specific and individualized based on the diagno-

sis or procedure of the case management plan. An institution may elect to use a generic tool (Figure 11-3) that is applicable to any case management plan regardless of the diagnosis or procedure. In both situations, the tool is not made a permanent part of the medical record. It is dealt with as defined in the institutional policy/procedure for variance data collection and analysis.

Providing feedback regarding the effectiveness of case management plans is important. Integral to any strategy for improving patient care is a provision for feedback to the clinicians and administrators who are involved in patient care processes and activities. A formal mechanism for communicating important and appropriate data must be in place in each institution. Reporting variance data should also be done on regular basis with specific time intervals. Variance data reports should be distributed to members of the interdisciplinary team that was involved in the development of the case management plan and to the related administrators for initiating relevant quality improvement projects.

Patient care monitoring and timely variance identification and resolution are keys to the success of case management plans and are crucial for the delivery of cost-effective and quality care. However, establishing a

Long Island College Hospital
Variance Tracking Tool: Adult Inpatient Community Acquired Pneumonia
Please place a check mark (✓) in the appropriate box

☐	Less severe pneumonia
☐	Severe pneumonia

☐	Initial antibiotic therapy did not meet guideline for severity class
☐	_____
	Drug/Dosage

☐	Conversion to oral antibiotic did not occur because of failure to meet:
	☐ Two consecutive oral temperature readings of < 100°F are obtained at least 8 hours apart in the absence of antipyretics
	☐ Decrease in leukocytosis to < 12,000
	☐ Improved pulmonary signs and symptoms
	☐ Able to tolerate oral medications
☐	Orders were not written to switch antibiotic
☐	Other:
	_____

☐	Oral antibiotic conversion did not meet the guideline selection
☐	_____
	Drug/Dosage

☐	Repeat chest x-ray necessary as per guideline
☐	Repeat chest x-ray is NOT necessary as per guideline

☐	Discharge did not occur within 24 hours of conversion to oral antibiotic
☐	Reason documented:
	_____
☐	Reason NOT documented

☐	Length of stay
☐	Readmission within 30 days due to failed outpatient management

Fig. 11-2 A variance tracking tool specific to a case management plan. (Redrawn from Long Island College Hospital, Long Island, NY. Used with permission.)

standardized process for variance data analysis and management remains the best strategy for improving patient care outcomes. In addition, feedback among health care administrators and direct care providers is extremely important in refining the use and the effectiveness of case management plans.

KEY POINTS

1. Outcomes can be used as indicators of quality.
2. Outcomes can be defined as the goals of health care delivery and can be directly or indirectly related to the patient's health.
3. Length of stay is an indicator of the success of a case management model and is often tracked to determine its effectiveness.
4. Clinical outcome indicators give the case manager a guide for progressing the patient from day to day, episode to episode, or toward discharge.
5. Variance data should be collected using variance tracking tools specific to the institution.
6. Variances should be classified and coded for ease of tracking. The same classifications should be used across the various care settings.
7. Variance data collection may be made the responsibility of the interdisciplinary team members or the nurse case manager only. Each institution may decide which mechanisms to be followed.
8. Variance data should be tracked, collated, analyzed, and evaluated for improvement opportunities.
9. Results of variance data analysis should be tied into a quality improvement system.
10. Reporting variance data and providing feedback to clinicians and administrators are important and integral to case management systems.

MERCY MEDICAL CENTER

Variance Key:
#1—Patient
#2—Process/System
#3—Practitioner
#4—Planning/Discharge

Diagnosis: _____
Date Pathway Initiated: ___/___/___
Date Pathway Completed: ___/___/___
Patient Discharge Date: ___/___/___

Addressograph

DATE	UNIT	TIME	PATHWAY DAY#	VARIANCE DESCRIPTION (SEE KEY)	ACTION TAKEN	SIGNATURE

Fig. 11-3 Generic variance tracking tools. (Redrawn from Mercy Medical Center, Rockville Center, New York. Used with permission.)

MERCY MEDICAL CENTER

A. PATIENT
A1. Patient refusal/noncompliance

A2. Communication barrier
A3. Adverse effects/complications
A4. Comorbidities
A5. Altered mental status
A6. Progression ahead of pathway

B. FAMILY/LIFESTYLE
B1. Noncompliance/unavailability

B2. Environmental barrier
B3. Socioeconomic concerns
B4. Others

C. SYSTEM
C1. Interdisciplinary/transfer issues

C2. Treatment delays
C3. Delayed results reporting
C4. Others

D. CARE GIVER
D1. Physician availability/response time

D2. Physician documentation/orders
D3. Nursing delays
D4. Ancillary delays
D5. Progression ahead of path
D6. Others

HOUSE OFFICER: _____   BEEPER NUMBER: _____

PATIENT NAME: _____   ROOM NUMBER: _____   MEDICAL RECORD NUMBER: _____

DATE OF REVIEW	DAY #	CODE	CRITICAL ELEMENT	VARIANCE EXPLANATION	ACTION IF TAKEN

Fig. 11-3, cont'd.

References

Bueno MM, Hwang RF: Understanding variances in hospital stay, *Nurs Manage* 24(11):51-57, 1993.

Cohen EL: Nursing case management: does it pay? *J Nurs Admin* 21(4):20-25, 1991.

Cohen EL, Cesta TG: *Nursing case management: from concept to evaluation,* ed 2, St Louis, 1997, Mosby.

Crosson FJ: Why outcomes measurement must be the basis for the development of clinical guidelines, *Managed Care Q* 3(2):6-11, 1995.

Granger CV, Gresham GE: *Functional assessment in rehabilitation medicine,* Baltimore, 1984, Williams & Wilkins.

Hampton DC: Implementing a managed care framework through care maps, *J Nurs Admin* 23(5):21-27, 1993.

Hinshaw A, Atwood J: A patient satisfaction instrument: precision by replication, *Nurs Res* 31(1):170-175, 1982.

Hoffman PA: Critical path method: an important tool for coordinating clinical care, *Joint Comm J Qual Improve* 19:235-246, 1993.

Ignatavicius DD, Bayne MV: *Medical-surgical nursing: a nursing process approach,* Philadelphia, 1991, WB Saunders.

Ignatavicius DD, Hausman KA: *Clinical pathways for collaborative practice,* Philadelphia, 1995, Saunders.

Mateo MA, Newton C: Managing variances in case management, *Nurs Case Manage* 1(1):45-51, 1996.

Pearson SD, Goulart-Fisher D, Lee TH: Critical pathways as a strategy for improving care: problems and potential, *Ann Intern Med* 123(12):941-948, 1995.

Schriefer J et al: Linking process improvement, critical paths, and outcomes data to increased profitability, *Surg Serv Manage* 2(6):46-50, 1996.

Strassner LF: The ABCs of case management: a review of the basics, *Nurs Case Manage* 1(1):22-30, 1996.

Tahan HA, Cesta TG: Evaluating the effectiveness of case management plans, *J Nurs Admin* 25(9):58-63, 1995.

Webster's third new international dictionary, vol III, Chicago, 1986, Encyclopedia Britannica, Inc.-

CHAPTER 12

LINKING JCAHO TO CASE MANAGEMENT

MARGUERITE WARD, MS, BSN, RN

OVERVIEW OF THE JCAHO STANDARDS

The Joint Commission on Accreditation of Healthcare Organizations (JCAHO) is a private enterprise that sets industry standards for health care. These standards are based on current acceptable practice within health care with direction toward future industry objectives. The JCAHO is comprehensive in its approach to institutional quality assessment and bases its requirements on extensively researched material. It is a regulatory agency in its establishment of standards, but it holds no direct authority over institutions. A JCAHO accreditation of an institution means recognition to reimbursement intermediaries, consumers, and the health care industry that acceptable quality standards are maintained and quality patient care is delivered.

The JCAHO conducts nation-wide assessments of many types of facilities, (e.g., acute care, long-term care, ambulatory care, home care, subacute care, and mental health care), pointing to a comprehensive approach in evaluating a national standard for review. Each survey incorporates specialty requirements into the overall JCAHO standards to enable the most complete review of a specific health care facility.

The JCAHO approaches its review with a focus on outcomes. These are measured and evaluated in the following three specific areas:
- Individual: patient/practitioner
- Structure: facility/environment
- Process: delivery of service/systems

The intent is to broadly assess the overall institutional performance in meeting quality standards. By weaving its review throughout the many facets of the facility, the JCAHO takes the opportunity to survey if and how well the institution manages itself.

The JCAHO has centered itself around the measurement of quality in a facility. It has defined for health care appropriate indications of quality by establishing standards reflective of the best-possible practice and providing guidelines to indicate the acceptable compliance measures.

The JCAHO standards require an organization to assess and evaluate its performance on all levels. This begins with the organization's vision and structure; it encompasses its actual day-to-day operations and departmental roles. It continues with communication at and between all levels, with careful examination of adequate and planned use of resources and the inspection of the general plant facilities.

The JCAHO has organized its standards into two broad categories and a third section dealing with specific health care components. There are eleven standards and four structures with functions within these three categories, as outlined in Box 12-1.

Patient-Focused Standards

The JCAHO's patient-focused standards are grouped to reflect the appropriate care and treatment phases for the patient rather than the caregiver. The standards cross all departments or divisions. The standards are judged to be met when information is obtained and shared by and with other disciplines and appropriate actions are taken based on the data collected.

The JCAHO urges caregivers to reduce the amount of duplication currently present within the health care system. In an effort to promote both efficient use of resources (staff and time) and customer satisfaction, they encourage the use of interdisciplinary communication and documentation tools. What is most important is that accurate, validated data be used to plan and evaluate care. Collection may be delegated to the most appropriate caregivers and used by other disciplines once validated (Case Manager's Tip 12-1).

The patient-focused standards guide the patient through an episode of illness back to the most appropriate care setting. The intent is to efficiently move the patient through the system while meeting the needs of the patient, family, and significant other. Past ideas of only seeing the patient through an episode of illness are gone. The industry has recognized the need to employ a comprehensive approach to care and treat-

case manager's tip	**12-1**	**Promoting Efficient Resource Use and Customer Satisfaction**

JCAHO encourages the use of interdisciplinary communication and documentation tools. What is most important is that accurate, validated data be used to plan and evaluate care. Once data are validated, collection may be delegated to the most appropriate caregivers and used by other disciplines.

---

box 12-1

JCAHO Standards and Functions

STANDARDS

Patient Focused

1. Patient rights and organization ethics
2. Assessment of patients
3. Care of patients
4. Education
5. Continuum of care

Organization Functions

1. Improving organization performance
2. Leadership
3. Management of the environment of care
4. Management of human resources
5. Management of information
6. Surveillance, prevention, and control of infection

STRUCTURES WITH FUNCTIONS

1. Governance
2. Management
3. Medical staff
4. Nursing

Joint Commission on Accreditation of Healthcare Organizations: *1996 comprehensive accreditation manual for hospitals*, Oakbrook Terrace, Ill, 1995, JCAHO.

---

ment. The introduction of cost containment by reimbursement parties with payment denials has cautioned the industry to plan appropriately and well but within reason.

Cognizant of these trends, the JCAHO recommends developing an efficient, effective treatment plan for the patient/family/significant other across the continuum of care. Point of entry into the health care system, whether hospital, primary care center, or physician office, is the point of initiation for discharge planning and return to the most appropriate care setting. Fundamental in this approach is strong, timely communication of information between and among the various entry points. Meeting the patient-focused JCAHO standards means putting the patient in the center and allowing the established institutional processes and systems to flow around the patient. The patient should experience hospitalization or an episode of illness in the most seamless way possible. Hospital rules and procedures should smoothly facilitate this flow. Return to the community care setting should be timely and well planned. Education and medical follow-up care to ensure the patient's ability to manage needed life-style adjustments should be outlined and appropriate. Necessary considerations for the diversity of the patient, family, and significant other must be addressed. Each patient must be allowed to participate in planning care and treatments and in addressing specific needs. These include cultural, ethnic, and spiritual considerations.

Organization Functions

The JCAHO patient-focused standards do place the patient at the heart of the delivery of services. They clearly delineate the need to adopt a holistic approach in providing care and meeting institutional objectives. In the next group of standards, "organization functions," the JCAHO (1995) establishes requirements to ensure that the facility adheres to the following:

- Designs efficient processes/systems
- Examines practice in an organized, planned, ongoing manner
- Identifies opportunities for improvements
- Implements cost-effective measures to ensure smooth operations
- Establishes job requirements and measurable criteria for staff performance
- Maintains a safe, clean, and appropriate environment for all: patient, employee, and visitor
- Develops effective methods to facilitate the communication of information

This second group of standards focuses on the institution's development of working relationships and systems that allow it to place the patient at the center. The intent in the measurement of these six standards is to see strong interdisciplinary teams that are knowledgeable of their individual departmental requirements and those institutional objectives that guide the operation of the facility, always with the patient at the center of the team.

Structures With Functions

The last set of standards governs "structures with functions." These four areas, governance, management, medical staff, and nursing, set the tone for the direction, guidance, and operation of the facility. The JCAHO (1995) requires the organization to clearly define the following:

- The mission, vision, and ethical code of operations
- The scope of services provided and the type of populations served
- The requirements of the practitioners and leaders of the facility, including education, experience, and clinical privileges
- The involvement of each leader in planning future services of the facility and developing operating budgets
- The relationship of the governing board in strategic planning, day-to-day operations, and the flow of information within the organization

It is easy to see how the JCAHO has focused and developed its own action plan in guiding organizations toward quality endeavors. It presents the standards manual in order of importance in the same way:

1. Patient-focused standards
↓
2. Organization functions
↓
3. Structures with functions

CONTINUOUS SELF-EVALUATION AND IMPROVEMENT

In addition to defining the quality standards, JCAHO has set an expectation for the organization to continuously evaluate itself and implement measures to improve the delivery of services. It has outlined a 10-step approach that may be used in developing quality review programs (Box 12-2). This process is the basis for defining and examining what an individual department/service does. It asks that each component be examined and defined in relation to the type and amount of services provided, the type of customers served, and the most important pieces of the services delivered. Once the components of service have been outlined, consideration can then be given to assessing and establishing expected performance measures.

Moving through the process, data are gathered, displayed, and analyzed to determine if performance is satisfactory or needs improvement. If improvement is warranted, a plan is developed, implemented, and measured for success. All this work is then shared within the facility/department to document improvement strides.

---

box 12-2

JCAHO 10-Step Process

1. Assign responsibility.
2. Delineate scope of care and service.
3. Identify important aspects of care.
4. Identify indicators.
5. Establish thresholds for evaluation.
6. Collect and organize data.
7. Evaluate data.
8. Take actions to improve care.
9. Assess effectiveness of actions and document improvement.
10. Communicate the results.

Joint Commission on Accreditation of Healthcare Organizations: *1996 comprehensive accreditation manual for hospitals,* Oakbrook Terrace, Ill, 1995, JCAHO.

The JCAHO further asks the organization to examine the many facets or dimensions of performance inherent in "doing the right thing" and "doing the right thing well." These include appropriateness, efficacy, timeliness, availability, effectiveness, continuity, safety, efficiency, and respect and caring (Joint Commission on Accreditation of Healthcare Organizations, 1995).

Finally, it asks that the personnel with the most knowledge and those with the ability to implement changes work together in teams to improve performance and effect better outcomes. Certainly this indicates a most-comprehensive approach to reviewing and determining how well an organization meets quality industry standards.

The JCAHO invests resources in developing standards that are future oriented. They strive to incorporate the very best of current practice while anticipating the needs of tomorrow. They are careful to balance the requirements of the future with the abilities of today. Perhaps the best illustration is in the information management standard. Recognizing the need for organizations to process a large volume of information coupled with the industry trend toward a lifetime medical record, JCAHO developed a quality standard relating to the use of computerization. The objective was to set an industry standard to decrease duplication, facilitate communication, improve the availability of information, encourage the use of comparative databases for benchmarking, and increase customer satisfaction—both patient and practitioner.

During field testing of this standard that incorporated feedback from a wide variety of organizations and practitioners, a harsh reality was discovered. Introducing computerization to a facility was a major financial investment/risk, and many organizations were wary of investing the required capital or could not allocate the needed funds at the time. Listening to all these views, JCAHO revised their requirements.

The information management standard now requires organizations to have a 5-year plan to adopt computerization (Case Manager's Tip 12-2).

This standard is the common thread among all eleven standards and the four structures with functions. At the heart of any organization, group, or team lies the ability to communicate and to share and process information. Examining the requirements to meet this standard awakens a realization that systems, processes, manuals, policies, and medical records are not enough to position the organization to achieve the quality **outcomes** it desires. What is needed is a well-developed cohesive and interactive approach by the organization and its employees toward accomplishing its stated goals, objectives, and mission. Adoption of a model and commitment to that model are the first steps in realizing success. Support and encouragement of the model and education regarding the need for change are the next logical steps. Finally, allowing the change to occur by empowering those individuals who need to make the change with the ability to do so establishes the model as a working concept. Continually evaluating and improving the model maintains its original intent—to improve care and services.

The JCAHO standards direct organizations to consider their primary focus first—the patient, family, and significant other. They proceed with the organizational functions needed to achieve the goal of quality patient care and end with the requirements for knowledgeable, progressive leaders who will demonstrate the ability to encourage and produce change within the organization. However, this is certainly easier to describe than to achieve.

RELATIONSHIP OF CASE MANAGEMENT TO JCAHO STANDARDS

The **case management** model embodies the same principles as the JCAHO standards. It uses the patient-focused care standards as its base and builds on with the addition of the organization functions. It is completed by the commitment and acknowledgment by the structures with functions as to its appropriateness, timeliness, effectiveness, efficiency, continuity, efficacy, availability, safety, and attention to respect and caring. The model complements the intent of the JCAHO standards and introduces a practical working approach to ensuring quality in a cost-conscious environment.

Case management reinforces the commitment to doing the right thing and doing the right thing well. Careful assessment and evaluation of patient needs allow appropriate selection of those patients requiring special attention to move through the system. Determining complexity of needs allows caregivers to tailor plans of care to meet customer, institutional, and regulatory expectations.

Case management focuses on getting the patient, family, and significant other through the system in the most efficient way possible. An expectation of this is to begin the process on entry into the system. By beginning with a careful needs assessment on admission, potential patients needing case management services can be identified. Point of entry may be physician's office, hospitalization, ambulatory care, or managed care enrollment. Taking a proactive approach to identifying care needs allows provisions to be made for a smooth experience through an episode of illness.

Case management, by design, sets expectations for a specified diagnosis or procedure for a specific time frame. It establishes the norm based on industry standards to treat approximately 80 % of those patients with the same diagnosis. By defining the norm and establishing sound care paths with delineated outcomes, efficient

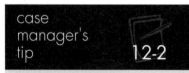

case manager's tip **12-2** **JCAHO's Information Management Standard**

When reviewing the organization's 5-year plan to adopt computerization, the JCAHO (1995) looks to see the following:
1. What has been planned?
2. Who has been involved in the planning?
3. Have financial considerations been addressed?
4. Is the facility positioned to incorporate this major change?
5. Has consideration been given to the use of outside comparative databases?
6. Has education of employees started?
7. What is the facility's vision of computerization?

and appropriate management of patient care is outlined and can thus be measured. Establishing structure allows caregivers to maintain control and prepare the patient for the anticipated experience. It makes provisions to begin postdischarge education early during the hospital stay. Allowing for time to evaluate and reinforce critical instructions ensures sound preparation in returning the patient to the appropriate care setting. The intent of case management is to move the patient through the system (acute care, ambulatory care, or home care) with minimal effort, reduced cost, and maximum efficiency. Well-defined outcomes accomplish the following:

- Provide caregivers an objective determination mark to move the patient to the next level
- Allow objective measures for quality and variance measurement
- Address the overall care needs of the patient while allowing for individualization

The patient remains the focus—the center of case management services. Patient care objectives may include the following:

- The smooth transition of the patient from one phase to the next
- Providing needed care and treatments in a timely, efficient manner
- Appropriate resource utilization: time, staff, supplies, costs, and length of stay
- Appropriate, timely, and safe discharge planning and preparation
- Ensuring that patient, family, and significant other have the right tools (equipment, education) to manage life-style adjustments in the community
- Addressing a holistic approach in planning delivery of care by involving the necessary members of the interdisciplinary team

Looking at the JCAHO standards and the case management objectives, it is apparent how well the use of one satisfies the requirements of the other.

The JCAHO has strongly urged health care organizations to take a hard look at themselves and how they provide services. The overall objective was to outline current processes and systems and assess how well they function. Implicit in the JCAHO intent was to review these functions from the patient's perspective. Organizations were asked to place themselves in the patient's shoes and walk through the process of hospitalization, experiencing it from the consumer's viewpoint. Many hospitals chose to diagram the steps and found many steps had been added over time to meet departmental needs. Often these additions made the process a little longer and more confusing to the patient. A commit-

ment to improving services and the quality of care delivered led organizations to ask the following questions:

- Why are things done this way?
- How can the process be streamlined to eliminate steps and improve efficiency?

Their goal was a smooth transition for the patient from one phase of care to the next, each step along the way. Their goal was improved customer satisfaction, a decrease in duplication of services, timely delivery of appropriate services, improved efficiency, reduced cost, and an improved overall hospital image.

Examining the development of case management, the same principles are seen. A review of current practice outlines the various steps of treatment and care for the patient. Looking at current practice for a diagnosis, outlined by day of stay, allows practitioners to review and decide if services could be scheduled sooner or less frequently. It ensures that practitioners plan needed care efficiently, with attention to cost-effective solutions. It further enables a standard of practice to be developed that addresses care needs in a timely manner. This allows each discipline the time to interact with the patient, family, and significant other and to meet specific outcomes for discharge.

The flow of hospitalization from one phase/day to the next and from one discipline to the other must be seamless to the patient. If the goal of the developed case management model is to place the patient at the center, then the work, care, and treatments must flow around the patient. Using the case management model to facilitate the process of hospitalization maps out a plan for care and services to be delivered to the patient rather than the patient to the care and services. The communication and planning processes developed by the hospital are the necessary investments in transitioning from an adopted model to a working plan. This model is a perfect illustration of how to implement the JCAHO standards. The case management model then is an operational approach to meeting the following (JCAHO, 1995):

- Customer expectations by providing well-planned, seamless management of care
- Institutional needs by addressing cost-effective solutions to the management of care
- Practitioner needs by allowing timely interventions for the delivery of care within a structured framework
- Regulatory needs by encompassing the principles and standards of the JCAHO in outlining the management of care

The case manager is responsible for moving patients with a range of needs through the system in a seamless manner. **Case management plans,** proactively developed as baseline tools, facilitate and arrange for an array of care, treatment, and services required in caring for highly complex patients. The benefit of the case management model is the provision of an individual practitioner to do this. The JCAHO does not set different standards for different types of patients. Rather, they outline high-quality standards for all. The ability to meet the standards for the group of patients with complex needs is challenging. The case management model recognizes this challenge and meets it by placing that complex population in the hands of a dedicated practitioner. The case manager is an additional investment by the organization to meet the increasing demands of today's health care population.

Using all the creativity and know-how necessary to maintain patients "on track" toward discharge, the case manager must plan and intervene as necessary to meet the unique needs of the complex patient. The case management model provides the necessary vehicle to accomplish this task. Its ability to organize care and treatments, coupled with its outlined progression to outcome achievement, makes it a natural approach toward managing care for the patient holistically while meeting regulatory standards. The ability of case managers to facilitate the process of care for those patients with complex needs is crucial to meeting the needs of the patient, practitioner, institution, and JCAHO standards.

Documentation Standards

The JCAHO (1995) has challenged health care providers to accomplish the following tasks:
- Design and implement efficient patient journeys through the continuum of care
- Decrease duplication through interdisciplinary team work
- Manage information and communication
- Remain cognizant of resource utilization, fiscal responsibilities, and length of stay issues
- Provide quality care based on sound current principles

Taken at face value it is easy to see how case management tools fit into the overall scheme of the JCAHO

standards. Examining each charge separately reinforces the importance and necessity of carefully developing interdisciplinary plans to outline specific outcomes to be achieved within specific time frames.

After reviewing the overall intent of the JCAHO standards and seeing the relationship between these standards and case management, it is necessary to look at the documentation tools and their relationship to the standards. This provides further evidence of the efficacy of case management in meeting the JCAHO requirements.

The familiar saying, "If it's not documented, it's not done," holds true when fiscal intermediaries and regulatory agencies review medical records. Any type of retrospective review that is used to evaluate the quality of care and services provided to patients relies heavily on the evaluation of documentation. Appearances count. Little can be said to give credence to sloppy, illegible, contradictory entries in a patient record. One of the assumptions made when records are not neat, consistent, or complete is that the care rendered is less than adequate, inconsistent, and lacking.

One should always remember that the JCAHO during its survey reviews both concurrent medical and retrospective closed records. Their objective is to see the care and treatment currently rendered and documented and compare this to past completed documentation (Case Manager's Tip 12-3). Specific diagnoses are chosen for review. The diagnoses chosen usually have high-risk, high-volume, and problem-prone issues or concerns surrounding them and require added interventions—either physical, emotional, ethical, or spiritual. This part of the JCAHO survey evaluates the quality of the documentation reflecting the holistic and seamless approach to needed care and treatments for the patient, family, and significant other.

The JCAHO uses a comparison to describe the closed medical record review. They liken the completed record to a book that details a story of patient care. The aim is to see a beginning (the assessment and planning for patient care), a middle (the interventions, outcomes, and patient responses to the care rendered), and an end (evaluation of services and goals and evidence of a thoughtful and safe discharge plan and preparation).

---

case manager's tip **12-3**

Evaluating the Quality of Documentation: Review of Records

Keep in mind that the JCAHO reviews both concurrent medical and retrospective closed records during its survey. The objective is to compare the care and treatment currently rendered and documented with past completed documentation.

Each phase is necessary in assessing the overall patient outcomes of hospitalization.

The JCAHO has provided structure to assist organizations in resolving issues/concerns related to documentation. They begin by requiring practitioners to base clinical practice on standards of care. These may be in many forms, including policy, procedure, and protocol. The key is that they are based on established and accepted practice. JCAHO requires periodic review and update of care standards to reflect current practice. Changes made must be substantiated with sound reasoning (e.g., regulatory changes, new scientific research).

Once standards have been developed and accepted, staff must be educated to expected practice, and the documents must be accessible as reference guides for practitioners. Use of the standard becomes the established norm, and variations in practice must be documented and explained. Once the standard is established and applied in the clinical setting, accountability for individual practice may be enforced with practitioners.

The documentation tools (e.g., case management plans) developed for the case management model are formulated on the same principles. They serve several purposes (Case Manager's Tip 12-4) and are developed with input from all health care providers who will use them. Representation is usually from the various disciplines. They outline current practice for the practitioner based on actual retrospective medical record review and current published standards and guidelines. They are designed to facilitate communication by condensing each discipline's plan of care into one document, thereby decreasing duplication and improving timely communication. By outlining care and treatments in an organized manner, an immediate flag is activated when patients deviate from predetermined case management plans. These variations may lead to the following:

- Increased costs and length of stay
- Indication of a need to revise the plan to reflect changes in practice

The basic premise of outlining the pathway and scheduling interventions correlated to **length of stay** supports the seamless approach to care. Using the outline, services can be activated for the patient as needed when required. This type of preplanning allows the work to flow around the patient and enhances the patient/family's view of appropriate holistic care. This creates a positive perception of the health care team and contributes to improved customer satisfaction.

Another contribution to improve satisfaction with the delivery of care is to decrease paperwork and duplication of data collection. Case management documentation tools support this charge by the JCAHO. Objective documentation on the case management plan lets each discipline review what has been done for and accomplished by the patient. Practitioners can then validate required information and patient responses rather than asking redundant questions. Several practitioners all performing the same assessment and data collection suggests to the patient that nobody talks to each other and each discipline must have to complete their work separate and apart from the rest. Certainly this is neither the intent nor the objective of a team effort. It is, however, a distinct impression imparted to the patient, family, and significant other.

To meet the documentation requirement by the JCAHO of decreasing duplication, documentation tools may be developed for disciplines to build on data collected by the team. Initial assessments may be gathered by one care team member, then reviewed by and added to by the next. The purpose is to accomplish the following:

- Reduce duplication
- Organize data logically to support collaboration and access to information for the interdisciplinary team
- Delegate to the appropriate caregiver the appropriate function
- Prepare practitioners for the computerization of clinical data

---

case manager's tip | 12-4 | Purposes Served by Documentation Tools

A key point to remember is that the documentation tool (e.g., case management plan) does more than just meet documentation requirements for the JCAHO and other regulatory agencies. It serves several purposes, and it acts as the following:

1. The patient map of care through the system
2. The practitioner guide to stay on track in providing necessary care and treatments
3. The communication tool for the multidisciplinary team
4. An evaluation tool for quality management to ascertain variations in practice and project fiscal and quality of care implications
5. A standard of practice for regulatory agencies, particularly the JCAHO

Building and refining old principles of documentation standards have led health care providers to creative solutions for complex issues. Case management is one of those creative solutions. Its ability to meet and support such a wide variety of concerns—fiscal, regulatory, and quality—make it a natural selection as a complete model for delivery of care. It blends into the JCAHO philosophy and addresses the requirements of the JCAHO standards. Its intrinsic value may be seen in its ability to place the patient at the center of the team while supporting collaboration of the interdisciplinary team in meeting stated outcomes. This may be not only one of its most valuable assets but also one of its most difficult to attain.

INTERDISCIPLINARY APPROACH TO PATIENT CARE

Another relationship between case management and the JCAHO to examine is the one involving the interdisciplinary team. How does the organization get individuals and/or departments to move beyond their separate spaces and work together? The answer is to break down the barriers and direct united energies into the delivery of quality patient care. The organization must continuously educate each department (no matter how far removed from the actual delivery of patient care) to the overall hospital mission. This involves commitment and dedication by the leadership to allow and support necessary collaboration to achieve cohesion among the team.

When the JCAHO revamped and reorganized its approach to the accreditation standards, it collapsed individual departmental requirements into patient-focused and organization functions. The immediate change was felt by all. No longer could nursing or radiology open to a chapter and measure only their individual performance. It was now necessary to work with other disciplines, to know what they did, to determine how and where they overlapped, and to assess the overall organizational performance. The JCAHO pressured hospitals to refocus on their ultimate mission and seek ways to point each department in the direction of meeting the organizational objectives.

Knowing this to be the sound, correct way for organizations to position themselves, the JCAHO was savvy enough to know that this would require intentional and undivided efforts to achieve. The incentive, however, was the same for each group—to meet the hospital mission. At the center of the hospital mission lie the patient, family, and significant other and the delivery of quality care.

Introduction of quality management and performance improvement concepts enabled organizations to educate staff. These ideas fueled the growth of working teams to assess, evaluate, and improve services; delivery of care; systems; and processes within the organization. What the JCAHO did by refocusing its quality assessment was to refocus the organization's way of thinking. It asked hospitals to consider that no matter how well each separate piece of the facility performed, without communication, collaboration, and the ability to work together, inefficiencies and bottlenecks would occur. The ability to deliver quality services efficiently would be hindered by duplication and miscommunication. What would remain at the center as focus would be the work or the job rather than the patient.

If that approach were moved to the level of the interdisciplinary team, each team member would reiterate the goal of quality patient care, but without necessary communication and planning to meet patient care needs, only the immediate needs of the individual disciplines are met. This picture is a fragmented approach and does not support a cohesive team image to the patient, family, and significant other.

Case management is a solution to bridge the multidisciplinary team. Case management provides the walkway or direction the patient needs to take to complete the course through an episode of illness. All team members have the opportunity to identify where and when they need to intervene to accomplish their care goals. Each team member knows who, how, and when to communicate with other team members as progression of the patient along the path takes place. Each member is aware of the involvement of the rest of the team and has access to the specific outcomes and the associated patient responses. The case management model facilitates a holistic approach to patient care. It recognizes the need for the many disciplines to contribute in directing the patient plan of care appropriately and efficiently. It recognizes the need to attend to details, to deal with unexpected issues, and to allow each team member to participate. Case management reinforces the commitment, responsibility, and accountability of the individual disciplines and the interdisciplinary team as a whole to efficient and timely delivery of care and treatments.

In addition, the case management model assists in educating the interdisciplinary team to necessary concepts and principles for survival in today's health care arena. It introduces discussion of the following:

- Cost issues and treatment efficacy
- Appropriate resource utilization and cost containment
- Standard requirements and regulatory needs
- Patient-focused care, reengineering, and redesign
- Care settings and appropriate levels of care

The "team" that previously allowed the members to interact independently with the patient, family, and significant other must now interact with each other in assisting the patient through hospitalization. Based on the developed case management plans, all members contribute their interventions and evaluations, allowing the next phase of care to occur and the work to flow around the patient. This approach is most necessary in providing quality patient care services and keeping all practitioners focused on the seamless transition of the patient through the system.

The case management model provides a strong working model to accomplish many objectives efficiently. It meets patient, practitioner, team, fiscal, and JCAHO needs with its effective and appropriate approach to delivery of quality patient care services. It allows organizations to put action into theory and theory into action.

Implementing a case management model puts a process in place at the level of patient care that parallels the JCAHO standards. It provides a sound baseline to move the organization forward in its vision and attainment of delivery of quality services. It recognizes the need to develop patient-centered systems and processes to meet patient needs and institutional objectives. Case management provides the interdisciplinary team with a way to organize standards of care and practice into cost-effective plans that move the patient through the various health care settings efficiently. It positions the patients at the center and prepares them for discharge appropriately into the community and helps them become ready to adopt necessary adjustments. It positions the team and organization around the patient, supporting them through the episode of illness and preparing where to use documented data regarding practice and outcomes to shape its future.

KEY POINTS

1. The use of interdisciplinary communication and documentation tools is encouraged by JCAHO. Case management provides a foundation for both of these.
2. Case management models embody the same principles as those outlined in the JCAHO standards.
3. The interdisciplinary team, such as the case management team, is a focus of the JCAHO standards.

Reference

Joint Commission on Accreditation of Healthcare Organizations: *1996 comprehensive accreditation manual for hospitals,* Oakbrook Terrace, Ill, 1995, JCAHO.

CHAPTER 13

LEGAL ISSUES IN CASE MANAGEMENT

TONIA DANDRY AIKEN, RN, BSN, JD

JULIA W. AUCOIN, MSN

Health care organizations, in conjunction with the federal government, have been struggling with ways to reduce the cost of health care, including costs related to medical malpractice insurance and litigation. Among the efforts pursued has been the implementation of **case management** systems for patient care delivery and services across the health care continuum. These systems, when fully implemented, rely heavily on the role of nurse **case managers,** discussed in Chapter 4, and the use of **case management plans** (CMPs), discussed in Chapter 9. This chapter, however, will discuss the legal liabilities and malpractice litigation associated with the components of case management systems.

CASE MANAGEMENT SYSTEMS, THE NURSE CASE MANAGER, AND THE LEGAL PROCESS

Case management has many wide-reaching effects on patients and their families. Enhanced communication and education of the patients and families allow for a better plan and more fully informed decisions about the care to be rendered. Because communication is more effective in case management systems, there can be an earlier identification of patients' discharge needs, which may result in the development of improved CMPs to troubleshoot potential problem areas or barriers. Nurse case managers can identify potential problems and barriers within a desired time frame that can be addressed proactively rather than retroactively. They can prevent overlapping and overutilization of many health care services through management, coordination, and facilitation of patient care activities, thereby minimizing or eliminating delays in treatments, care, and tests required by patients. Nurse case managers can facilitate changes in the provision of care, which may improve cost, quality, effectiveness, and efficiency of the health care system.

Today, nurse case managers are found to assume responsibilities in all care settings (Box 13-1). They are obligated to actively participate in ensuring that patients receive the best health care in the most effective and efficient manner. Their autonomy, accountability, and responsibility toward management, planning, delivery, coordination, brokering, facilitation, and evaluation of patient care practices put them at higher risk for **malpractice litigation** (Nichols, 1996). Because of their position at the hub of the interdisciplinary care team and their role as **gatekeepers** of care, they find themselves increasingly involved in complex situations that require subtle decisions and present higher legal accountability, therefore increasing the chances for malpractice and liability.

Several causes of litigation appear repetitively in lawsuits, such as discourteous behavior, communication failures, lack of patient understanding, and lack of information given to the patient and family. For example, patients and/or their families may sue when common complications occur and they claim they were not told or informed that such problems could occur.

If the patient is involved in a lawsuit, the nurse case manager may encounter legal terminology that is not commonly used by the layperson. Nurse case managers should become familiar with the legal terminology (e.g., plaintiff, defendant, malpractice suit, standard of care, and **negligence**) they may come across in the case of a legal claim. The **plaintiff** is the person who brings a claim or lawsuit into court. If the case involves the death of a patient, the plaintiff is the next of kin or the appropriate legal guardian. The defendant in a lawsuit is the person or entity against whom a claim is brought by the plaintiff (i.e., the provider of health care services; e.g., the hospital, physician, nurse case manager, registered nurse, nurse manager).

Most health care institutions have provided nurse case managers with the responsibility of managing patient care in collaboration with members of the interdisciplinary health care team. Such responsibility increases the risk for malpractice lawsuits against nurse case managers. Malpractice suits are suits filed in court against professional people (e.g., nurse case managers or physicians) who have a level of skill and knowledge that exceeds that of a lay or ordinary person. These suits are usually filed against professionals who practice health care below the *common* standards.

STANDARDS OF CARE

In medical malpractice claims, the nurse case manager's care and treatment is judged based on the standards of care applied by other case managers with the same knowledge and experience and who are practicing under similar circumstances in a case management setting. The standard of care is then defined as a measuring scale by which the provider's (i.e., nurse case manager's) conduct is compared to determine if there is negligence or malpractice that has caused damage or injury to the plaintiff and if the provider acted "reasonably" (Nichols, 1996). To avoid malpractice litigation, nurse case managers are advised to practice their duties in a manner consistent with their skills and knowledge, job description, standards, policies, and procedures defined by their institutions.

The sources of standards of care for nurse case managers may include any or all of those issued by professional societies such as the following:

- National Association of Geriatric Care Managers
- National Institute of Community Based Long Term Care
- American Nurses Association's Steering Committee on the National Case Management Task Force
- Association of Rehabilitation Nurses
- American Managed Care and Review Association
- Agency for Health Care Policy and Research

- National Institutes of Health
- Health Care Financing Administration

Nurse case managers may also apply the clinical practice guidelines that have been developed by national organizations and associations such as the American Medical Association, American College of Physicians, American College of Cardiology, and American Diabetes Association. If nurse case managers receive certifications, they will be held to the standards of care of the society sponsoring the certification (e.g., the certified case manager [CCM], advance competency continuity of care [ACCC], certified rehabilitation registered nurse [CRRN], certified insurance rehabilitation specialist [CIRS], occupational health nurse [OHN], and certified rehabilitation counselor [CRC]). Other sources of standards include the following:

- The facility/hospital policies, procedures, and protocols
- Statutes
- Regulations
- Nurse practice act
- Equipment manuals
- Job descriptions
- Guidelines
- Authoritative textbooks
- Expert witnesses

In situations where the patient is involved in litigation, nurse case managers may be called to testify in court, or the CMP applied for the care of the patient and the medical record may be used to demonstrate the standard of care. Documentation (discussed in Chapter 8) that is thorough, factual, and concrete is essential to aid in the defense of the nurse case manager and to provide a proper "picture" of the care and treatment rendered to the patient.

Negligence

If there is a claim involving allegations of negligence or breaches of the standard of care, nurse case managers will be held to the standard that was in effect *at the time of the alleged incident.* They will be judged by the "reasonable person's" standard, not the highest standard of care required under the same circumstances.

If there is an allegation of a breach of a standard based on negligence, then several areas must be evaluated. Negligence is the failure to act as an ordinary, prudent, or "reasonable person" would do under similar circumstances. To determine a successful claim against a nurse case manager four elements of negligence must be evident (Box 13-2).

For example, if a nurse case manager fails to obtain and review pertinent patient's records with the managed care organization and as a result the patient is denied the **certification** for surgery or extended hospital

---

box 13-2

The Four Elements of Negligence*

1. A duty (standard of care) is owed to the patient by the practitioner or health care organization
2. A breach of duty or a breach of the standard of care by the provider
3. A proximate cause or connection exists between the breach of duty and the patient
4. Damages or injuries incurred by the patient

---

*Holzer, 1990; Merz, 1993; Nichols, 1996; West, 1994.

---

box 13-3

Elements of Disclosure

1. The type of procedure(s) to be performed (e.g., debridement of knee wound)
2. The material risks and hazards inherent in the procedures (e.g., infection, bleeding)
3. The projected/desired outcome(s) hoped for (e.g., elimination of infected tissue and revitalization of new tissue)
4. Available alternatives, if any (e.g., medication)
5. Consequences of no treatment (e.g., continuation of pain, necrosis, sepsis, or possible amputation)

---

stay, causing serious injuries (further complications/deterioration in condition), the nurse case manager and the managed care organization are held liable. The four elements of negligence are evident in this case. The case manager has a duty to obtain and evaluate all medical data so that the patient can receive the appropriate treatment based on needs. By failing to do so, the case manager demonstrated negligence and proximately caused additional injuries to the patient. Breach of the standard of care is also evident. The patient has a valid case.

Damages or injuries can include such things as loss of love and affection; pain and suffering; mental anguish; emotional distress; disfigurement; loss of consortium; past, present, and future medical expenses or lost wages; loss of guidance; loss of nurturance; loss of chance for survival; exacerbation of a preexisting condition; and premature death.

Malpractice

If the nurse case manager is involved in a professional allegation of misconduct or negligent care, then the term *malpractice* is used. Malpractice is defined as professional misconduct; negligent care and treatment; or failure to meet the standard of care, which results in harm to others.

Claims of malpractice or negligence against providers must be brought to the court's attention within a certain period of time (statute of limitation). The *statute of limitation* is known as a specific time limit allowed to file a lawsuit. In personal injury, medical malpractice, and breach of contract claims, state and federal laws vary. Claims should be reviewed to determine the appropriate time period within which a claim can be brought against the potential defendant.

INFORMED CONSENT

Nurse case managers are often involved in some way in the process of informed consent. Informed consent is consent given by a patient or the next of kin, legal guardian, or designated person in the medical durable

power of attorney after the provision of sufficient information by the provider. The elements of disclosure (Box 13-3) are those items that must be discussed with the patient by the health care provider performing the treatment, procedure, or surgery.

There are several exceptions to obtaining informed consent and discussing all of the elements of disclosure with the patient. The first exception is if there is an emergency situation and/or a situation in which the client is unconscious or incompetent (e.g., the patient is in a life-threatening situation and there is no time to have a discussion). Second, a therapeutic privilege may be invoked if it is medically contraindicated to disclose the risk and hazards to the patient or if it may result in illness, emotional distress, serious psychological damage, or failure on the part of the patient to receive lifesaving treatment. Third, the patient may waive the right to informed consent. Finally, the patient may have had the procedure performed once before and waives the right of informed consent because he or she has already received the information. This information must be documented appropriately in the medical record to protect health care providers against malpractice litigation.

LEGAL AND ETHICAL DILEMMAS FOR THE NURSE CASE MANAGER

Common legal and ethical issues that are potential areas of exposure and litigation in the area of case management may or may not involve nurse case managers directly. Examples of such issues include the following:

- **Third-party payors** and health care facilities can be held legally accountable when inappropriate decisions regarding medical services result from defects in design or implementation of cost-containment mechanisms instituted by the facility or insurance company.
- Physicians can be held liable if they comply with the limitations imposed by third-party payors and do not protest when the patient can be

harmed by these decisions. Physicians are ultimately responsible.

- Breach of contract, bad faith, and refusal to provide services and pay **benefits** or claims are also issues that may be litigated. A *contract* is an agreement consisting of one or more legally enforceable promises between two or more parties. The elements of a contract are offer, acceptance, consideration, and breach.
- If there is a breach of implied covenant or good faith and fair dealing, legal actions may be taken.
- Clients may also allege a failure to exercise due care in the discharge of the contractual duties.
- A failure to properly investigate an insider's claim is a potential litigation.
- If standards of medical necessity that are significantly at **variance** with community standards are applied, there may be legal exposure.
- Failure to properly document care activities and/or **outcomes.**
- An allegation of good faith violation of duty may be alleged when a subscriber's claim for hospital benefits is denied and the subscriber (an **enrollee** of a managed care company) is not informed of his or her contractual right to impartial review and arbitration of the disputed claim.
- Failure to obtain all of the necessary documents/medical records can result in the denial of care needed, which then exerts potential liability.

- Allegations of negligent referral claims may be filed if there is evidence of failure to properly investigate the qualifications and competencies of the providers and/or facilities to which nurse case managers refer patients for treatment. In addition, if it can be shown that nurse case managers were not reasonable in making a referral to that particular facility or provider, the allegation of negligent referral can be made.
- Failure of nurse case managers to act as patients' advocates or in their interest.
- Failure to apply the "reasonable" standard to the care of patients.
- Any type of "kickback" or "incentive" program with a provider/payor and the nurse case manager. Such practices are considered illegal (conflict of interest). They also are unethical behaviors that may result in the patient not be receiving the best possible care by the most appropriate provider.

A list of suggestions to help prevent or minimize malpractice litigation appears in Case Manager's Tip 13-1.

Health care organizations and nurse case managers should be aware of the reputation and operations of other providers to whom patients are referred for further treatment. Decisions should be made in the best interest of patients and their families. Several considerations should be reviewed to determine if the providers to whom patients are referred are appropriate and meet the interests and needs of patients.

---

case manager's tip 13-1 **Suggestions for Preventing Malpractice Litigation**

To prevent malpractice litigation, the health care organization and the nurse case manager should do the following:
1. Delineate a referral process for community services and care provision that is in the best interest of the patient and family. The referral process should be accessible in writing to all those involved (i.e., health care providers). It should be clear and concise.
2. Ensure that corrective measures are taken and action plans are developed immediately if a health care issue arises or if care is questionable. Evaluation and follow-up on such plans should be reflected in the patient's medical record or hospital's administrative reports as needed.
3. Develop and implement policies and procedures regarding the process of developing case management plans that are easily understood and applied. They should reflect the best interest of the patient and family. In addition, the procedure for documentation of care activities and variance identification and collection should be made easy and explicit.

To minimize malpractice litigation, the nurse case manager should do the following:
1. On admission, and in collaboration with the patient and family and the interdisciplinary team, individualize the case management plan to meet the patient's and family's needs.
2. Always consult the treating physician.
3. Review the patient's medical record thoroughly before contacting the representative of managed care organizations.
4. Ensure that **precertifications** for treatments have been obtained in a timely manner.
5. Comply with the law (e.g., patient privacy and confidentiality procedures).
6. Make certain that the patient and family consent to the indicated treatment plan and procedures.
7. Advocate for the patient and family.

Examples of these considerations include the following:

- Types of services provided and current practices
- Reports of patient and staff satisfaction scores
- Resource utilization practices
- Practices of quality assurance, assessment, monitoring, and improvement
- Timeliness of delivery of services
- Billing practices (e.g., how do they bill, what types of insurance do they accept)
- Insurance coverage (i.e., are they properly and adequately insured)
- Records of any settlements and/or judgments against the facility or health care provider (check the courthouse records; do a computer search)
- The allegations of the breaches of the standard of care found in the medical malpractice settlements or judgments (do the allegations pertain to the type of care that would be rendered to the patients to be referred for services)
- Current licensure (check with the state boards)
- Current accreditation (check with the appropriate agencies)
- Reports on outcomes of care of patients with similar problems to the ones to be referred

NONCOMPLIANCE/MISMANAGEMENT

If it can be proven that there has been noncompliance with the plan of care (case management plan) agreed on by the family, nurse case manager, and members of the interdisciplinary team, then there may be a claim of mismanagement. It is important for providers, including nurse case managers, to explain to the patient and family that certain complications or undesired outcomes may occur regardless of the efforts made to prevent them. It is also helpful to avoid providing false guarantees regarding outcomes of care, particularly when the situation at hand is considered to be high risk. False guarantees of this kind may be viewed as noncompliance with or mismanagement of the standards. When guarantees are provided but not met, and the patient and/or family are able to prove that guarantees were not met, the situation results in potential breach.

Nurse case managers must practice within the realm of the responsibilities defined by the professional license they hold and must not infer in any way that they are developing medical treatment plans for their patients. Any evident noncompliance with the regulations governing the practice of nursing may present potential problems, which may result in medical malpractice litigation. It may also be a potential problem wherein the nurse case manager is viewed as practic-

ing medicine. This can result in a disciplinary action and an impingement on the license (e.g., revocation, suspension, or probation).

DOCUMENTATION

A nurse case manager must act as the patient's advocate and look out for what is in the patient's best interest. If it is determined that the physician and/or facility that the patient has been referred to is not properly performing or providing the services needed, then action to change the situation must be taken and should be documented so as to protect the provider. Documentation should occur when reviewing and evaluating credentials and performance of practitioners and facilities that patients have been referred to so that the nurse case manager can determine if they are providing the appropriate levels of care needed by patients and families. In addition, follow-up documentation regarding actions taken to correct any identified problems must be evident, along with subsequent documentation of the outcomes of these corrective measures. Case Manager's Tip 13-2 presents some areas in which accurate and thorough documentation is considered critical in reducing malpractice litigation. Documentation serves multiple purposes, including the following:

- Evidence of the provision of care
- Justification of the need for referrals to specific providers
- Evaluation of the patient's condition in light of treatment
- Evidence that proper investigation of the qualifications, credentials, and competencies of health care providers is completed
- Communicating the plan of care of individual patients to the various health care team members
- Protection against litigation
- Assistance in determining whether the resources are being used appropriately
- Clarification of continuity of care after the hospital stay
- Summary of nursing and medical history for use in future admissions
- Reporting of data for quality of care review and risk management
- Reporting of data for continuing education and research
- Review of data for billing and reimbursement purposes
- Recording care that forms the basis of evaluation by regulatory agencies (e.g., the Joint Commission on Accreditation of Healthcare Organizations [JCAHO], state health departments)

Areas in Which Documentation is Critical

1. Plan of care agreed on with the patient and family
2. Medical stability of patient within 24 hours of discharge
3. Falls
4. Restraints
5. Third-party (insurance) reimbursement
6. JCAHO accreditation of facility
7. Discharge planning and patient's readiness for discharge
8. Patient and family teaching
9. Informed consent
10. Disclosure of information
11. Advance directives
12. Living wills
13. Medical durable power of attorney
14. Reportable events (e.g., violent injuries, communicable diseases, abuse)
15. Do not resuscitate orders

- Legal evidence for use by the hospital, other health care providers, the patient and/or family, and members of the judicial system

CASE MANAGEMENT PLANS

Health care providers have raised concerns regarding the admissibility of CMPs as evidence in case of malpractice litigation. It has been noted by lawyers that when CMPs are used for documenting the provision of care (planning, implementing, and evaluating) and are made a permanent part of the patient's medical record, it is most certain that they will be admitted into court as evidence (Nolin and Lang, 1992).

A CMP is an interdisciplinary proactive set of daily prescriptions that has been prepared following a particular time line to facilitate the care of a specific patient population from preadmission to postdischarge. The CMP identifies patient care activities that are thought to be required for providing care for a specific patient population. These activities are categorized as the assessments, treatments, teaching, discharge planning, diagnostic tests, consultations, and interventions that should be completed for the patient's optimal recovery (see Chapter 9 for detailed discussion). The CMP holds valuable evidence, because it includes information (data and evidence) about the patient's projected and actual course of treatment. It includes the following:

- Patient's actual and potential problems
- Patient's projected and actual outcomes
- Medical interventions
- Nursing and other interventions

- Projected discharge times/target times
- Intermediate and discharge care outcomes

Case management plans are usually developed by professional societies, health care institutions, insurance companies, or federal agencies. Sometimes they are called "clinical practice guidelines" or "practice parameters." Professional societies and governmental agencies have developed practice guidelines to counteract or reduce the risk for liability and litigation (Holzer, 1990; Zweig and Witte, 1993). They are developed and used to improve the quality of care and reduce cost through standardizing practice. They are also helpful in reducing the cost of and risk for malpractice litigation through delineating the standard of care (West, 1994).

Once a CMP is admitted into court as evidence, it is thought to be an extremely powerful evidentiary tool used by the jury to determine the sequence of events (treatments and outcomes). If the provider was noted to have been compliant with the projections of the CMP and the documentation justifies the deviation from the CMP's recommendations, then the chances are that the provider's actions will be deemed appropriate and in compliance with the standard of care (Nolin and Lang, 1992). The key in this case is appropriate documentation of variances from the CMP.

The procedure followed in the development of CMPs affects the degree of its consideration by the jury and its reliability in the lawsuit. It is recommended that procedures be based on expert opinion, research, and the latest advents of treatment as recommended by professional societies and governmental agencies (Case Man-

case
manager's
tip

13-3

Points to Remember About Case Management Plans

1. Can be presented as evidence if they are made part of the patient's medical record.
2. Improve communication among members of the health care team, thus reducing the risk for liability or litigation.
3. Can be determined by the jury as the standards of care.
4. Should allow for deviations. However, documentation in the medical record of variances related to the plan of care, including the medical and nursing plans, is important for reducing liability.
5. Help the jury describe the sequence of events (treatments and outcomes).
6. Developed by one health care organization may be inappropriate for another organization.
7. Will not be admitted as evidence unless proven relevant to the case in question.
8. Should be flexible prescriptions and allow for deviations as long as they are justified.
9. Should be developed following a scientific method.
10. Standardize the care provided by multiple providers.

---

box 13-4

Patient Rights

1. Right to access to needed health and social services
2. Right to treatment with dignity and respect
3. Right to confidentiality
4. Right to privacy
5. Right to know cost of services
6. Right to self-determination
7. Right to comprehensive and fair assessment
8. Right to notification of discharge, termination, or change of service
9. Right to withdraw from a case management program
10. Right to a grievance procedure
11. Right to choose a particular community services agency or long-term care provider

---

ager's Tip 13-3 contains a list of suggestions for CMPs). However, if they are developed poorly and arbitrarily, the CMPs will hold no power in court and will be judged as inappropriate care standards. Therefore the care provider will not be able to defend the case.

PATIENT CONFIDENTIALITY

Like any health care provider, nurse case managers are obligated to safeguard the patient's privacy and confidentiality. Unauthorized disclosure of information is considered breach of confidentiality and may result in litigation. It is important for nurse case managers to seek the guidance of a legal counsel before disclosing any information. In spite of confidentiality laws, reporting of certain events such as elder or child abuse, contagious diseases, deaths, births, and animal bites is mandatory and protected by federal laws. Some information requires the patient's permission for release

(written and signed release). The release should delineate the name(s) of the party the information is to be released to. Examples of such information include the following:

- Drug or alcohol abuse treatment
- Mental health/psychiatric care
- Sexually transmitted diseases
- HIV or AIDS status
- Abortion
- Specific medical or surgical history

It is important for nurse case managers to remember and respect patients' rights every time they face a legal or ethical dilemma or any challenges related to the provision of care. The patient has several rights that must not be forgotten (Box 13-4).

The nurse case manager can play an important role in advocating on behalf of the patient and family. During such situations, the nurse case manager should always remain aware of the patient's legal rights, as well as issues of confidentiality pertaining to patient care.

Case management plans can serve an important function in protecting the rights of both the patient and the health care provider. Special attention should be paid to the process of their development, their use, and the way documentation is incorporated into them.

KEY POINTS

1. Nurse case managers can be held liable. They should be aware of the legal process and the legal terminology used.
2. Case management plans are admissible in court. They can be reviewed by the jury to determine the standard of care followed at the time care was provided.

3. Case management plans should be developed following a scientific process.
4. The use of case management systems in patient care delivery may reduce the cost of malpractice litigation.
5. Thorough documentation in the medical record is extremely important. The patient's medical record and the case management plan used can be admissible in court as evidence.

References

Holzer JF: The advent of clinical standards for professional liability, *Qual Rev Bull* 16(2):71-79, 1990.

Merz SM: Clinical practice guidelines: policy issues and legal implications, *J Qual Improve* 19(8):306-311, 1993.

Nichols DJ: Legal liabilities in case management. In Flarey DL, Smith-Blancett S: *Handbook of nursing case management,* Gaithersburg, Md, 1996, Aspen.

Nolin CE, Lang CG: *An analysis of the use and effect of caremap tools in medical malpractice litigation,* South Natick, Mass, 1992, The Center for Case Management, Inc.

West JC: The legal implications of medical practice guidelines, *J Health Hosp Law* 27(4):97-103, 1994.

Zweig FM, Witte HA: Assisting judges in screening medical practice guidelines for health care litigation, *J Qual Improve* 19(8):342-353, 1993.

Case Management Plans

Appendixes A through G present some examples of case management plans (CMPs) that pertain to different care settings. The significance of these plans is that they represent an interdisciplinary approach to the plan of care of patients with particular diagnoses or surgical procedures. CMPs usually delineate the standards of care; identify patients' actual and potential problems, the goals of treatment, and the necessary patient care activities; and establish the projected outcomes of care.

The following examples of CMPs are included here:
- Appendix A: MAP, Asthma (p. 170)
- Appendix B: MAP, Chemotherapy (days 1 and 2 only) (p. 180)
- Appendix C: MAP, Peritoneal dialysis, post-catheter replacement (p. 182)
- Appendix D: MAP, Rehab protocol, total hip replacement (p. 191)
- Appendix E: Visit guidelines, hip fracture, open reduction internal fixation: physical therapy (p. 215)
- Appendix F: Directly observed therapy (DOT) MAP, Tuberculosis (p. 216)
- Appendix G: MAP, Well newborn (p. 220)

Things to Remember When Developing Case Management Plans

Keep the following guidelines in mind when developing a CMP:
- Establish an interdisciplinary team.
- Identify team members based on the diagnosis or surgical procedure in question. Members should be chosen based on their clinical experiences, leadership skills, communication skills, tolerance to hard work, and commitment to the institution and the project.
- Identify a team leader and a facilitator.
- Provide the team with administrative and clerical support.
- Establish a project work plan (time line of activities) before the team's first meeting.
- Train team members in the process of developing CMPs.
- Team members should prepare their work in between meetings. Meetings should be held to review the work and determine the next steps.
- Regardless of the format of the CMP, it should always include the patient care elements as identified by the

organization, the patient problems, projected length of stay and outcomes of care, a variance tracking form, and patient care activities and interventions.
- Time line the CMP as indicated by the care setting. For example, minutes to hours in emergency departments, number of visits in clinics and home care, days in acute care, weeks in areas of longer length of stay such as neonatal intensive care area, and months in nursing homes and group homes. The time line of CMPs in subacute care and rehabilitation centers can be established based on the length of stay, goals of treatment, and intensity of activities. For the most part, it is daily or weekly.
- Preestablish the expected (acceptable) length of stay.
- Determine the mechanism for tracking variances and define the variance categories to be evaluated.
- Ensure that the CMP is the standard of care applied by all health care providers, including physicians.
- Include patient and family teaching and discharge planning activities in all CMPs.
- Determine whether CMPs are a permanent part of the medical record.
- Maximize documentation on the CMP. Require all patient care services to use the CMP for documentation.
- Develop CMPs based on the latest recommendations of research and professional societies.
- Avoid being rigid in recommending treatments. For example, use words like "consider" when including treatments, medications, or interventions that may not be applicable to every patient, completion may not always be possible within the indicated time frame, or progress may be dependent on patient's condition.
- Identify the intermediate and discharge outcomes of care in each CMP.
- Delineate the ICD-9 code or the DRG number of the CMP on the cover page.
- Include all disciplines involved in the care of patients as indicated by the diagnosis or surgical procedure considered.
- Stress the importance of patient care activities that historically were identified as problem areas or requiring improvement.
- Establish a time frame for reviewing and revising the CMP.

CASE MANAGER'S JOB DESCRIPTION AND PERFORMANCE APPRAISAL

Appendix H presents a job description and a performance appraisal of a nurse case manager as established by one institution. The case manager's job description should delineate the power and the level of independence granted in the role. It provides a clear description of the roles, functions, and responsibilities of nurse case managers. The performance appraisal should always be criteria based. Evaluating performance is important for determining the effectiveness of the nurse case manager in the role. Institutions are advised to incorporate reviewing the job description and the process of evaluating performance in the training and education of nurse case managers when they assume the new role. Goals and objectives of the role and the institution can be also shared. A detailed example of the case manager's job description and appraisal can be found in Appendix H (p. 231).

Things to Remember About the Nurse Case Manager Job Description

- Define the scope of practice and describe the roles, functions, and responsibilities of the nurse case manager.
- Delineate the power provided in the role. Define the reporting relationship and indicate to whom the nurse case manager is accountable.
- Define the minimum educational background and experience required for the role.
- Specify the licensure or certification requirements.
- Identify the skills required for the role.
- Establish a job description that fits the institution's operations, systems, and standards of care and practice.
- Establish a job description that reflects the mission, values and beliefs, and philosophy of the institution.
- Specify if it is necessary to belong to professional nursing societies.

Things to Remember About Performance Appraisal

- Develop a performance appraisal that is criteria based and reflective of the job description.
- Define the rating system used in the performance appraisal.
- Specify the minimum acceptable rating (performance).

- Make expectations known.
- Include the skills, knowledge, and abilities required for the job in the performance appraisal.
- Delineate the frequency of evaluating performance.
- Identify the competencies related to the role.

CASE MANAGER'S MONTHLY REPORTS

Appendix I presents the case manager's monthly report. It should summarize the nurse case manager's progress and activities and identify the problems encountered during the month. Requiring nurse case managers to submit such a report to their superiors helps them plan their monthly work and responsibilities and encourages them to be goal oriented. It also helps them be more focused in their work. An example of the case manager's monthly report can be found in Appendix I (p. 244).

Contents of the Case Manager's Report

- The number of case management plans implemented.
- The number of patients followed/case managed.
- Consultations performed.
- Problems identified or faced during the month and action plans developed for resolving such problems.
- Projects involved in, such as developing of patient and family education materials or case management plans.
- Committees or task forces attended.
- Goals for next month.
- Continuing education sessions held or attended.
- Outstanding variances that require immediate attention and/or referral for quality improvement task forces.

CASE MANAGER'S DATA FLOW RECORD

Appendix J presents the Case Management Data Flow Record. The Case Management Data Flow Record could be used as a log for keeping track of patients for whom a case management plan was applied for their care, for whom care was managed by a nurse case manager, or both. This report could be used in an automated (i.e., spread sheet) or paper-and-pencil format. The information collected with this record is important for developing administrative reports such as productivity of the various nurse case managers, length of stay, cost of care, and resource utilization. Reports generated based on the data flow record could include productivity of nurse case managers, length of stay, cost, and resource utilization. An example of the Case Management Data Flow Record can be found in Appendix J (p. 245).

Things to Remember When Developing a Case Management Data Flow Record

- Identify the purpose(s) of the data flow record first, and then determine the number and types of data fields needed.
- Limit the number of data fields to those deemed necessary.
- Maximize automation of such record.
- Include demographics such as the patient's name and medical record number.
- Include information regarding admission and discharge dates if you desire to generate a specific report on length of stay.
- Include information on whether the care of the patient was case managed by a nurse case manager and whether a case management plan was applied.
- Maximize the use of previously existing patient databases such as those used in admitting offices or medical record departments.
- Minimize unnecessary duplication of efforts.
- Consult with personnel from information systems departments when developing such records.
- Do not reinvent the wheel. Evaluate what is already available in the market.
- Generate monthly administrative reports based on data from the flow record.

APPENDIX A-1

Beth Israel Medical Center

MULTIDISCIPLINARY ACTION PLAN

|||||||||||| |||| || ||| |||| ||| ||
2200

DIAGNOSIS: <u>ASTHMA</u>

UNIT: _____

ADMISSION DATE: _____/____/_____ **TIME:**_____:_____ am/pm

DATE MAP INITIATED: _____/____/_____ **TIME:**_____:_____ am/pm

DRG #: <u>96/97</u>

EXPECTED LENGTH OF STAY: <u>4 DAYS</u>

SHORT TRIM POINT: <u>2 DAYS</u>

FOLLOWED BY PATIENT CARE MANAGER/CASE MANAGER: YES ☐ NO ☐
(If Yes) Name: _____

SOCIAL WORKER: _____

GOALS MUTUALLY SET WITH PATIENT AND/OR FAMILY

_____ YES

_____ NO EXPLAIN _____

PRIOR MEDICAL HISTORY: _____

PATIENT ALLERGIES:	_____	YES / NO	DATE
	_____		
	_____	DNR:	

HEALTH CARE PROXY

MAP 029 (Rev 12/94)
Copyright Beth Israel
Medical Center 1992.
All rights reserved

OR LIVING WILL:_____

APPENDIX A-2

Beth Israel Medical Center
MULTIDISCIPLINARY ACTION PLAN
DAY 1
MD: _____

DIAGNOSIS: <u>ASTHMA</u> _____

RN/MD REVIEW: _____

DATE: _____

MAP DOES NOT REPLACE MD ORDERS

NOTES

TESTS/ PROCEDURES/ TREATMENTS:	Peak flow daily.	

MEDICATION:	1. Methylprednisolone 40mg. Q6H IVSS x24 hours (minimum dose).
	2. Triamcinolone (Azmacort MDI) 10 puffs BID with spacer.
	3. Aminophylline may be discontinued when above medications are ordered unless there is clear clinical indication for its use.
	4. Albuterol (Proventil/Ventolin) 4 puffs Q4H and PRN with spacer.
	  • MDI's and spacer given to each patient immediately on admission to floor.
	  • If patient is trained and able to use spacer all nebulized medications should be discontinued.	

ACTIVITY:	As tolerated.	
NUTRITION:	Diet as tolerated. Encourage fluids.	
CONSULTS:	Asthma team if indicated.	

PATIENT EDUCATION:	1. Each pt given an MDI & spacer with specific instructions by house staff and retraining on a daily basis.
	2. Each patient receives daily visit by house staff/asthma team that emphasizes:
	  A. Proper use of MDI with spacer.
	  B. Pathophysiology of disease.
	  C. Differences in medication types.
	  D. Possible side effects.	

SOCIAL WORK:	Consult with RN and MD to screen for hi-risk/ psychosocial and discharge planning needs; document decision.	
DISCHARGE PLANNING:	Specific care provider and appointment identified to patient with earliest possible F/U in Chest and/or Medical Clinic. RN to consult with social work to determine if patient requires social work intervention, if social work is not required, determine if Home Health Care evaluation is needed.	

SHIFT	INITIALS	PRINT NAME	SIGNATURE

MAP 029 (Rev 12/94). Copyright Beth Israel Medical Center 1992. All rights reserved

APPENDIX A-3

Beth Israel Medical Center
MULTIDISCIPLINARY ACTION PLAN
DAY 1: NURSING DOCUMENTATION

MD: _____

DIAGNOSIS: <u>ASTHMA</u>_____

DATE: _____

|||||| 2200

PATIENT PROBLEM AND NURSING INTERVENTIONS	EXPECTED PATIENT OUTCOME AND/OR DISCHARGE OUTCOME	ASSESSMENT/ EVALUATION		
1. IMPAIRED BREATHING DUE TO HYPERACTIVE AIRWAY AND AIRWAY INFLAMMATION	**1. BREATHING PATTERN WILL BE NORMAL OR NEAR NORMAL**			
A. Lung auscultation every 8 hours and PRN.	A. Improved breath sounds by auscultation (decrease in wheezing).	A.	A.	A.
B. Vitals/temperature Q8H and PRN.	B. Vital signs near normal.	B.	B.	B.
C. Monitor ABG values, if applicable.	C. ABGs near normal.	C.	C.	C.
D. Encourage adequate hydration to enhance expectoration.	D. Good hydration, able to expectorate sputum.	D.	D.	D.
E. Administer O₂ as per MD order.	E. Improved breathing.	E.	E.	E.
F. Administer asthma medications, as per MD order.	F. Respiratory rate near normal. Less chest tightness, wheezing.	F.	F.	F.
G. Be alert for impending respiratory failure (s/s pulse paradoxes, extreme distress, impaired consciousness, severe wheezes) notify MD.	G. Absence of distress.	G.	G.	G.
H. Measure peak flow pre/post albuterol QD and PRN.	H. Improved peak flow with albuterol use.	H.	H.	H.
2. SLEEP AND REST DEPRIVATION DUE TO FREQUENT COUGH	**2. IMPROVED SLEEP/REST**			
A. Comfort measures: position of comfort he/she chooses, tissues/kidney basin within patient's reach.	A. Verbalize comfort and rest.	A.	A.	A.
B. Encourage adequate hydrations.	B. Good hydration.	B.	B.	B.
C. Administer bronchodilator inhalers (proventil/ventolin) prior to bedtime and PRN.	C. Improved breathing, able to sleep/rest, minimal coughing spells.	C.	C.	C.
D. Enhance feeling of security by Call Bell within reach, easy access to inhalers, softer lightings and minimize noise level.	D. Verbalizes feeling of security.	D.	D.	D.
3. KNOWLEDGE DEFICIT ACTUAL OR POTENTIAL R/T ASTHMA	**3. INCREASED KNOWLEDGE OF DISEASE AND TREATMENT**			
A. Teach patient the following:	A.	A.	A.	A.
1. Asthma pathophysiology.	1. Verbalize understanding.	1.	1.	1.
2. Asthma medication dose, frequency, purpose, expected effect and it's side effects.	2. Verbalize understanding.	2.	2.	2.
3. Differentiation in function of inhalers.	3. Return demonstration.	3.	3.	3.
4. Emphasize proper MDI use with spacer.	4. Verbalize understanding.	4.	4.	4.
5. Proper maintenance and care of spacer.	5. Verbalize understanding.	5.	5.	5.
B. Assist patient in identifying specific asthma triggers.	B. Patient able to identify at least 3 triggers.	B.	B.	B.
C. Instruct patient on management of asthma triggers.	C. Patient able to verbalize appropriate management of asthma triggers.	C.	C.	C.
D. Review treatment plan.	D. Verbalize understanding.	D.	D.	D.
E. Review projected discharge plan with patient and/or significant other.	E. Verbalize understanding.	E.	E.	E.
F. Discuss importance of keeping follow-up appointment.	F. Verbalize understanding.	F.	F.	F.

APPENDIX A-4

Beth Israel Medical Center
MULTIDISCIPLINARY ACTION PLAN
DAY 2

MD: _____

DIAGNOSIS: ASTHMA _____

RN/MD REVIEW: _____

DATE: _____

MAP DOES NOT REPLACE MD ORDERS

		NOTES
TESTS/ PROCEDURES/ TREATMENTS:	Peak flow daily.	
MEDICATION:	1. Prednisone 40mg. po daily when PF >200 or >40% predicted in combination with clinical improvement. Asthma team will aid in decision as to timing of switch from Methylprednisolone IVSS to Prednisone P.O. 2. Triamcinolone (Azmacort MDI) 10 puffs BID with spacer. 3. Albuterol (Proventil/Ventolin) 4 puffs Q4H and PRN with spacer. 4. If patient is trained and able to use spacer all nebulized medications should be discontinued ASAP.	
ACTIVITY:	Encourage ambulation.	
NUTRITION:	Diet as tolerated.	
CONSULTS:		
PATIENT EDUCATION:	1. The following teaching reinforcement by house staff/asthma team as needed: A. Proper use of MDI teaching with spacer. B. Pathophysiology of disease. C. Differences in medication types. D. Possible side effects.	
SOCIAL WORK:	For patients requiring social work intervention, initiate psychosocial assessment and project discharge plan.	
DISCHARGE PLANNING:	Specific care provider and appointment identified to patient with earliest possible F/U in Chest and/or Medical Clinic. (BIMC APC Friday (Asthma clinic) Ext. 4313, 7th floor, Fierman Hall). RN to determine if new information or patient's response to treatment warrants social work intervention if not proceed with home health care evaluation as appropriate.	

SHIFT	INITIALS	PRINT NAME	SIGNATURE

Beth Israel Medical Center
MULTIDISCIPLINARY ACTION PLAN
DAY 2: NURSING DOCUMENTATION

MD: _____

DIAGNOSIS: ASTHMA _____

DATE: _____

2200

PATIENT PROBLEM AND NURSING INTERVENTIONS	EXPECTED PATIENT OUTCOME AND/OR DISCHARGE OUTCOME	ASSESSMENT/ EVALUATION		
1. IMPAIRED BREATHING DUE TO HYPERACTIVE AIRWAY AND AIRWAY INFLAMMATION	**1. BREATHING PATTERN WILL BE NORMAL OR NEAR NORMAL**			
A. Lung auscultation every 8 hours and PRN.	A. Improved breath sounds by auscultation (minimal or decrease in wheezing).	A.	A.	A.
B. Vitals/temperature Q8H and PRN.	B. Vital signs near normal.	B.	B.	B.
C. Ensure adequate hydration to enhance expectoration.	C. Good hydration, able to expectorate sputum.	C.	C.	C.
D. Reassess need for O$_2$.	D. Minimal to no SOB, minimal wheezing.	D.	D.	D.
E. Administer asthma medications, as per MD order.	E. Respiratory rate near normal. Less chest tightness, wheezing.	E.	E.	E.
F. Notify MD for any signs of deterioration.	F. Improved respiratory status.	F.	F.	F.
G. Measure peakflow pre/post Albuterol use.	G. Improved peakflow.	G.	G.	G.
2. SLEEP AND REST DEPRIVATION DUE TO FREQUENT COUGH	**2. IMPROVED SLEEP/REST**			
A. Administer bronchodilator inhaler (proventil/ventolin) prior to bedtime and PRN.	A. Improved breathing, able to sleep/rest, minimal coughing spells.	A.	A.	A.
B. Comfort measures: position of comfort he/she chooses, tissue/kidney basin at patient's reach.	B. Verbalize comfort and rest.	B.	B.	B.
C. Enhance feeling of security by Call Bell within reach, easy access to inhalers.	C. Verbalizes feeling of security.	C.	C.	C.
3. KNOWLEDGE DEFICIT ACTUAL OR POTENTIAL R/T ASTHMA	**3. INCREASED KNOWLEDGE OF DISEASE AND TREATMENT**			
A. Review the following teachings:	A.	A.	A.	A.
1. Asthma pathophysiology.	1. Verbalize understanding.	1.	1.	1.
2. Asthma medication dose, frequency, purpose, expected effect and it's side effects.	2. Verbalize understanding.	2.	2.	2.
3. Differentiation in function of inhalers.	3. Return demonstration.	3.	3.	3.
4. Emphasize proper MDI use with spacer.	4. Verbalize understanding.	4.	4.	4.
5. Maintenance and care of spacer.	5. Verbalize understanding.	5.	5.	5.
B. Assist patient in identifying specific asthma triggers.	B. Patient able to identify at least 3 triggers.	B.	B.	B.
C. Instruct patient on management of asthma triggers.	C. Patient able to verbalize appropriate management of asthma triggers.	C.	C.	C.
D. Review ongoing treatment plan.	D. Verbalize understanding.	D.	D.	D.
E. Review discharge plan.	E. Verbalize understanding.	E.	E.	E.
F. Discuss follow-up appointment as per asthma teams recommendation.	F. Verbalize understanding.	F.	F.	F.

APPENDIX A-6

Beth Israel Medical Center
MULTIDISCIPLINARY ACTION PLAN
DAY 3

MD: _____
DIAGNOSIS: <u>ASTHMA</u>_____
RN/MD REVIEW: _____
DATE: _____

MAP DOES NOT REPLACE MD ORDERS

NOTES

TESTS/ PROCEDURES/ TREATMENTS:	Peak flow daily.
MEDICATION:	1. Prednisone 40mg. po daily when PF >200 or >40% predicted in combination with clinical improvement. Asthma team will aid in decision as to timing of switch from Methylprednisolone IVSS to Prednisone P.O. 2. Triamcinolone (Azmacort MDI) 10 puffs BID with spacer. 3. Albuterol (Proventil/Ventolin) 4 puffs Q4H and PRN with spacer. 4. If patient is trained and able to use spacer all nebulized medications should be discontinued ASAP.
ACTIVITY:	Encourage ambulation.
NUTRITION:	Diet as tolerated.
CONSULTS:	
PATIENT EDUCATION:	1. The following teaching reinforcement by house staff/asthma team as needed: A. Proper use of MDI teaching with spacer. B. Pathophysiology of disease. C. Differences in medication types. D. Possible side effects.
SOCIAL WORK:	Continued assessment intervention and planning with RN and MD; ensure that necessary forms and referrals have been completed and that necessary services are available.
DISCHARGE PLANNING:	Specific care provider and appointment identified to patient with earliest possible F/U in Chest and/or Medical Clinic. (**BIMC APC Friday (Asthma clinic) Ext. 4313, 7th floor, Fierman Hall**). RN to confirm plans for Home Health Care if indicated if social work not involved verify patient's readiness for discharge.

SHIFT	INITIALS	PRINT NAME	SIGNATURE

APPENDIX **A-7**

Beth Israel Medical Center
MULTIDISCIPLINARY ACTION PLAN
DAY 3: NURSING DOCUMENTATION

MD: _____

DIAGNOSIS: ASTHMA _____

DATE: _____

2200

PATIENT PROBLEM AND NURSING INTERVENTIONS	EXPECTED PATIENT OUTCOME AND/OR DISCHARGE OUTCOME	ASSESSMENT/ EVALUATION		
1. IMPAIRED BREATHING DUE TO HYPERACTIVE AIRWAY AND AIRWAY INFLAMMATION	**1. BREATHING PATTERN WILL BE NORMAL OR NEAR NORMAL**			
A. Lung auscultation every 8 hours and PRN.	A. Improved breath sounds by auscultation (absence or minimal wheezes).	A.	A.	A.
B. Vitals/temperature Q8H and PRN.	B. Vital signs within normal.	B.	B.	B.
C. Ensure adequate hydration to enhance expectoration.	C. Good hydration, able to expectorate sputum.	C.	C.	C.
D. Reassess need for O_2.	D. Minimal to no SOB, minimal wheezing.	D.	D.	D.
E. Administer asthma medications, as per MD order.	E. Respiratory rate near normal. Less chest tightness, wheezing.	E.	E.	E.
F. Notify MD for any signs of deterioration.	F. Improved respiratory status.	F.	F.	F.
G. Measure peak flow pre/post albuterol use.	G. Improved peak flow.	G.	G.	G.
2. SLEEP AND REST DEPRIVATION DUE TO FREQUENT COUGH	**2. IMPROVED SLEEP/REST**			
A. Administer bronchodilator inhaler (proventil/Ventolin) prior to bedtime and PRN.	A. Improved breathing, able to sleep/rest, minimal coughing spells.	A.	A.	A.
B. Comfort measures: position OI comfort he/she chooses, tissue/kidney basin at patient's reach.	B. Verbalize comfort and rest.	B.	B.	B.
C. Enhance feeling of security by Call Bell within reach, easy access to inhalers.	C. Verbalizes feeling of security.	C.	C.	C.
3. KNOWLEDGE DEFICIT ACTUAL OR POTENTIAL R/T ASTHMA	**3. INCREASED KNOWLEDGE OF DISEASE AND TREATMENT**			
A. Review the following teachings: 1. Asthma pathophysiology. 2. Asthma medication dose, frequency, purpose, expected effect and it's side effects. 3. Differentiation in function of inhalers. 4. Emphasize proper MDI use with spacer. 5. Maintenance and care of spacer.	A. 1. Verbalize understanding. 2. Verbalize understanding. 3. Return demonstration. 4. Verbalize understanding. 5. Verbalize understanding.	A. 1. 2. 3. 4. 5.	A. 1. 2. 3. 4. 5.	A. 1. 2. 3. 4. 5.
B. Assist patient in identifying specific asthma triggers.	B. Patient able to identify at least 3 triggers.	B.	B.	B.
C. Instruct patient on management of asthma triggers.	C. Patient able to verbalize appropriate management of asthma triggers.	C.	C.	C.
D. Review ongoing treatment plan.	D. Verbalize understanding.	D.	D.	D.
E. Review discharge plan.	E. Verbalize understanding.	E.	E.	E.
F. Provide follow-up appointment.	F. Verbalize understanding.	F.	F.	F.

APPENDIX A-8

Beth Israel Medical Center
MULTIDISCIPLINARY ACTION PLAN
DAY 4

MD: _____
DIAGNOSIS: ASTHMA _____
RN/MD REVIEW: _____
DATE: _____

MAP DOES NOT REPLACE MD ORDERS

NOTES

TESTS/ PROCEDURES/ TREATMENTS:	Peak flow daily.
MEDICATION:	1. Prednisone 40mg. po daily when PF >200 or >40 predicted in combination with clinical improvement. Asthma team will aid in decision as to timing of switch from Methylprednisolone IVSS to Prednisone P.O. 2. Triamcinolone (Azmacort MDI) 10 puffs BID with spacer. 3. Albuterol (Proventil/Ventolin) 4 puffs Q4H and PRN with spacer.
ACTIVITY:	Encourage ambulation.
NUTRITION:	Diet as tolerated.
CONSULTS:	
PATIENT EDUCATION:	1. The following teaching reinforcement by house staff/asthma team as needed: A. Proper use of MDI teaching with spacer. B. Pathophysiology of disease. C. Differences in medication type. D. Possible side effects.
SOCIAL WORK:	Re-confirm patient's readiness with RN and MD provide patient with written social work discharge plan.
DISCHARGE PLANNING:	Specific care provider and appointment identified to patient with earliest possible F/U in Chest and/or Medical Clinic. (BIMC APC Friday (Asthma clinic) Ext. 4313, 7th floor, Fierman Hall). Re-confirm with MD and social work. Provide patient with written instructions and discharge teaching form.

SHIFT	INITIALS	PRINT NAME	SIGNATURE

MAP 029 (Rev 12/94). Copyright Beth Israel Medical Center 1992. All rights reserved

APPENDIX A-9

Beth Israel Medical Center
MULTIDISCIPLINARY ACTION PLAN
DAY 4: NURSING DOCUMENTATION

MD: _____

DIAGNOSIS: ASTHMA _____

DATE: _____

2200

PATIENT PROBLEM AND NURSING INTERVENTIONS	EXPECTED PATIENT OUTCOME AND/OR DISCHARGE OUTCOME	ASSESSMENT/ EVALUATION		
1. IMPAIRED BREATHING DUE TO HYPERACTIVE AIRWAY AND AIRWAY INFLAMMATION	**1. BREATHING PATTERN WILL BE NORMAL OR NEAR NORMAL**			
A. Lung auscultation every 8 hours and PRN.	A. Improved breath sounds by auscultation (absence or minimal wheezes).	A.	A.	A.
B. Vitals/temperature Q8H and PRN.	B. Vital signs within normal.	B.	B.	B.
C. Ensure adequate hydration to enhance expectoration.	C. Good hydration, able to expectorate sputum.	C.	C.	C.
D. Reassess need for O$_2$.	D. No SOB, minimal wheezing.	D.	D.	D.
E. Administer asthma medications, as per MD order.	E. Respiratory rate near or normal. Less chest tightness.	E.	E.	E.
F. Notify MD for any signs of deterioration.	F. Improved respiratory status.	F.	F.	F.
2. SLEEP AND REST DEPRIVATION DUE TO FREQUENT COUGH	**2. IMPROVED SLEEP/REST**			
A. Administer bronchodilator inhaler (proventil/ventolin) prior to bedtime and PRN.	A. Improved breathing, able to sleep/rest.	A.	A.	A.
B. Comfort measures: position Ol comfort he/she chooses, tissue/kidney basin at patient's reach.	B. Verbalize comfort and rest.	B.	B.	B.
C. Enhance feeling of security by Call Bell within reach, easy access to inhalers.	C. Verbalizes feeling of security.	C.	C.	C.
3. KNOWLEDGE DEFICIT ACTUAL OR POTENTIAL R/T ASTHMA	**3. INCREASED KNOWLEDGE OF DISEASE AND TREATMENT**			
A. Review the following teachings:	A.	A.	A.	A.
1. Asthma pathophysiology.	1. Verbalize understanding.	1.	1.	1.
2. Asthma medication dose, frequency, purpose, expected effect and it's side effects.	2. Verbalize understanding.	2.	2.	2.
3. Differentiation in function of inhalers.	3. Return demonstration.	3.	3.	3.
4. Emphasize proper MDI use with spacer.	4. Verbalize understanding.	4.	4.	4.
5. Maintenance and care of spacer.	5. Verbalize understanding.	5.	5.	5.
B. Assist patient in identifying specific asthma triggers.	B. Patient able to identify at least 3 triggers.	B.	B.	B.
C. Instruct patient on management of asthma triggers.	C. Patient able to verbalize appropriate management of asthma triggers.	C.	C.	C.
D. Provide follow-up appointment.	D. Verbalize understanding.	D.	D.	D.

APPENDIX A-10

Beth Israel Medical Center

MULTIDISCIPLINARY ACTION PLAN

DATE/TIME	PROGRESS NOTES

A P P E N D I X B-1

Beth Israel Medical Center
MULTIDISCIPLINARY ACTION PLAN
DAY 1

MD: _____

DIAGNOSIS: CHEMOTHERAPY (5 DAY PROTOCOL)

DATE: _____

PATIENT PROBLEM AND NURSING INTERVENTIONS	EXPECTED PATIENT OUTCOME AND/OR DISCHARGE OUTCOME	ASSESSMENT/EVALUATION		
1. KNOWLEDGE DEFICIT/ANXIETY	**1. INCREASED KNOWLEDGE OF TREATMENT PLAN/ DIMINISHED ANXIETY**			
A. Orient to room, unit and routine. B. Discuss chemotherapy & premed. C. Encourage PO fluids. D. Explain reason for strict I&O. E. Offer & discuss with pt "Chemotherapy & You" (NIH) booklet. F. Refer to support groups. G. Review treatment plan and projected date of discharge with pt and/or significant other.	A. Diminished anxiety. B. Verbalizes understanding. C. Verbalizes understanding. D. Verbalizes understanding. E. Verbalizes understanding. F. Participates in support group. G. Understanding of treatment and discharge plans.	A. B. C. D. E. F. G.	A. B. C. D. E. F. G.	A. B. C. D. E. F. G.
2. NUTRITION ALTERATION: LESS THAN BODY REQUIREMENT RELATED TO NAUSEA, VOMITING STOMATITIS, DYSPHAGIA	**2. MAINTAIN OPTIMAL NUTRITIONAL STATUS**			
A. Assess pt's height and weight. B. Assess oral cavity. C. Assess for special dietary needs. D. Assess for history of N&V related to chemotherapy. E. Assess pt's tolerance of meals. F. Discuss frequent mouth care. G. Eval. effectiveness of antiemetics.	 B. Clear and intact. D. N&V will be minimal or controlled. E. Tolerates well. F. Complies with mouth care. G. No nausea or vomiting.	A.See Adm Assmt B. C. D. E. F. G.	A.See Adm Assmt B. C. D. E. F. G.	A.See Adm Assmt B. C. D. E. F. G.
3. FLUID VOLUME DEFICIT RELATED TO TREATMENT AND DISEASE PROCESS	**3. FREE OF SIGNS OF DEHYDRATION OR RENAL DYSFUNCTION**			
A. Assess I&O Q8H. B. Assess for dehydration: lethargy; dark & decreased urine output; poor skin turgor;dry & cracked mucous membrane C. Monitor vital signs Q8H. D. Evaluate appropriate lab values (CBC, PLT, BUN/Creat Mag. Potassium) prior to chemo adm. E. Institute IV fluids order.	A. Balanced I&O. B. No signs of dehydration. C. Vital signs WNL. D. Lab values are acceptable parameters for treatment.	A. See I&O Record B. C. See Flowsheet D. E.	A. See I&O Record B. C. See Flowsheet D. E.	A. See I&O Record B. C. See Flowsheet D. E.
4. ALTERATION IN COMFORT RELATED TO DISEASE PROCESS	**4. EXPERIENCE DIMINISHED PAIN**			
A. Ask pt to rate pain using 0-10 pain scale provided on Daily Pt Care Flowsheet (Refer to pain guidelines). B. Medicate patient as ordered. C. Eval. effec. of pain med.2H after PO/PRadm 1H after parenteral adm. D. Provide quiet environment. E. Position patient for comfort. F. Discuss distraction relaxation techs. (ex. breathing, exercises).	A. Verbalize pain relief. B. Taken as needed. C. Relate relief. D. Feels relaxed & comfortable. E. Feels relaxed & comfortable. F. Feels relaxed & comfortable.	A. See Flow Sheet B. C. See Flow Sheet D. E. F.	A. See Flow Sheet B. C. See Flow Sheet D. E. F.	A. See Flow Sheet B. C. See Flow Sheet D. E. F.

MAP 046 (Rev 7/94)

Beth Israel Medical Center
MULTIDISCIPLINARY ACTION PLAN
DAY 2

MD: _____

DIAGNOSIS: CHEMOTHERAPY (5 DAY PROTOCOL)

RN/MD REVIEW: _____

DATE: _____

MAP DOES NOT REPLACE MD ORDERS

CHRONIC PAIN MANAGEMENT	Assess pain Q8H. Score pain using the Pain/Relief scale. Follow chronic pain management guidelines. Assess effectiveness of pain medication. Consider changing pain medication, if no relief.		
PAIN GUIDELINES	I **IF PAIN SCORE <5** A. **ASSESS IF THIS IS AN ACCEPTABLE LEVEL OF PAIN FOR PATIENT.** B. **ASSESS FOR COMFORT MEASURES: PHARMACOLOGICAL, POSITIONING, RELAXATION, DISTRACTION.**	II **IF PAIN SCORE >5** A. **REVIEW LAST PRN DOSE OF PAIN MED.** B. **IDENTIFY IF PATIENT HAS STANDING PAIN MEDICATION ORDERED.** C. **EVALUATE IF PAIN IS RELATED TO ANY RECENT ACTIVITY OR PROCEDURE.** D. **ASSESS PAIN LOCATION (OLD VS NEW).** E. **ASSESS SEDATION LEVEL USING THE 0-5 SEDATION SCALE PROVIDED ON THE DAILY PT CARE FLOW SHEET.** F. **ASSESS FOR NAUSEA OR VOMITING.**	III. **IF 2 CONSECUTIVE PAIN SCORES >5** A. **NOTIFY MD** B. **DOCUMENT IN PROGRESS NOTES.**
TESTS/ PROCEDURES/ TREATMENTS:			**NOTES**
MEDICATION	Premedications: Chemotherapy: Antiemetic therapy: Compazine 10mg IVPB/PO/IM PRN Consider (pain control). Consider MAGIC mouthwash		
ACTIVITY	Out of bed ad lib.		
NUTRITION	Regular diet and supplemental feedings as tolerated.		
CONSULTS	Pain team (if indicated).		
SOCIAL WORK	Continued assessment, intervention and planning with RN and MD as well as patient and family.		
DISCHARGE PLANNING	Interdisciplinary consultation regarding patient's clinical status and discharge needs.		

SHIFT	INITIALS	PRINT NAME	SIGNATURE

MAP 046 (Rev 7/94)

APPENDIX C-1

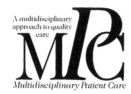

BETH ISRAEL MEDICAL CENTER

MULTI-DISCIPLINARY ACTION PLAN

DIAGNOSIS: <u>PERITONEAL DIALYSIS:</u>
<u>POST-CATHETER PLACEMENT</u>

UNIT: _____

ADMISSION DATE: _____/_____/_____ **TIME:** _____:_____ AM/PM

DATE MAP INITIATED: _____/_____/_____ **TIME:** _____:_____ AM/PM

DRG #: <u>468</u>

EXPECTED LENGTH OF STAY: <u>4 DAYS</u>

SHORT TRIM POINT: <u>3 DAYS</u>

FOLLOWED BY PATIENT CARE MANAGER: YES ☐   NO ☐
(If Yes) Name: _____

SOCIAL WORKER: _____

GOALS MUTUALLY SET WITH PATIENT AND/OR FAMILY

_____ YES

_____ NO   EXPLAIN _____

_____

PRIOR MEDICAL HISTORY: _____

_____

_____

PATIENT ALLERGIES: _____   YES/NO   DATE

_____

_____   DNR: _____

HEALTH CARE PROXY

OR LIVING WILL:_____

<u>Beth Israel Medical Center</u>
MULTIDISCIPLINARY ACTION PLAN
DAY 1 OF 4

MD: _____

DIAGNOSIS: <u>PERITONEAL DIALYSIS:</u>
             <u>POST CATHETER PLACEMENT</u>

RN/MD REVIEW: _____

DATE: _____

MAP DOES NOT REPLACE MD ORDERS   **NOTES**

HISTORY/PHYSICAL EXAM/TESTS/ PROCEDURES/ TREATMENTS:	Complete medical history/physical assessment by MD. Daily weight. I&O. CXR, EKG. CBC with DIFF. SMAC 20. <u>PD Orders:</u> Dialyzing solution, volume, sequence, percentage dextrose to be determined by renal MD. Only renal MD may write orders for PD, including any additives. PD fluid for cell count and C&S.	
MEDICATION:	Review pre-admission medications intake and order as necessary. If patient did not receive prophylactic antibiotics prior to catheter insertion, please give vancomycin 1 gram, IV and tobramycin 80 mg. IV. Vitamins, calcium, colace, iron, erythropoietin, anti-hypertensive medications. Intraperitoneal medication as determined by renal MD. (e.g. Heparin 1000 units/exchange if evidence of fibrin like fluid/blood tinged).	
ACTIVITY:	As tolerated.	
NUTRITION:	Determined by medical condition. <u>Consider:</u> Adequate protein intake, low sodium, low potassium, modified fluid restriction (approximately 1 ½ quarts per day - advise patient to drink only when thirsty). Daily weight.	
CONSULTS:	CAPD Nurse Clinician, extension 4070, when PD catheter is placed (if patient is going to be followed up at CAPD clinic). Nutritionist to see patient.	
SOCIAL WORK:	Consult with medical and nursing staff regarding patient's psychosocial needs and begin discharge planning assessment if indicated.	
DISCHARGE PLANNING:	RN and MD to refer to social work if indicated.	

SHIFT	INITIALS	PRINT NAME	SIGNATURE

Map 069-5-94

Beth Israel Medical Center
MULTIDISCIPLINARY ACTION PLAN
DAY 1 OF 4
MD: _____
DIAGNOSIS: PERITONEAL DIALYSIS:
           POST CATHETER PLACEMENT
DATE: _____

PATIENT PROBLEM AND NURSING INTERVENTIONS	EXPECTED PT OUTCOME AND/OR DISCHARGE OUTCOME	ASSESSMENT/EVALUATION		
1. POTENTIAL FOR FLUID AND ELECTROLYTE IMBALANCE R/T RENAL FAILURE.	1. MAINTAIN FLUID & ELECTROLYTE BALANCE			
1A. Daily wts, after draining the peritoneal cavity. B. Record Intake and Output Q8H. C. Maintain peritoneal dialysis record. Record time of beginning & end of each exchange, amt. of solution instilled & amount drained. Fluid balance. Number each exchange. Meds in dialyzing solution as per MD.	A. B. C.	A. See Flowsheet B. See I&O Sheet C. See PD Record	A. See Flowsheet B. See I&O Sheet C. See PD Record	A. See Flowsheet B. See I&O Sheet C. See PD Record
D. Assess for fluid overload and report to MD: HTN, rales, dyspnea, distended neck veins, pounding pulse, peripheral edema.	D. No fluid overload noted.	D.	D.	D.
E. Assess for fluid volume deficit & report: Headache, dizziness, hypotension, tachycardia, poor skin turgor, wt loss.	E. No fluid volume deficit noted.	E.	E.	E.
F. Evaluate outflow of dialysis fluid for obstruction, tubing kinks or drainage around cath site.	F. Dialysis fluid outflows freely.	F.	F.	F.
G. Monitor electrolytes and report abnormal values or signs and symptoms of imbalance.	G. Electrolytes are normal or near normal.	G.	G.	G.
2. POTENTIAL FOR INFECTION	2. FREE OF INFECTION			
A. Maintain sterile tech when connecting or disconnecting catheter during dialysis and when adding medications to solution.	A. Infection free.	A.	A.	A.
B. Report to MD and culture drainage if presence of fibrin, cloudy or bloody.	B. Done as needed.	B.	B.	B.
C. Assess catheter exit site for redness, swelling, or leakage. Change dressing if saturated.	C. No changes in exit site.	C.	C.	C.
D. Be certain catheter tube is securely anchored; avoid tension.	D. Catheter is safe.	D.	D.	D.
3. KNOWLEDGE DEFICIT.	3. INCREASED KNOWLEDGE OF DISEASE & TREATMENT			
A. Assess knowledge of renal disease and teach patient as needed.	A. Verbalize understanding of disease process.	A.	A.	A.
B. Teach pt about the need for peritoneal dialysis. Have pt watch first 4 exchanges demonstrated & explained by nurse performing peritoneal dialysis.	B. Verbalize understanding of peritoneal dialysis procedure.	B.	B.	B.
C. Instruct pt to report undesirable signs & symptoms post discharge to Peritoneal Dialysis Team: fever, abdominal pain or distension, nausea, vomiting, vertigo, edema or rapid wt gain, signs of infection at catheter site or dialysis drainage.	C. Verbalize symptoms to report to Dialysis Team.	C.	C.	C.
D. Review discharge plan & projected date of discharge with pt and/or significant other.	D. Verbalize understanding of discharge plan.	D.	D.	D.

APPENDIX C-4

Beth Israel Medical Center
MULTIDISCIPLINARY ACTION PLAN

DAY 2 OF 4

MD: _____

DIAGNOSIS: PERITONEAL DIALYSIS: _____

POST CATHETER PLACEMENT _____

RN/MD REVIEW: _____

DATE: _____

MAP DOES NOT REPLACE MD ORDERS

NOTES

HISTORY/PHYSICAL EXAM/TESTS/ PROCEDURES/ TREATMENTS:	Follow PD instructions for volume, sequence, percentage dextrose. Only renal MD may write orders for PD. PD fluid for cell count and C&S (only if fluid cloudy, presence of fibrin or bloody). Daily weights. I&O.	
MEDICATION:	Vitamins, calcium, colace, iron, erythropoietin. Anti-hypertensive medications. Intraperitoneal medication as determined by renal MD (e.g. Heparin 1000 units/exchange if evidence of fibrin like fluid/blood tinged).	
ACTIVITY:	As tolerated.	
NUTRITION:	Determined by medical condition. <u>Consider:</u> Adequate protein intake, low sodium, low potassium, modified fluid restriction (approximately 1 ½ quarts per day daily weight - advise patient to drink only when thirsty).	
CONSULTS:	CAPD Nurse Clinician. Ensure that nutritionist screened patient.	
SOCIAL WORK:	Assess future needs, prepare and formulate social work intervention plan; consider referral to HHIC for home care, if appropriate.	
DISCHARGE PLANNING:	RN and MD to advise social work regarding patient's response to treatment and preliminary discharge needs.	

SHIFT	INITIALS	PRINT NAME	SIGNATURE

Map 069-5-94

APPENDIX C-5

Beth Israel Medical Center
MULTIDISCIPLINARY ACTION PLAN
DAY 2 OF 4

MD: _____

DIAGNOSIS: PERITONEAL DIALYSIS:
POST CATHETER PLACEMENT

DATE: _____

PATIENT PROBLEM AND NURSING INTERVENTIONS	EXPECTED PT OUTCOME AND/OR DISCHARGE OUTCOME	ASSESSMENT/EVALUATION		
1. POTENTIAL FOR FLUID AND ELECTRO- LYTE IMBALANCE R/T RENAL FAILURE.	**1. MAINTAIN FLUID AND ELECTROLYTE BALANCE.**			
1A. Daily weights, after draining the peritoneal cavity.	A.	A. See Flowsheet	A. See Flowsheet	A. See Flowsheet
B. Record Intake and Output Q8H.	B.	B. See I&O Sheet	B. See I&O Sheet	B. See I&O Sheet
C. Maintain peritoneal dialysis record. Record time of beginning and end of each ex- change, amt of solution instilled and amount drained. Fluid balance. Number each exchange. Meds in dialyzing solution as per MD.	C.	C. See PD Record	C. See PD Record,	C. See PD Record
D. Assess for fluid overload and report to MD: HTN, rales, dyspnea, distended neck veins, pounding pulse, peripheral edema.	D. No fluid overload noted.	D.	D.	D.
E. Assess for fluid volume deficit and report: Headache, dizziness, hypotension, tachycardia, poor skin turgor, weight loss.	E. No fluid volume deficit noted.	E.	E.	E.
F. Evaluate outflow of dialysis fluid for obstruction, tubing kinks or drainage around catheter site.	F. Dialysis fluid outflows freely.	F.	F.	F.
G. Monitor electrolytes and report abnormal values or signs & symptoms of imbalance.	G. Electrolytes are normal or near normal.	G.	G.	G.
2. POTENTIAL FOR INFECTION	**2. FREE OF INFECTION.**			
A. Maintain sterile technique when connecting or disconnecting catheter during dialysis and when adding medications to solution.	A. Infection free.	A.	A.	A.
B. Report to MD and culture drainage if presence of fibrin, cloudy or bloody.	B. Done as needed.	B.	B.	B.
C. Assess catheter exit site for redness, swelling, or leakage. Change dressing if saturated.	C. No changes in exit site.	C.	C.	C.
D. Be certain catheter tube is securely anchored; avoid tension.	D. Catheter is safe.	D.	D.	D.
3. KNOWLEDGE DEFICIT.	**3. VERBALIZE INSTRUC- TIONS PROVIDED**			
3A. Teach procedure for peritoneal dialysis. Have patient participate in exchanges as nurse performing peritoneal dialysis talks patient through procedure.	A. Understanding of peri- toneal dialysis procedure.	A.	A.	A.
B. Teach patient about strength of solution being used for exchange.	B. Understanding of fluid used for dialysis.	B.	B.	B.
C. Teach names of medications, dosage, purpose, schedule and side effects.	C. Understanding of medications instructions.	C.	C.	C.
D. Reinforce disease process, signs and symptoms, to report to Peritoneal Dialysis Team as needed.	D. Understanding of disease process and symptoms to report to Dialysis Team.	D.	D.	D.

A P P E N D I X **C-6**

Beth Israel Medical Center
MULTIDISCIPLINARY ACTION PLAN

DAY 3 OF 4

MD: _____

DIAGNOSIS: <u>PERITONEAL DIALYSIS:</u>
                     <u>POST CATHETER PLACEMENT</u>

RN/MD REVIEW: _____

DATE: _____

MAP DOES NOT REPLACE MD ORDERS   NOTES

HISTORY/PHYSICAL EXAM/TESTS/ PROCEDURES/ TREATMENTS:	Daily weights. Intake and Output. SMA7, PD fluid for cell count and C&S. Continue Peritoneal Dialysis as ordered.	
MEDICATION:	Vitamins, calcium, colace, iron, erythropoietin. Anti-hypertensive medication. Intraperitoneal medication as determined by renal MD (e.g. Heparin 1000 units/exchange if evidence of fibrin like fluid/blood tinged).	
ACTIVITY:	As tolerated.	
NUTRITION:	Determined by medical condition. <u>Consider:</u> Adequate protein intake, low sodium, low potassium, modified fluid restriction (approximately 1 ½ quarts per day daily weight - advise patient to drink only when thirsty).	
CONSULTS:	Ensure that patient is evaluated by CAPD Nurse Clinician.	
SOCIAL WORK:	Finalize discharge plan. Confirm discharge plan with patient and family. Arrange transportation if needed.	
DISCHARGE PLANNING:	MD to confirm discharge with patient and social work. RN to insure that prescriptions are completed by MD.	

SHIFT	INITIALS	PRINT NAME	SIGNATURE

Map 069-5-94

APPENDIX **C-7**

<u>Beth Israel Medical Center</u>
MULTIDISCIPLINARY ACTION PLAN
DAY 3 OF 4
MD: _____
DIAGNOSIS: <u>PERITONEAL DIALYSIS:</u>
<u>POST CATHETER PLACEMENT</u>
DATE: _____

PATIENT PROBLEM AND NURSING INTERVENTIONS	EXPECTED PT OUTCOME AND/OR DISCHARGE OUTCOME	ASSESSMENT/EVALUATION		
1. **POTENTIAL FOR FLUID AND ELECTROLYTE IMBALANCE R/T RENAL FAILURE.**	1. **MAINTAIN FLUID AND ELECTROLYTE BALANCE.**			
A. Daily wts, after draining peritoneal cavity. B. Record Intake and Output Q8H. C. Maintain peritoneal dialysis record. Record time of beginning & end of each ex-change, amt of solution instilled & amount drained. Fluid balance. # each exchange. Meds in dialyzing solution per MD. D. Assess for fluid overload & report to MD: HTN, rales, dyspnea, distended neck veins, pounding pulse, peripheral edema. E. Assess fluid volume deficit & report: Headache, dizziness, hypotension, tachycardia, poor skin turgor, wt loss. F. Evaluate outflow of dialysis fluid for obstruction, tubing kinks or drainage around catheter site. G. Monitor electrolytes & report abnormal values or signs & symptoms of imbalance.	A. B. C. D. No fluid overload noted. E. No fluid volume deficit noted. F. Dialysis fluid outflows freely. G. Electrolytes are normal or near normal.	A. See Flowsheet B. See I&O Sheet C. See PD Record D. E. F. G.	A. See Flowsheet B. See I&O Sheet C. See PD Record D. E. F. G.	A. See Flowsheet B. See I&O Sheet C. See PD Record D. E. F. G.
2. **POTENTIAL FOR INFECTION**	2. **FREE OF INFECTION**			
A. Maintain sterile tech. when connecting or disconnecting catheter during dialysis & when adding meds to solution. B. Report to MD and culture drainage if presence of fibrin, cloudy or bloody. C. Assess catheter exit site for redness, swelling, or leakage. Change dressing if saturated. D. Be certain catheter tube is securely anchored; avoid tension.	A. Infection free. B. Done as needed. C. No changes in exit site. D. Catheter is safe.	A. B. C. D.	A. B. C. D.	A. B. C. D.
3. **KNOWLEDGE DEFICIT.**	3. **INCREASED KNOWLEDGE OF DISEASE PROCESS & TREATMENT**			
A. Teach procedure for peritoneal dialysis by having pt do peritoneal dialysis exchange, as nurse responsible for peritoneal dialysis reinforces as needed. B. Teach skin & peritoneal catheter care: Protect catheter from damage. Keep sterile cap & dressing in place. Teach pt to perform exit site dressing change, after bath/shower. Cover site with sterile dressing. C. Instruct pt to avoid over-the-counter meds unless approved by M.D. D. Reinforce disease process, signs and symptoms, to report to Peritoneal Dialysis Team as needed.	A. Able to perform peritoneal dialysis procedure successfully. B. Able to perform exit site care successfully. C. Verbalize understanding of instructions. D. Verbalize understanding of disease process & symptoms to report to Dialysis Team.	A. B. C. D.	A. B. C. D.	A. B. C. D.

Map 069-5-94

Beth Israel Medical Center
MULTIDISCIPLINARY ACTION PLAN
DAY 4 OF 4

MD: _____

DIAGNOSIS: PERITONEAL DIALYSIS:
POST CATHETER PLACEMENT

RN/MD REVIEW: _____

DATE: _____

MAP DOES NOT REPLACE MD ORDERS   NOTES

HISTORY/PHYSICAL EXAM/TESTS/ PROCEDURES/ TREATMENTS:	Daily weights. Intake and Output. PD fluid for cell count and C&S (only if fluid is fibrin like, bloody or cloudy). Continue Peritoneal Dialysis as ordered. Schedule patient for follow-up in the CAPD out-patient clinic (if indicated).	
MEDICATION:	Vitamins, calcium, colace, iron, erythropoietin. Anti-hypertensive medications. Prescriptions to patient.	
ACTIVITY:	As tolerated.	
NUTRITION:	Determined by medical condition. Consider: Adequate protein intake, low sodium, low potassium, modified fluid restriction (approximately 1 ½ quarts per day daily weight - advise patient to drink only when thirsty). Ensure that patient has diet copy/instructions from dietician.	
CONSULTS:	Notify CAPD out-patient clinic of discharge.	
SOCIAL WORK:	Re-confirm medical clearance for discharge. Provide patient with written instructions and discharge form.	
DISCHARGE PLANNING:	All follow-up appointments and prescriptions are given to patient.	

SHIFT	INITIALS	PRINT NAME	SIGNATURE

Map 069-5-94

APPENDIX C-9

Beth Israel Medical Center
MULTIDISCIPLINARY ACTION PLAN
DAY 4 OF 4
MD: _____
DIAGNOSIS: PERITONEAL DIALYSIS: _____
            POST CATHETER PLACEMENT _____
DATE: _____

PATIENT PROBLEM AND NURSING INTERVENTIONS	EXPECTED PT OUTCOME AND/OR DISCHARGE OUTCOME	ASSESSMENT/EVALUATION		
1. POTENTIAL FOR FLUID AND ELECTRO-LYTE IMBALANCE R/T RENAL FAILURE	1. MAINTAIN FLUID & ELECTROLYTE BALANCE			
1A. Daily weights, after draining the peritoneal cavity.	A.	A. See Flowsheet	A. See Flowsheet	A. See Flowsheet
B. Record Intake and Output Q8H.	B.	B. See I&O Sheet	B. See I&O Sheet	B. See I&O Sheet
C. Maintain peritoneal dialysis record. Record time of beginning & end of each exchange, amount of solution instilled and amount drained. Fluid balance. Number each exchange. Meds in dialyzing solution as per MD.	C.	C. See PD Record	C. See PD Record	C. See PD Record
D. Assess for fluid overload & report to MD: HTN, rales, dyspnea, distended neck veins, pounding pulse, peripheral edema.	D. No fluid overload noted.	D.	D.	D.
E. Assess for fluid volume deficit & report: Headache, dizziness, hypo-tension, tachycardia, poor skin turgor, wt. loss.	E. No fluid volume deficit noted.	E.	E.	E.
F. Evaluate outflow of dialysis fluid for obstruction, tubing kinks or drainage around catheter site.	F. Dialysis fluid outflows freely.	F.	F.	F.
G. Monitor electrolytes & report abnormal values or signs&symptoms of imbalance	G. Electrolytes are normal or near normal.	G.	G.	G.
2. POTENTIAL FOR INFECTION	2. FREE OF INFECTION			
A. Maintain sterile technique when connecting or disconnecting catheter during dialysis and when adding medications to solution.	A. Infection free.	A.	A.	A.
B. Report to MD and culture drainage if presence of fibrin, cloudy or bloody.	B. Done as needed.	B.	B.	B.
C. Assess catheter exit site for redness, swelling, or leakage. Change dressing if saturated.	C. No changes in exit site.	C.	C.	C.
D. Be certain catheter tube is securely anchored; avoid tension.	D. Catheter is safe.	D.	D.	D.
3. KNOWLEDGE DEFICIT.	3. INCREASED KNOW-LEDGE RELATED TO DISEASE PROCESS AND TREATMENT.			
A. Evaluate pt's competency on performing CAPD exchanges and exit site care. Have pt demonstrate ability to do PD exchange without assistance.	A. Able to perf peritoneal dialysis procedure & exit site care successfully.	A.	A.	A.
B. Reinforce previous teachings as needed (medication, signs and symptoms of complications, PD catheter care).	B. Verbalize understanding of instructions.	B. See D/C Instruc.	B. See D/C Instruc.	B. See D/C Instruc.
C. Teach importance of follow-up care with CAPD out-patient clinic.	C. Verbalize understanding of discharge instructions.	C. See D/C Instruc.	C. See D/C Instruc.	C. See D/C Instruc.

Map 069-5-94

APPENDIX **D-1**

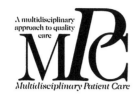

BETH ISRAEL MEDICAL CENTER

MULTI-DISCIPLINARY ACTION PLAN

DIAGNOSIS: <u>REHAB PROTOCOL</u>
<u>TOTAL HIP REPLACEMENT</u>

UNIT: <u>3 KARPAS</u>
DRG #: <u>DRG EXEMPT</u>
EXPECTED LENGTH OF STAY: <u>10 DAYS</u>

ADMISSION DATE TO 3 KARPAS: _____ / _____ / _____   **TIME:** _____ : _____ am/pm

DATE MAP INITIATED: _____ / _____ / _____   **TIME:** _____ : _____ am/pm

ATTENDING PHYSICIAN: _____ **RESIDENT PHYSICIAN:** _____

FOLLOWED BY PATIENT CARE MANAGER: ☐ YES   ☐ NO
    (If Yes) Name: _____

SOCIAL WORKER: _____

GOALS MUTUALLY SET WITH PATIENT AND/OR FAMILY
_____ YES _____ NO, EXPLAIN _____

ORTHOPEDIC SURGEON: _____ **INTERNIST:** _____

DATE OF SURGERY: _____ / _____ / _____

TYPE OF PROSTHESIS: _____ **CEMENTED:** ☐ **NONCEMENTED:** ☐

WEIGHT BEARING STATUS: _____ **PRIOR FUNCTIONAL STATUS (at home):**

UNTIL: _____ _____

PRIOR THERAPY: ☐ YES   ☐ NO   _____

THERAPIST: _____ **DATE INITIATED:** _____ / _____ / _____

STATUS: _____

PRIOR MEDICAL HISTORY: _____
_____

PATIENT ALLERGIES: _____   YES / NO   DATE

_____

_____   DNR:

HEALTH CARE PROXY

OR LIVING WILL: _____

APPENDIX **D-2**

<u>Beth Israel Medical Center</u>
MULTIDISCIPLINARY ACTION PLAN
DAY 1
MD: _____
DIAGNOSIS: <u>REHAB PROTOCOL - TOTAL HIP</u>
<u>REPLACEMENT</u>
RN/MD REVIEW: _____
DATE: _____

MAP DOES NOT REPLACE MD ORDERS

NOTES

TESTS/ PROCEDURES/ TREATMENTS:	Review x-ray films if not available, order lateral and frog leg films of affected hip. If no labs for 7 days: CBC, SMA7, UA, Clean Catch PT (keep 15-18) seconds Evaluate incision line and DC dressing if dry Obtain weight bearing status from Orthopedics Consider eggcrate mattress.	
MEDICATION	Maintain all prior medications for 24 hours Discontinue IV if no IV meds ordered. SC Heparin 5000U q12 hours if not on Coumadin If on Coumadin continue If high risk (obese, immobile, hypercoaguable): Coumadinize: 10mg QHS x 3 day Bowel program: Senokot 1-2 tabs PO QHS. Colace 100 mg TID (Glycerin suppository PRN). Patient to commode after breakfast	
ACTIVITY ROM LIMITATIONS	Weight bearing status per orthopedics; Out of bed; No hip flexion beyond 90°; No adduction beyond neutral; No internal rotation beyond neutral	
NUTRITION	As tolerated	
CONSULTS		
PATIENT EDUCATION	1. View rehab orientation video. 2. Instruct patient not to cross legs. 3. Keep abduction pillow between legs at all times. 4. Sit on high chair. 5. Use elevated toilet seat. 6. No injections in the affected leg.	
SOCIAL WORK	Initiate psychosocial and financial assessment.	
DISCHARGE PLANNING	RN to refer to social work and determine if Home Care Services were provided prior to admission	
PHYSICAL THERAPY	Physical therapy evaluation including: Range of motion Assessment of wound Strengthening Develop treatment plan including Function exercises and activities Mental status appropriate to func. STG & LTG. Sensation Initiate home exercise program Balance	**PHYSICAL THERAPY COMMENTS:** See Progress Notes for Initial Evaluation.
OCCUPATIONAL THERAPY	Occupational therapy evaluation including: Upper extremity function, basic self-care activities/instrumental ADL, physical demands of lifestyle, home accessibility, and support available in home.	**OCCUPATIONAL THERAPY COMMENTS:** See Progress Notes for Initial Evaluation

SHIFT	INITIALS	PRINT NAME	SIGNATURE	SHIFT	INITIALS	PRINT	SIGNATURE

Map 062 (Rev 6/94)

Beth Israel Medical Center
MULTIDISCIPLINARY ACTION PLAN
DAY 1
MD: _____

DIAGNOSIS: REHAB PROTOCOL - TOTAL HIP
REPLACEMENT

DATE: _____

MAP DOES NOT REPLACE MD ORDERS

PATIENT PROBLEM AND NURSING INTERVENTIONS	EXPECTED PATIENT OUTCOME AND/OR DISCHARGE OUTCOME	ASSESSMENT/EVALUATION		
1. KNOWLEDGE DEFICIT	**1. INCREASED KNOWLEDGE OF TREATMENT AND DISCHARGE PLAN**			
A. Orient to room and unit. B. Welcome to 3 Karpas letter. C. Orientation video. D. Teach activities per patient education section. E. Review plan of care & projected date of discharge with patient and/or significant other.	A. Diminished anxiety. B. Diminished anxiety. C. Verbal understanding. D. Verbalize understanding/demonstrate E. Verbalize understanding.	A. B. C. D E.	A. B. C. D. E.	A. B. C. D. E.
2. PAIN	**2. RELIEVED/DIMINISHED PAIN**			
A. Assess for verbal and nonverbal signs of pain. B. Assess pain score using pain/relief scale on the Daily Patient Care flowsheet. C. Administer analgesics as ordered D. Assess effectiveness of meds. E. Enc. relax techniques & diversional activities.	A. Relay symptoms. B. Low scores. C. Taken as needed. D. Pain relief. E. Pain relief.	A. B. See Flowsheet C. See MAR D. E.	A. B. See Flowsheet C. See MAR D. E.	A. B. See Flowsheet C. See MAR D. E.
3. IMPAIRED MOBILITY	**3. MAINTAIN OPTIMAL ACTIVITY**			
A. Review hip precautions B. Reinforce and instruct pt to keep abduction pillow between legs/use of raised toilet seat. C. Encourage OOB to high hip chair. D. TED stockings.	A. Apply/verbalize understanding. B. Follows instructions. C. Tolerate/use hip chair. D. No complications.	A. B. C. D.	A. B. C. D.	A. B. C. D.
4. POTENTIAL FOR ELIMINATION PROBLEMS	**4. MAINTAIN BASELINE PATTERN**			
A. Assess bowel and bladder status q8 hours. B. Institute "routines" as necessary. C. Use of raised toilet seat. D. Follow bowel program.	A. Resume normal pattern B. Resume normal pattern C. Able to use seat. D. Resume normal pattern	A. See Flowsheet B. C. D.	A. See Flowsheet B. C. D.	A. See Flowsheet B. C. D.
5. POTENTIAL FOR SKIN BREAKDOWN	**5. MAINTAIN SKIN INTEGRITY**			
A. Padded seat and mattress overlay (eggcrate). B. Check suture line q 8 hours. C. Evaluate pressure points. D. Assess patient's ability to reposition.	A. Intact skin. B. Clean and dry. C. Intact skin. D. Position self well.	A. B. See Flowsheet C. See Flowsheet D.	A. B. See Flowsheet C. See Flowsheet D.	A. B. See Flowsheet C. See Flowsheet D.
6. POTENTIAL FOR NEURO-VASCULAR IMPAIRMENT	**6. MAINTAIN INTACT NEURO-VASCULAR**			
A. Check N/V Status to affected extremity Q8H. B. Evaluate pulses, color, temperature, sensation and capillary refill. C. Instruct patient about signs and symptoms that need to be reported to staff/MD: numbness, weakness.	A. No changes. B. Normal status. C. Verbalize understanding.	A. See Flowsheet B. See Flowsheet C.	A. See Flowsheet B. See Flowsheet C.	A. See Flowsheet B. See Flowsheet C.

Map 062 (Rev 6/94)

APPENDIX D-4

Beth Israel Medical Center
MULTIDISCIPLINARY ACTION PLAN

DAY 2

MD: _____

DIAGNOSIS: REHAB PROTOCOL - TOTAL HIP
                        REPLACEMENT

RN/MD REVIEW: _____

DATE: _____

MAP DOES NOT REPLACE MD ORDERS   NOTES

TESTS/ PROCEDURES/ TREATMENTS:	PT if on Coumadin	
MEDICATION	Review medications, switch from IM/IV analgesia to PO pain medications D/C IV or saline lock if no IV meds If on Coumadin (keep patient 15-18 seconds) SC Heparin 5000U Q12 hours Continue bowel program per day 1	
ACTIVITY ROM LIMITATIONS	Weight bearing status per orthopedics Out of bed No hip flexion beyond 90° No adduction beyond neutral No internal rotation beyond neutral	
NUTRITION	As tolerated	
CONSULTS		
PATIENT EDUCATION	Instruct Patient: 1. Do not bend at the waist. 2. Do not bend hip greater than 90°. 3. Do not stoop, kneel or squat. 4. Use assistive device as instructed by therapist.	
SOCIAL WORK	Continued assessment, intervention and planning with RN and MD as well as patient and family. Project discharge plan and provide psychosocial counseling as needed.	
DISCHARGE PLANNING	Interdisciplinary conference regarding patients response to treatment and projected discharge plan. Consult with Social Work regarding initial screening and projected discharge plan.	
PHYSICAL THERAPY	Continue patient evaluation Develop treatment plan	PHYSICAL THERAPY COMMENTS: See Progress Notes for Initial Evaluation.
OCCUPATIONAL THERAPY	Complete OT evaluation and develop treatment plan. Address weight-bearing status, precautions and contraindications to be utilized during functional activities. Instruct patient in hip precautions and provide with handout on safety during performance of ADL. Complete overbed ADL board	OCCUPATIONAL THERAPY COMMENTS: See Progress Notes for Initial Evaluation.

SHIFT	INITIALS	PRINT NAME	SIGNATURE	SHIFT	INITIALS	PRINT	SIGNATURE

Map 062 (Rev 6/94)

APPENDIX **D-5**

<u>Beth Israel Medical Center</u>
MULTIDISCIPLINARY ACTION PLAN
DAY 2
MD: _____
DIAGNOSIS: <u>REHAB PROTOCOL - TOTAL HIP</u>
               <u>REPLACEMENT</u>
DATE: _____

PATIENT PROBLEM AND NURSING INTERVENTIONS	EXPECTED PATIENT OUTCOME AND/OR DISCHARGE OUTCOME	ASSESSMENT/EVALUATION		
1. KNOWLEDGE DEFICIT	**1. INCREASED KNOWLEDGE OF TREATMENT AND DISCHARGE PLAN**			
A. Reinforce rehab orientation. B. Explain therapy schedule. C. Reinforce weight bearing status and use of abduction pillow. D. Teach activities per patient education section.	A. Diminished anxiety. B. Verbal understanding. C. Verbal understanding. D. Verbalize under-standing/demonstrate	A. B. C. D.	A. B. C. D.	A. B. C. D.
2. PAIN	**2. RELIEVED/DIMINISHED PAIN**			
A. Assess for verbal and nonverbal signs of pain. B. Assess pain score using pain/relief scale on the Daily Patient Care flowsheet. C. Administer analgesics as ordered D. Assess effectiveness of meds. E. Enc. relaxation techniques & diversional activities.	A. Relay symptoms. B. Low scores. C. Taken as needed. D. Pain relief. E. Pain relief.	A. B. See Flowsheet C. See MAR D. E.	A. B. See Flowsheet C. See MAR D. E.	A. B. See Flowsheet C. See MAR D. E.
3. IMPAIRED MOBILITY	**3. MAINTAIN OPTIMAL ACTIVITY**			
A. Reinforce weight bearing status. B. Assist with transfers and ADL as necessary C. Assess for calf tenderness. D. TED stockings. E. Use high hip chair.	A. Follow instructions. B. Perform ADLs with minimal assistance. C. No tenderness. D. No complications. E. Tolerate/use chair.	A. B. C. D. E.	A. B. C. D. E.	A. B. C. D. E.
4. POTENTIAL FOR ELIMINATION PROBLEM	**4. MAINTAIN BASELINE PATTERN**			
A. Assess bowel and bladder status q8 hours. B. Institute "routines" as necessary. C. Use of raised toilet seat.	A. Resume normal pattern. B. Resume normal pattern. C. Able to use seat.	A. B. C.	A. B. C.	A. B. C.
5. POTENTIAL FOR SKIN BREAKDOWN	**5. MAINTAIN SKIN INTEGRITY**			
A. Use W/C seat cushion as necessary B. Check suture line q8 hours, document, report to MD. C. Evaluate pressure points. D. Assess patient's ability to reposition.	A. Intact skin. B. Clean and dry. C. Intact skin. D. Position self well.	A. B. See Flowsheet C. See Flowsheet D.	A. B. See Flowsheet C. See Flowsheet D.	A. B. See Flowsheet C. See Flowsheet D.
6. POTENTIAL FOR NEURO-VASCULAR IMPAIRMENT	**6. MAINTAIN INTACT NEURO-VASCULAR**			
A. Check N/V Status to affected extremity Q8H. B. Eval. pulses, color, temperature, sensation, and capillary refill. C. Instruct patient about signs and symptoms that need to be reported to staff/MD: numbness, weakness.	A. No changes. B. Normal status. C. Verbalize understanding.	A. See Flowsheet B. See Flowsheet C.	A. See Flowsheet B. See Flowsheet C.	A. See Flowsheet B. See Flowsheet C.

APPENDIX D-6

Beth Israel Medical Center
MULTIDISCIPLINARY ACTION PLAN
DAY 3

MD: _____

DIAGNOSIS: <u>REHAB PROTOCOL - TOTAL HIP</u>
<u>REPLACEMENT</u>

RN/MD REVIEW: _____

DATE: _____

MAP DOES NOT REPLACE MD ORDERS

NOTES

TESTS/ PROCEDURES/ TREATMENTS:	PT if on Coumadin Assess suture line Inform patient of tentative discharge date	
MEDICATION	Assess pain relief; If on Coumadin (keep PT 15-18 seconds); SC Heparin 5000U q12 hours; Continue bowel program per day 1	
ACTIVITY ROM LIMITATIONS	Weight bearing status per orthopedics Out of bed No hip flexion beyond 90° No adduction beyond neutral No internal rotation beyond neutral	
NUTRITION	As tolerated	
CONSULTS		
PATIENT EDUCATION	Instruct patient about medications. Reinforce positioning and use of adaptive devices.	
SOCIAL WORK	Follow-up on specific problems as indicated. Cont. consult with MD, PT and begin to formulate discharge plan. Refer to CCMU if plan is LTC or Medicaid Home Care.	
DISCHARGE PLANNING	Request Home Health Care evaluation. Monitor progress on discharge plan. Consult with Social Work, MD, and HHIC.	**PHYSICAL THERAPY COMMENTS:**
PHYSICAL THERAPY Evaluate FIM I FIM Level _____ Date of Evaluation ___ / ___ / ___	Goal 1: Transfer from wheelchair to standing FIM: 1-2: Strengthening training and re-evaluate appropriateness of rehab. 3-5: Reinforce transfer training and proceed to ambulation. 6-7: Proceed to ambulation training Initiate exercise program, initiate group	
OCCUPATIONAL THERAPY Evaluate FIM F, I & J FIM Level _____ Date of Evaluation ___ / ___ / ___	Goal: Patient will transfer to bed, wheelchair, chair, and toilet, and will be assessed for toileting skills. FIM: 3-6: Strengthening and balance training. Provide transfer training. Re-evaluate appropriateness for rehabilitation. Assist with transfers. 7-12: Reinforce precautions and safety techniques. Provide transfer training. Advise patient to request for assistance when transferring. Assist with transfers. 13-21: Ensure patient has proper setup for safe transfers. Begin to incorporate safe use of walking device into transfers, as indicated.	**OCCUPATIONAL THERAPY COMMENTS:** Address environmental set up, adaptive equipment, judgment regarding safety, adjustment to disability, caregiver involved in treatment program.

SHIFT	INITIALS	PRINT NAME	SIGNATURE	SHIFT	INITIALS	PRINT	SIGNATURE

Map 062 (Rev 6/94)

Beth Israel Medical Center
MULTIDISCIPLINARY ACTION PLAN

DAY 3

MD: _____

DIAGNOSIS: <u>REHAB PROTOCOL - TOTAL HIP</u>
                    <u>REPLACEMENT</u>

DATE: _____

PATIENT PROBLEM AND NURSING INTERVENTION	EXPECTED PATIENT OUTCOME AND/OR DISCHARGE OUTCOME	ASSESSMENT/EVALUATION		
1. KNOWLEDGE DEFICIT/ANXIETY	**1. INCREASED KNOW- LEDGE OF TREAT- MENT & D/C PLAN/ REDUCED ANXIETY**			
A. Reinf. abduction pillow use & wt bearing status B. Instruct pt not to adduct legs beyond neutral. C. Discuss with MD if mental status or anxiety is interfering with therapy or patient care. D. Teach activities per patient education section.	A. Verbal understanding. B. Verbal understanding. C. Verbal understanding. D. Verbalize under- standing/demonstrate	A. B. C. D.	A. B. C. D.	A. B. C. D.
2. PAIN	**2. RELIEVED/DIMINISHED PAIN**			
A. Assess for verbal and nonverbal signs of pain. B. Assess pain score using pain/relief scale on the Daily Patient Care flowsheet. C. Administer analgesics as ordered D. Assess effectiveness of meds. E. Enc. relax techniques & diversional activities.	A. Relay symptoms. B. Low scores. C. Taken as needed. D. Pain relief. E. Pain relief.	A. B. See Flowsheet C. See MAR D. E.	A. B. See Flowsheet C. See MAR D. E.	A. B. See Flowsheet C. See MAR D. E.
3. IMPAIRED MOBILITY	**3. MAINTAIN OPTIMAL ACTIVITY**			
A. Reinforce weight bearing status. B. TED stockings. C. Evaluate functional ADL status. D. Assist with ADL and transfers as needed E. Encourage the use of adaptive device.	A. Follow instructions. B. No complications. C. Perform ADLs with minimal assistance. D. Perform ADLs with minimal assistance. E. Utilize devices as needed.	A. B. C. D. E.	A. B. C. D. E.	A. B. C. D. E.
4. POTENTIAL FOR ELIMINATION PROBLEMS	**4. MAINTAIN BASELINE PATTERN**			
A. Assess bowel and bladder status Q8H. B. Institute "routines" as necessary. C. Use raised toilet seat. D. Confine bowel program.	A. Resume normal pattern B. Resume normal pattern C. Able to use seat. D. Resume normal pattern	A. B. C. D.	A. B. C. D.	A. B. C. D.
5. POTENTIAL FOR SKIN BREAKDOWN	**5. MAINTAIN SKIN INTEGRITY**			
A. Assess skin Q8H. B. Check suture line Q8H. C. Teach patient symptoms of wound infection: fever, pain, drainage from suture line D. Encourage the use of high hip chair.	A. Intact skin. B. Clean and dry. C. Infection free. D. Tolerate/use chair.	A. See Flowsheet B. See Flowsheet C. D.	A. See Flowsheet B. See Flowsheet C. D.	A. See Flowsheet B. See Flowsheet C. D.
6. POTENTIAL FOR NEURO-VASCULAR IMPAIRMENT	**6. MAINTAIN INTACT NEURO-VASCULAR**			
A. Check N/V Status to affected extremity Q8H. B. Evaluate pulses, color, temperature, sensation, & capillary refill. C. Instruct pt about signs&symptoms that need to be reported to staff/MD: numbness, weakness.	A. No changes. B. Normal status. C. Verbalize understanding.	A. See Flowsheet B. See Flowsheet C.	A. See Flowsheet B. See Flowsheet C.	A. See Flowsheet B. See Flowsheet C.

Map 062 (Rev 6/94)

APPENDIX D-8

Beth Israel Medical Center
MULTIDISCIPLINARY ACTION PLAN
DAY 4

MD: _____

DIAGNOSIS: REHAB PROTOCOL - TOTAL HIP
            REPLACEMENT

RN/MD REVIEW: _____

DATE: _____

MAP DOES NOT REPLACE MD ORDERS

		NOTES
TESTS/ PROCEDURES/ TREATMENTS:	Team evaluation and conference to assess goals, nursing problems and discharge needs. Date of evaluation _____ / _____ / _____ Consider family conference	
MEDICATION	Assess pain relief obtained from PO meds; SC Heparin 5000U Q12 hours; If on Coumadin, (keep PT 15-18 seconds); continue bowel program per day 1	
ACTIVITY ROM LIMITATIONS	Weight bearing status per orthopedics; Out of bed; No hip flexion beyond 90°; No adduction beyond neutral; No internal rotation beyond neutral.	
NUTRITION	As tolerated	
CONSULTS		
PATIENT EDUCATION	Reinforce positioning and use of adaptive devices.	
SOCIAL WORK	Monitor HC evaluation if it was requested. Follow-up on completion and submission of all required forms.	
DISCHARGE PLANNING	Continue to monitor patient progress and status of discharge plan.	**PHYSICAL THERAPY COMMENTS:** <u>Gait Deviations:</u>
PHYSICAL THERAPY Evaluate FIM L FIM Level _____ Date of Evaluation _____ / _____ / _____	Goal 2: Ambulation with walker FIM: 1-2: Have MD re-evaluate appropriateness of rehab 3-4: Ambulation training in parallel bars 5: Continue ambulation training; increase 20 feet as tolerated 6-7: Proceed to cane and increase ambulation as tolerated if weight bearing Continue exercise program; update over the bed boards.	<u>Patient Ability to Weight Bear on Affected LE (if applicable):</u>
OCCUPATIONAL THERAPY Evaluate FIM C FIM Level _____ Date of Evaluation _____ / _____ / _____	Goal: Patient will utilize adaptive equipment safely when bathing, incorporating use of assistive devices for lower extremity self-care. FIM: 1-2: If score low, re-evaluate appropriateness of rehabilitation. Instruct in sponge bathing at sink. 3-5: Train in use of assistive devices for washing lower extremities at sink. 6-7: Proceed to training in tub transfers with adaptive equipment.	**OCCUPATIONAL THERAPY COMMENTS:** Address need for assistive devices/adaptive equipment. Instructions for carryover on unit. Review handout on hip precautions during ADL.

SHIFT	INITIALS	PRINT NAME	SIGNATURE	SHIFT	INITIALS	PRINT	SIGNATURE

Map 062 (Rev 6/94)

APPENDIX **D-9**

<u>Beth Israel Medical Center</u>
MULTIDISCIPLINARY ACTION PLAN
DAY 4
MD: _____

DIAGNOSIS: <u>REHAB PROTOCOL - TOTAL HIP</u>
<u>REPLACEMENT</u>

DATE: _____

PATIENT PROBLEM AND NURSING INTERVENTIONS	EXPECTED PATIENT OUTCOME AND/OR DISCHARGE OUTCOME	ASSESSMENT/EVALUATION		
1. **KNOWLEDGE DEFICIT**	1. **INCREASED KNOWLEDGE OF TREATMENT AND DISCHARGE PLAN**			
A. Provide question and answer period for pt. B. Pt will participate in D/C plans. C. Reinforce teaching re: hip precautions, ADL, transfer, & impairment of neurovascular status. D. Teach activities per pt education section.	A. Diminished anxiety. B. Diminished anxiety. C. Verbal understanding. D. Verbal understanding.	A. B. C. D.	A. B. C. D.	A. B. C. D.
2. **PAIN**	2. **RELIEVED/DIMINISHED PAIN**			
A. Administer PO analgesics as ordered B. Assess effectiveness of meds. C. Teach patient about meds and side effects D. Enc. proper positioning of affected limb. E. Instruct patient regarding use of medication in relation to activity.	A. Taken as needed. B. Pain relief. C. Verbal understanding. D. Follow instructions. E. Verbal understanding.	A. See MAR B. C. D. E.	A. See MAR B. C. D. E.	A. See MAR B. C. D. E.
3. **IMPAIRED MOBILITY**	3. **MAINTAIN OPTIMAL ACTIVITY**			
A. Assist with transfer, ADL as needed. B. Encourage use of assistive devices. C. OOB with assistance. D. Progressive ambulation with assistive device. E. Discuss functional status at Team Conference & est. team goals, instructions. F. Precautions sheets at bedside in place and complete.	A. Perform ADLs with minimal assistance. B. Utilize device approp. C. Able to get OOB. D. Ambulates with device.	A. B. C. D. E. F.	A. B. C. D. E. F.	A. B. C. D. E. F.
4. **POTENTIAL FOR ELIMINATION PROBLEMS**	4. **MAINTAIN BASELINE PATTERN**			
A. Review dietary factors with patient (i.e. fiber, fluids). B. Enc. pt to report variations from "norm".	A. Verbal understanding. B. Relay any changes.	A. B.	A. B.	A. B.
5. **POTENTIAL FOR SKIN BREAKDOWN**	5. **MAINTAIN SKIN INTEGRITY**			
A. Have patient check suture line. B. Review symptoms of wound infection. C. Assess skin Q8H D. Encourage the use of high hip chair.	A. Clean and dry. B. Verbal understanding. C. Intact skin. D. Tolerate/use chair.	A. B. C. D.	A. B. C. D.	A. B. C. D.
6. **POTENTIAL FOR NEURO-VASCULAR IMPAIRMENT**	6. **MAINTAIN INTACT NEURO-VASCULAR**			
A. Chk N/V Status to affected extremity Q8H. B. Evaluate pulses, color, temperature sensation, and capillary refill. C. Instruct patient about signs and symptoms that need to be reported to staff/MD: numbness, weakness.	A. No changes. B. Normal status. C. Verbalize understanding.	A. See Flowsheet B. See Flowsheet C.	A. See Flowsheet B. See Flowsheet C.	A. See Flowsheet B. See Flowsheet C.

Map 062 (Rev 6/94)

APPENDIX D-10

Beth Israel Medical Center
MULTIDISCIPLINARY ACTION PLAN
DAY 5
MD: _____

DIAGNOSIS: <u>REHAB PROTOCOL - TOTAL HIP</u>
<u>REPLACEMENT</u>

RN/MD REVIEW: _____

DATE: _____

MAP DOES NOT REPLACE MD ORDERS   NOTES

TESTS/ PROCEDURES/ TREATMENTS:		
MEDICATION	Assess pain relief P.O. PRN's for pain D/C Coumadin and Heparin if ambulatory If on Coumadin (keep PT 15-18 seconds) SC Heparin 5000U Q12 hours. Continue bowel program per day 1	
ACTIVITY ROM LIMITATIONS	Weight bearing status per orthopedics Out of bed No hip flexion beyond 90° No adduction beyond neutral No internal rotation beyond neutral	
NUTRITION	As tolerated	
CONSULTS		
PATIENT EDUCATION	Review positioning and use of adaptive devices. Plan for discharge planning conference group.	
SOCIAL WORK	Continue consultation with MD, PT, RN as to patient progress.	
DISCHARGE PLANNING	Consult with HHIC as indicated.	**PHYSICAL THERAPY COMMENTS:** <u>Patient Ability to Perform Closed Chain Exercises (if applicable):</u>
PHYSICAL THERAPY Evaluate FIM L FIM Level _____ Date of Evaluation ____/____/____	Goal 2: Ambulation with walker FIM: 1-2: Have MD re-evaluate appropriateness of rehab 3-4: Ambulation training in parallel bars 5: Continue ambulation training; increase 20 feet as tolerated 6-7: Proceed to cane and increase ambulation as tolerated Increase repetitions on home exercise program	
OCCUPATIONAL THERAPY Evaluate FIM K FIM Level _____ Date of Evaluation ____/____/____	Goal: Patient will perform bathtub transfer with tub bench/seat, utilizing safety techniques during use of devices. FIM: 1-2: Re-evaluate appropriateness of rehab. Focus on transfers to bed, wheelchair and toilet. 3-5: Train in safe tub transfers, using adapted seating and use of handheld shower. 6-7: Evaluate skill and safety during actual shower. Encourage follow-through in AM routine.	**OCCUPATIONAL THERAPY COMMENTS:** Address ability to lift legs into bathtub and maintain standing, reach faucets and control water temperature.

SHIFT	INITIALS	PRINT NAME	SIGNATURE	SHIFT	INITIALS	PRINT	SIGNATURE

Map 062 (Rev 6/94)

APPENDIX D-11

<u>Beth Israel Medical Center</u>
MULTIDISCIPLINARY ACTION PLAN
DAY 5

MD: _____

DIAGNOSIS: <u>REHAB PROTOCOL - TOTAL HIP</u>
<u>REPLACEMENT</u>

DATE: _____

PATIENT PROBLEM AND NURSING INTERVENTIONS	EXPECTED PATIENT OUTCOME AND/OR DISCHARGE OUTCOME	ASSESSMENT/EVALUATION		
1. KNOWLEDGE DEFICIT A. Provide question & answer period for pt. B. Encourage participation of "significant others" C. Reinforce teaching re: hip precautions, ADL, transfer, and impairment of neurovascular status. D. Teach activities per patient education section.	**1. INCREASED KNOWLEDGE OF TREATMENT AND DISCHARGE PLAN** A. Diminished anxiety. B. Diminished anxiety. C. Verbal understanding. D. Verbal understanding.	A. B. C. D.	A. B. C. D.	A. B. C. D.
2. PAIN A. Reinforce teaching patient about meds and side effects. B. Teach patient use of medication in relation to activity. C. Assess pain score using the pain/relief scale on the patient daily flowsheet. D. Medicate patient as needed. E. Assess effectiveness of pain meds.	**2. RELIEVED/DIMINISHED PAIN** A. Taken as needed. B. Pain relief. C. Verbal understanding. D. Follow instructions. E. Verbal understanding.	A. B. C. See Flowsheet D. See MAR E.	A. B. C. See Flowsheet D. See MAR E.	A. B. C. See Flowsheet D. See MAR E.
3. IMPAIRED MOBILITY A. Encourage independence in ADL with assistive devices. B. Encourage transfer, ambulation as needed using assistive device. C. Maintain status as reported by OT/PT. D. Encourage dressing in street clothes.	**3. MAINTAIN OPTIMAL ACTIVITY** A. Perform ADLs with minimal assistance. B. Utilize device approp. C. Utilize device approp.	A. B. C. D.	A. B. C. D.	A. B. C. D.
4. POTENTIAL FOR ELIMINATION PROBLEMS A. Review "routines" with patient B. Continue bowel program.	**4. MAINTAIN BASELINE PATTERN** A. Verbal understanding. B. Resume normal pattern.	A. B.	A. B.	A. B.
5. POTENTIAL FOR NEURO-VASCULAR IMPAIRMENT A. Check N/V status to affected extremity Q8H. B. Evaluate pulses, color, temperature sensation, and capillary refill. C. Instruct patient about signs and symptoms that need to be reported to staff/MD: numbness, weakness.	**5. MAINTAIN NEURO-VASCULAR** A. No changes B. Normal status C. Verbal understanding.	A. See Flowsheet B. See Flowsheet C.	A. See Flowsheet B. See Flowsheet C.	A. See Flowsheet B. See Flowsheet C.

Map 062 (Rev 6/94)

APPENDIX **D-12**

<u>Beth Israel Medical Center</u>
MULTIDISCIPLINARY ACTION PLAN
DAY 6

MD: _____

DIAGNOSIS: <u>REHAB PROTOCOL - TOTAL HIP</u>
<u>REPLACEMENT</u>

RN/MD REVIEW: _____

DATE: _____

MAP DOES NOT REPLACE MD ORDERS

NOTES

TESTS/ PROCEDURES/ TREATMENTS:	PT if on coumadin	
MEDICATION	Assess pain relief; P.O. PRN's for pain D/C Coumadin and Heparin if patient ambulatory For non-ambulatory patients: Coumadin (keep PT 15-18 seconds); SC Heparin 5000U Q12 hours; Continue bowel program per day 1	
ACTIVITY ROM LIMITATIONS	Weight bearing status per orthopedics; Out of bed; No hip flexion beyond 90°; No adduction beyond neutral; No internal rotation beyond neutral	
NUTRITION	As tolerated	
CONSULTS		
PATIENT EDUCATION	Instruct patient in tub transfers if cleared by O.T. Review positioning and use of adaptive devices Instruct patient that sex may be resumed adopting a passive position.	
SOCIAL WORK	Ensure that necessary forms and referrals have been completed and that necessary services are available if plan is for patient to return home.	
DISCHARGE PLANNING	Continue to monitor patient's progress in preparation for discharge.	**PHYSICAL THERAPY COMMENTS:** <u>Number of steps achieved:</u>
PHYSICAL THERAPY Evaluate FIM M FIM Level _____ Date of Evaluation ____/____/____	Goal 3: Negotiate stairs and elevated surfaces <u>FIM:</u> 1-2: Continue strengthening and activities from Day 4&5 3-5: Stair training 6-7: Initiate community re-entry Increase difficulty home exercise program	
OCCUPATIONAL THERAPY Evaluate FIM D and E FIM Level _____ Date of Evaluation ____/____/____	Goal: Patient will dress in street clothing, utilizing assistive devices for lower extremities. FIM 2-4: Re-evaluate appropriateness for rehab. Patient will perform upper extremity dressing and be trained in adapted lower extremity dressing strategies. Continue to focus on transfer training. 5-11: Dressing training utilizing assistive devices for lower extremity garments. 12-14: Review safety and precautions in use of assistive devices. Patient responsible for daily dressing in street clothing.	**OCCUPATIONAL THERAPY COMMENTS:** Address compliance, carryover in use of assistive devices.

SHIFT	INITIALS	PRINT NAME	SIGNATURE	SHIFT	INITIALS	PRINT	SIGNATURE

Map 062 (Rev 6/94)

APPENDIX D-13

<u>Beth Israel Medical Center</u>
MULTIDISCIPLINARY ACTION PLAN
DAY 6

MD: _____

DIAGNOSIS: <u>REHAB PROTOCOL - TOTAL HIP</u>
              <u>REPLACEMENT</u>

DATE: _____

PATIENT PROBLEM AND NURSING INTERVENTIONS	EXPECTED PATIENT OUTCOME AND/OR DISCHARGE OUTCOME	ASSESSMENT/EVALUATION		
1. KNOWLEDGE DEFICIT A. Provide question and answer period for patient. B. Assist patient to formulate questions for other disciplines (i.e. equipment, assistance at home...) C. Teach regarding meds and activity. D. Teach activities per patient education section.	**1. INCREASED KNOWLEDGE OF TREATMENT AND DISCHARGE PLAN** A. Diminished anxiety. B. Diminished anxiety. C. Verbal understanding. D. Verbal understanding.	A. B. C. D.	A. B. C. D.	A. B. C. D.
2. PAIN A. Instruct patient on use of medication in relation to activity. B. Medicate as needed. C. Assess effectiveness of meds.	**2. RELIEVED/DIMINISHED PAIN** A. Verbalize understanding. B. Taken as needed. C. Pain relief.	A. B. See MAR C.	A. B. See MAR C.	A. B. See MAR C.
3. IMPAIRED MOBILITY A. Maintain status as reported by OT/PT. B. Encourage patient to verbalize any concerns regarding ADL or ambulation. C. Encourage dressing in street clothes. D. Encourage transfer, ambulation, with assistive device as needed.	**3. MAINTAIN OPTIMAL ACTIVITY** B. Diminished anxiety/perform ADLs with minimal assistance. C. Dress in street clothes. D. Ambulate with device.	A. B. C. D.	A. B. C. D.	A. B. C. D.
4. POTENTIAL FOR NEURO-VASCULAR IMPAIRMENT A. Check N/V status to affected extremity Q8H. B. Evaluate pulses, color, temperature sensation, and capillary return. C. Instruct patient about signs and symptoms that need to be reported to staff/MD: numbness, weakness.	**6. MAINTAIN INTACT NEURO-VASCULAR** A. No changes. B. Normal status. C. Verbalize understanding.	A. See Flowsheet B. See Flowsheet C.	A. See Flowsheet B. See Flowsheet C.	A. See Flowsheet B. See Flowsheet C.

APPENDIX D-14

<u>Beth Israel Medical Center</u>
MULTIDISCIPLINARY ACTION PLAN
DAY 7
MD: _____
DIAGNOSIS: <u>REHAB PROTOCOL - TOTAL HIP</u>
                <u>REPLACEMENT</u>
RN/MD REVIEW: _____
DATE: _____

MAP DOES NOT REPLACE MD ORDERS

NOTES

TESTS/ PROCEDURES/ TREATMENTS:		
MEDICATION	Wean off narcotics, try oral NSAID if off Coumadin > 24 hours. Continue bowel program	
ACTIVITY ROM LIMITATIONS	Weight bearing status per orthopedics; Out of bed; No hip flexion beyond 90°; No adduction beyond neutral; No internal rotation beyond neutral	
NUTRITION	As tolerated	
CONSULTS		
PATIENT EDUCATION	Review positioning and use of adaptive device. Instruct patient to notify MD for: swelling, drainage, redness from incision line, swelling of affected leg. Increased pain or fever, shortness of breath or chest pain.	
SOCIAL WORK	Continue interdisciplinary coordination and monitor patient's progress with regard to discharger plan.	
DISCHARGE PLANNING	Advise social work and MD on any changes in patient that would impact on discharge.	**PHYSICAL THERAPY COMMENTS:** <u>Gait Deviation:</u>
PHYSICAL THERAPY Evaluate FIM M FIM Level _____ Date of Evaluation ___ / ___ / ___	Goal 3: Negotiate stairs and elevated surfaces <u>FIM</u> 1-2: Emphasize strengthening, continue activities from days 3-6 3-5: Continue stair training 6-7: Initiate community re-entry Communicate home needs with social worker Communicate equipment needs to occupational therapist	<u>Ability to Perform Closed Chain Exercises:</u> <u>Amb. Device Needed:</u>

OCCUPATIONAL THERAPY
Evaluate FIM N, O, P, Q, R
FIM Level _____
Date of Evaluation
 	
___ / ___ / ___
	Goal: Patient will be knowledgeable of precautions
	          during simple homemaking activities.
	<u>FIM</u>
	5-10: Ensure D/C home with Home Car Services and
	       24 hour supervision. Continue transfer training.
	11-25: Ensure D/C home with VNS referral for OT and
	       assistance at home as indicated. Evaluate light
	       meal preparation skills and safety in kitchen.
	26-35: Order durable medial equipment, review hip
	       precautions, body mechanics, and energy
	       conservation. Reinforce safety during simple
	       homemaking tasks.
		OCCUPATIONAL THERAPY COMMENTS:

SHIFT	INITIALS	PRINT NAME	SIGNATURE	SHIFT	INITIALS	PRINT	SIGNATURE

Map 062 (Rev 6/94)
Copyright Beth Israel Medical Center 1992. All rights reserved

APPENDIX D-15

<u>Beth Israel Medical Center</u>
MULTIDISCIPLINARY ACTION PLAN
DAY 7

MD: _____

DIAGNOSIS: <u>REHAB PROTOCOL - TOTAL HIP</u>
              <u>REPLACEMENT</u>

DATE: _____

PATIENT PROBLEM AND NURSING INTERVENTIONS	EXPECTED PATIENT OUTCOME AND/OR DISCHARGE OUTCOME	ASSESSMENT/EVALUATION		
1. KNOWLEDGE DEFICIT A. Provide question and answer period for patient. B. Assess remaining teaching needs regarding meds and activity and teach accordingly.. C. Encourage socialization with peers. D. Teach activities per patient education section.	**1. INCREASED KNOWLEDGE OF TREATMENT AND DISCHARGE PLAN** A. Diminished anxiety. B. Verbal understanding. C. Diminished anxiety. D. Verbal understanding.	A. B. C. D.	A. B. C. D.	A. B. C. D.
2. PAIN A. Review correct positioning to relieve or prevent pain. B. Review medication and timing of activities. C. Medicate for pain as needed.	**2. RELIEVED/DIMINISHED PAIN** A. Return demonstration. B. Verbalize understanding. C. Taken as needed/diminished pain.	A. B. C. See MAR	A. B. C. See MAR	A. B. C. See MAR
3. IMPAIRED MOBILITY A. Progressive ambulation with P.T. B. Assess independence with assistive devices for ADL. C. Provide time for observation by "significant other" and assist by "significant other" as needed.	**3. MAINTAIN OPTIMAL ACTIVITY** A. Ambulate well. B. Use device independently. C. Significant other involvement.	A. B. C.	A. B. C.	A. B. C.
4. POTENTIAL FOR NEURO-VASCULAR IMPAIRMENT A. Check N/V status to affected extremity Q8 hours. B. Evaluate pulses, color, temperature sensation, and capillary return. C. Instruct patient about signs and symptoms that need to be reported to staff/MD: numbness, weakness.	**6. MAINTAIN INTACT NEURO-VASCULAR** A. No changes. B. Normal status. C. Verbalize understanding.	A. See Flowsheet B. See Flowsheet C.	A. See Flowsheet B. See Flowsheet C.	A. See Flowsheet B. See Flowsheet C.

Beth Israel Medical Center
MULTIDISCIPLINARY ACTION PLAN
DAY 8
MD: _____
DIAGNOSIS: <u>REHAB PROTOCOL - TOTAL HIP</u>
<u>REPLACEMENT</u>
RN/MD REVIEW: _____
DATE: _____

MAP DOES NOT REPLACE MD ORDERS   NOTES

TESTS/ PROCEDURES/ TREATMENTS:	Consider staple removal if 2 weeks post-op. Arrange follow-up appointments 1 week after discharge with - Orthopedics, Internist	
MEDICATION	Wean off narcotics, try oral NSAID; Cont. bowel program	
ACTIVITY ROM LIMITATIONS	Weight bearing status per orthopedics; Out of bed; No hip flexion beyond 90°; No adduction beyond neutral; No internal rotation beyond neutral	
NUTRITION	As tolerated	
CONSULTS	Notify Orthopedics regarding D/C date	
PATIENT EDUCATION	Review positioning and use of adaptive device. Review symptoms that should be reported to MD. Encourage patient to maintain goal weight. Instruct patient about oral antibiotics before any dental work.	
SOCIAL WORK	Continue psychosocial counseling as indicated in preparation for transition back to community.	
DISCHARGE PLANNING	If pt is returning home, RN to ensure that prescriptions are completed by MD; PCM, PT/OT will coordinate ordering of necessary equipment and supplies as appropriate.	PHYSICAL THERAPY COMMENTS: <u>Amb. Device Needed:</u>
PHYSICAL THERAPY Evaluate Overall FIM (I, L, M) FIM Level ____ Date of Evaluation __/__/__	Goal 4: Community re-entry FIM: 1-7: Order wheelchair, continue stair training 7-14: Arrange for VNS, or outpatient P.T., continue stair training. 14-21: Continue with high level activities. Continue exercise program with patient demonstration of exercise program without verbal cues.	
OCCUPATIONAL THERAPY Evaluate FIM L, N, O, P, Q, and R FIM Level ____ Date of Evaluation __/__/__	Goal: Complete Durable Medical Equipment order form and have M.D. review and sign. PT. will participate in mobility activities within the hospital environment, using ambulation device or wheelchair. FIM 6-12: Familiarize caregiver and patient with mobility outside rehab unit. 13-30: Familiarize patient with architectural barriers and practice mobility on a variety of surfaces. 31-42: Review safety techniques when negotiating a variety of surfaces with walking device.	OCCUPATIONAL THERAPY COMMENTS: Address ability to surmount architectural barriers and safely negotiate ramps, inclines, steps and uneven surfaces, problem-solving skills, safety in negotiating ramps, inclines, steps, and uneven surfaces.

SHIFT	INITIALS	PRINT NAME	SIGNATURE	SHIFT	INITIALS	PRINT	SIGNATURE

Map 062 (Rev 6/94)

APPENDIX **D-17**

<u>Beth Israel Medical Center</u>
MULTIDISCIPLINARY ACTION PLAN
DAY 8

MD: _____

DIAGNOSIS: <u>REHAB PROTOCOL - TOTAL HIP</u>
<u>REPLACEMENT</u>

DATE: _____

PATIENT PROBLEM AND NURSING INTERVENTIONS	EXPECTED PATIENT OUTCOME AND/OR DISCHARGE OUTCOME	ASSESSMENT/EVALUATION		
1. **KNOWLEDGE DEFICIT** A. Continue to review hip precautions with patient and provide written information for patient to take home. B. Arrange MD follow-up appointments C. Review with S.W. and VNS patient's D/C arrangements. D. Teach activities per patient education section.	1. **INCREASED KNOWLEDGE OF TREATMENT AND DISCHARGE PLAN** A. Verbalize understanding/ return demonstration. D. Verbalize understanding.	A. B. C. D.	A. B. C. D.	A. B. C. D.
2. **IMPAIRED MOBILITY** A. Include S.O. and/or HHA in ADL techniques explaining amount of assistance needed and use of adaptive equipment. B. Assess patient progress with use of assistive devices. C. Review with PT/OT assistive devices to be ordered for patient's home use.	2. **MAINTAIN OPTIMAL ACTIVITY** A. S.O./HHA verbalize understanding. B. Use device independently. C. Ordered as needed.	A. B. C.	A. B. C.	A. B. C.
3. **POTENTIAL FOR NEURO-VASCULAR IMPAIRMENT** A. Check N/V status to affected extremity Q8 hours. B. Evaluate pulses, color, temperature sensation, and capillary return. C. Instruct patient about signs and symptoms that need to be reported to staff/MD: numbness, weakness.	3. **MAINTAIN INTACT NEURO-VASCULAR** A. No changes. B. Normal status. C. Verbalize understanding.	A. See Flowsheet B. See Flowsheet C.	A. See Flowsheet B. See Flowsheet C.	A. See Flowsheet B. See Flowsheet C.

Map 062 (Rev 6/94)

APPENDIX D-18

<u>Beth Israel Medical Center</u>
MULTIDISCIPLINARY ACTION PLAN
DAY 9

MD: _____

DIAGNOSIS: <u>REHAB PROTOCOL - TOTAL HIP</u>
<u>REPLACEMENT</u>

RN/MD REVIEW: _____

DATE: _____

MAP DOES NOT REPLACE MD ORDERS   **NOTES**

TESTS/ PROCEDURES/ TREATMENTS:	Consider staple removal Consider Doppler study to lower extremities (B.I. North patients)	
MEDICATION	Evaluate analgesics; Continue bowel program	
ACTIVITY ROM LIMITATIONS	Weight bearing status per orthopedics; Out of bed; No hip flexion beyond 90°; No adduction beyond neutral; No internal rotation beyond neutral.	
NUTRITION	As tolerated	
CONSULTS	Notify Orthopedics regarding D/C date	
PATIENT EDUCATION	Call for Ortho appointment 1 week after discharge. BI: 420-2462 BI North: 870-9000 Review: No driving for 6 weeks, sit on 2 pillows in car, enter car from street level, seat fully back before entering.	
SOCIAL WORK	On day prior to discharge; finalize discharge plan; verify personal belongings, keys, clothes, etc. Arrange transportation, notify family, confirm Home Care plans with SW, HHIC and CCMU. Coordinate preparation of required documents for transfer, PRI inter-institutional form. Arrange for transportation home and to clinic.	
DISCHARGE PLANNING		**PHYSICAL THERAPY COMMENTS:** <u>Amb. Device Needed:</u>
PHYSICAL THERAPY Evaluate Overall FIM (I, L, M) FIM Level _____ Date of Evaluation ___ / ___ / ___	Goal 4: Community re-entry <u>FIM:</u> 1-14: Continue stair training 14-21: Continue with high level activities Continue exercise program Ensure independence with home exercise program. Coordinate appropriate transportation home with social worker.	<u>Gait Deviations:</u>
OCCUPATIONAL THERAPY Evaluate FIM L, N, O, P, Q, and R FIM Level _____ Date of Evaluation ___ / ___ / ___	Goal: Patient will participate in community re-entry activities. <u>FIM</u> 6-12: Familiarize patient with traveling outside in wheelchair. 13-30: Instruct and assist patient with opening a variety of doors, crossing a street and/or entering a car. 31-42: Reinforce safety techniques and encourage independent problem-solving with confronted with an architectural barrier.	**OCCUPATIONAL THERAPY COMMENTS:** Address donning/doffing outerwear, caregiver participation, problem-solving, safety, and any limitations.

SHIFT	INITIALS	PRINT NAME	SIGNATURE	SHIFT	INITIALS	PRINT	SIGNATURE

Map 062 (Rev 6/94)

<u>Beth Israel Medical Center</u>
MULTIDISCIPLINARY ACTION PLAN
DAY 9

MD: _____

DIAGNOSIS: <u>REHAB PROTOCOL - TOTAL HIP</u>
 <u>REPLACEMENT</u>

DATE: _____

PATIENT PROBLEM AND NURSING INTERVENTIONS	EXPECTED PATIENT OUTCOME AND/OR DISCHARGE OUTCOME	ASSESSMENT/EVALUATION		
1. KNOWLEDGE DEFICIT A. Continue to review hip precautions with patient and provide written information for patient to take home. B. Arrange MD follow-up appointments C. Review with S.W. and VNS patient's D/C arrangements. D. Teach activities per patient education section.	**1. INCREASED KNOWLEDGE OF TREATMENT AND DISCHARGE PLAN** A. Verbalize understanding/return demonstration. D. Verbalize understanding.	A. B. C. D.	A. B. C. D.	A. B. C. D.
2. IMPAIRED MOBILITY A. Include S.O. and/or HHA in ADL techniques explaining amount of assistance needed and use of adaptive equipment. B. Assess patient's progress with use of assistive devices. C. D/C TEDS.	**2. MAINTAIN OPTIMAL ACTIVITY** A. S.O./HHA verbalize understanding. B. Use device independently.	A. B. C.	A. B. C.	A. B. C.
3. POTENTIAL FOR NEURO-VASCULAR IMPAIRMENT A. Check N/V status to affected extremity Q8 hours. B. Evaluate pulses, color, temperature sensation, and capillary return. C. Instruct patient about signs and symptoms that need to be reported to staff/MD: numbness, weakness.	**3. MAINTAIN INTACT NEURO-VASCULAR** A. No changes. B. Normal status. C. Verbalize understanding.	A. See Flowsheet B. See Flowsheet C.	A. See Flowsheet B. See Flowsheet C.	A. See Flowsheet B. See Flowsheet C.

Map 062 (Rev 6/94)

APPENDIX D-20

Beth Israel Medical Center
MULTIDISCIPLINARY ACTION PLAN
DAY 10

MD: _____

DIAGNOSIS: __REHAB PROTOCOL - TOTAL HIP__
_____REPLACEMENT_____

RN/MD REVIEW: _____

DATE: _____

MAP DOES NOT REPLACE MD ORDERS   NOTES

TESTS/ PROCEDURES/ TREATMENTS:	Discharge patient	
MEDICATION	Prescriptions to patient D/C bowel program	
ACTIVITY ROM LIMITATIONS	Weight bearing status per orthopedics Out of bed No hip flexion beyond 90° No adduction beyond neutral No internal rotation beyond neutral	
NUTRITION	As tolerated	
CONSULTS		
PATIENT EDUCATION	Review discharge instructions Answer all patient questions Review positioning and use of adaptive devices Review symptoms that should be reported to MD Maintain hip precautions 3-6 months	
SOCIAL WORK	Discharge Day	
DISCHARGE PLANNING	Discharge Day	
PHYSICAL THERAPY	Write discharge summary for VNS } Copy } to Confirm equipment ordered/received } patient Measure received equipment to fit patient	**PHYSICAL THERAPY COMMENTS:** See Discharge Summary Sheet in Progress Note Section of the Chart.
OCCUPATIONAL THERAPY	Write discharge summary and/or VNS referral, complete orange attendance sheet, customize equipment received to patient's specific needs and advise patient/caregivers of DME sent to home. Obtain M.D.'s signature on insurance form. Provide patient with copy of discharge summary.	**OCCUPATIONAL THERAPY COMMENTS:** See Discharge Summary Sheet in Progress Note Section of the Chart.

SHIFT	INITIALS	PRINT NAME	SIGNATURE	SHIFT	INITIALS	PRINT	SIGNATURE

Map 062 (Rev 6/94)

A P P E N D I X **D-21**

<u>Beth Israel Medical Center</u>
MULTIDISCIPLINARY ACTION PLAN
DAY 10

MD: _____

DIAGNOSIS: <u>REHAB PROTOCOL - TOTAL HIP</u>
            <u>REPLACEMENT</u>

DATE: _____

PATIENT PROBLEM AND NURSING INTERVENTION	EXPECTED PATIENT OUTCOME AND/OR DISCHARGE OUTCOME	ASSESSMENT/EVALUATION		
1. *KNOWLEDGE DEFICIT*	1. *INCREASED KNOWLEDGE OF TREATMENT AND DISCHARGE PLAN*			
A. Complete nursing D/C instruction sheet and review with patient/family. Provide copy for patient to take home.	A. Verbalize understanding.	A. See D/C Instruc.	A. See D/C Instruc.	A. See D/C Instruc.
B. Review with S.W. re: patient D/C arrangements HHA.	B. D/C needs in place.	B.	B.	B.
C. Finalize MD appointments and provide transportation through S.W.		C. See D/C Instruc.	C. See D/C Instruc.	C. See D/C Instruc.
D. Review signs and symptoms that should be reported to MD: i) fever ii) swelling iii) shortness of breath iv) drainage from incisions site v) activity	D. Verbalize understanding/ return demonstration.	D. See D/C Instruc.	D. See D/C Instruc.	D. See D/C Instruc.
E. Answer questions by patient or significant other.	E. Diminished anxiety.	E.	E.	E.

Map 062 (Rev 6/94)

APPENDIX D-22

Beth Israel Medical Center

**DEPARTMENT OF PHYSICAL MEDICINE
AND REHABILITATION**
INITIAL EVALUATION CONFERENCE
REPORT

IN ATTENDANCE

Physical Therapist: _____

Occupational Therapist: _____

Speech Pathologist: _____

Social Worker: _____

Nurse: _____

Nutritionist: _____

DIAGNOSIS ON ADMISSION

DISABILITY (Functional Losses and Medical Problems)

GOALS - SHORT TERM

GOALS - LONG TERM

PLAN

_____   _____
PHYSICIAN'S SIGNATURE   **DATE**

Map 062 (Rev 6/94)

APPENDIX D-23

Beth Israel Medical Center

DEPARTMENT OF PHYSICAL MEDICINE
AND REHABILITATION
RE-EVALUATION CONFERENCE REPORT

IN ATTENDANCE

Physical Therapist: _____

Occupational Therapist: _____

Speech Pathologist: _____

Social Worker: _____

Nurse: _____

Nutritionist: _____

PROGRESS

PROBLEM

PLAN

_____   _____
PHYSICIAN'S SIGNATURE   **DATE**

APPENDIX D-24

FUNCTIONAL INDEPENDENCE MEASURE
FIM

L E V E L S		
7 Complete Independence (Timely, Safely) 6 Modified Independence (Device)		NO HELPER

Modified Dependence
   5 Supervision
   4 Minimal Assist (Subject = 75% +)
   3 Moderate Assist (Subject = 50% +)
Complete Dependence
   2 Maximal Assist (Subject = 25% +)
   1 Total Assist (Subject = 0% +)
		HELPER

		ADMIT	DISCHARGE	FOLLOW-UP
	Self Care			
A.	Feeding	☐	☐	☐
B.	Grooming	☐	☐	☐
C.	Bathing	☐	☐	☐
D.	Dressing-Upper Body	☐	☐	☐
E.	Dressing-Lower Body	☐	☐	☐
F.	Toileting	☐	☐	☐
	Sphincter Control			
G.	Bladder Management	☐	☐	☐
H.	Bowel Management	☐	☐	☐
	Mobility Transfer			
I.	Bed, Chair, W/Chair	☐	☐	☐
J.	Toilet	☐	☐	☐
K.	Tub, Shower	☐	☐	☐
	Locomotion	W ☐ Both ☐	W ☐ Both ☐	W ☐ Both ☐
L.	Walk/wheelChair	C ☐	C ☐	C ☐
M.	Stairs	☐	☐	☐
	Communication	A ☐ Both ☐	A ☐ Both ☐	A ☐ Both ☐
N.	Comprehension	V ☐	V ☐	V ☐
O.	Expression	V ☐ Both ☐	V ☐ Both ☐	V ☐ Both ☐
		N ☐	N ☐	N ☐
	Social Cognition			
P.	Social Interaction	☐	☐	☐
Q.	Problem Solving	☐	☐	☐
R.	Memory	☐	☐	☐
	TOTAL	☐	☐	☐

APPENDIX **E-1**

VISIT GUIDELINES

HIP FRACTURE, OPEN REDUCTION INTERNAL FIXATION: PHYSICAL THERAPY

PATIENT OBJECTIVES	INTERVENTIONS	VISITS						
		1	2	3	4	5	6	7
7. THERAPEUTIC SELF CARE DEFICIT: GAIT TRAINING -- WEIGHT BEARS AS PRESCRIBED USING PROPER GAIT PATTERN								
1. Demonstrates weight bearing as prescribed	1. Assess ability to weight bear as prescribed							
	2. Teach proper weight bearing useing assistive device(s)							
2. Demonstrates correct gait pattern	1. Perform gait evaluation: ▪ cadence ▪ endurance ▪ swing/stance phase							
	2. Assess need for assistive device/equipment							
	3. Order assistive device/equipments as needed							
	4. Teach proper gait patterns while using assistive device(s) on level surfaces							
3. Demonstrates stair climbing with assistive device with minimal assistance	1. Assess environment: ▪ number of stairs ▪ railing ▪ stair height ▪ lighting							
	2. Assess ability to climb stairs: ▪ endurance ▪ UE/LE strength							
	3. Teach proper stair climbing techniques with weight bearing as prescribed							
	4. Contact MD following initial evaluation, report ongoing progress and any atypical patient response							
	5. Contact COC following initial evaluation, report ongoing progress and any atypical response							
8. PHYSICAL MOBILITY: AMBULATION -- AMBULATES INDEPENDENTLY USING ASSISTIVE DEVICE								
1. Ambulates independently indoors at least 250 feet	1. Assess ability to ambulate: ▪ distance ▪ endurance ▪ balance ▪ maneuver around obstacles							
	2. Instruct to ambulate 3x/day with assistance as needed							
	3. Teach to increase distance as tolerated							
	4. Contact MD following initial evaluation, report ongoing progress and any atypical patient response							
	5. Contact COC following initial evaluation, report ongoing progress and any atypical response							
2. Demonstrates community ambulation with minimal assistance	1. Teach how to manage doors/doorways and locks							
	2. Teach how to manage building access							
	3. Teach how to manage elevators, if applicable							
	4. Teach how to maneuver curbs and ramps							
	5. Teach how to access vehicles/public transportation with assistance as needed							

APPENDIX F-1

Beth Israel Medical Center

MULTIDISCIPLINARY ACTION PLAN (MAP)
DIRECTLY OBSERVED THERAPY (DOT)
DIAGNOSIS: *TUBERCULOSIS*
MMTP CLINIC: _____

Last Name:
First Name:
RUID:
MR:
DOB:

DATE OF TB DIAGNOSIS: _____
FACILITY OR MD MAKING DIAGNOSIS: _____
PRIMARY CARE PROVIDER: _____
ADDRESS: _____
CONTACT PERSON: _____ PHONE: ( )_____
NYC DOT CASE REGISTRY #: _____
TB DIAGNOSIS: ( ) Pulmonary   Site: _____
( ) Extrapulmonary   Date Smear +: _____
Date Culture +: _____

FIRST POSITIVE SPUTUM	DATE	POSITIVE OR NEGATIVE
SMEAR		
CULTURE		

LAST THREE SPUTUMS	DATE	POSITIVE OR NEGATIVE	DATE	POSITIVE OR NEGATIVE	DATE	POSITIVE OR NEGATIVE
SMEAR						
CULTURE						

IF ANY CULTURE IS POSITIVE, LIST DATE AND RESISTANT DRUGS: _____
MOST RECENT CXR RESULTS AND DATE: _____

DEVELOPMENT OF MULTIDISCIPLINARY ACTION PLAN FUNDED, IN PART, BY THE NEW YORK STATE DEPARTMENT OF HEALTH

APPENDIX F-2

Last Name:
First Name:
Ruid:
MR:
DOB:

DATE DOT STARTED:
EXPECTED DATE OF TREATMENT COMPLETION: _____
ANTI-TB MEDICATION/DRUG NAME/DOSAGE :
DAYS PER WEEK: ( )7 ( )5 ( )3 ( )2

( ) INH ____ mg.   ( ) ETH ____ mg.   ( ) FLOX ____ mg.

( ) RIF ____ mg.   ( ) CYC ____ mg.   ( ) Other (Specify)

( ) PZA ____ mg.   ( ) CIP ____ mg.   _____

( ) EMB ____ mg.   ( ) PAS ____ mg.   _____

TEAM: _____
TB COORDINATOR: _____
MD/RPA: _____
SOCIAL WORKER: _____
OUTREACH WORKER: _____
DATE MAP INITIATED: _____

APPENDIX F-3

Beth Israel Medical Center
MULTIDISCIPLINARY ACTION PLAN
DAY 1   Date:
DIAGNOSIS: *TUBERCULOSIS*

LAST NAME:
FIRST NAME:
RUID:
MR:
DOB:

MULTIDISCIPLINARY INTERVENTION	PATIENT GOALS OR EXPECTED OUTCOMES	ACHIEVED	IF NOT EXPLAIN ON REVERSE SIDE
ASSESSMENT			
A. RPA:			
1. Meet patient.	A. Patient understands diagnosis of Tuberculosis (TB), course of treatment, medical follow-up appointments and signs necessary releases.	A. ☐	A. ☐
2. Review patient chart and history.		1. ☐	1. ☐
3. Confer with primary care provider.		2. ☐	2. ☐
4. Obtain necessary releases.		3. ☐	3. ☐
5. Review medications.		4. ☐	4. ☐
6. Make follow-up appointments.		5. ☐	5. ☐
7. Reviews case with MD.		6. ☐	6. ☐
		7. ☐	7. ☐
B. RN:			
1. Organize Interdisciplinary Case Conference (ICC). Reg. Nurse (RN), Physician (MD), Registered Physician Assistant (RPA), Social Worker (SW), Counselor, Clinic Supervisor, HIV Health Coordinator and patient in attendance.	B. 1. Patient attends ICC for DOT Treatment Plan.	B. 1. ☐	B. 1. ☐
2. Review medicating procedure and prescriptions.	2. Patient agrees to medication schedule.	2. ☐	2. ☐
3. Begin Directly Observed Therapy (DOT) paper work: a. TB Treatment Face Sheet b. Medication and Dosage Progress Notes.	3.	3. ☐	3. ☐
4. Notify TB Services of newly enrolled DOT patient.	4. RN notifies TB Services of all newly diagnosed TB patients.	4. ☐	4. ☐
CONSENTS & CONSULTS			
A. RPA: Patient signs all consents.	A. All consents are signed.	A. ☐	A. ☐
B. RN:	B.	B.	B.
1. Ensure patient signs Consent for Pharmacy (Poison Prevention Safety Act) for the blister pack enrollment.	1. Patient signs Poison Prevention Safety Act form.	1. ☐	1. ☐
2. Notify BIMC Pharmacy of enrolled DOT patient.	2.	2. ☐	2. ☐
C. COUNSELOR/SUPERVISOR	C. Patient signs consents and contracts and understands NYCDOH is informed of diagnosis, treatment, and nonadherence.	C. ☐	C. ☐
Ensure patient signs consent to disclose TB information to the New York City Department of Health (NYCDOH).			
MEDICATIONS			
A. RPA:	A.	A. ☐	A. ☐
1. Review TB medication prescriptions for appropriateness.	1. Patient begins medication.	1. ☐	1. ☐
2. Discuss regimen appropriateness with primary care provider.		2. ☐	2. ☐
3. Consult with TB Services for direction when medication regimen is not appropriate.		3. ☐	3. ☐
4. When indicated, recommend change in the patient pick-up schedule.	4. Patient understands reason for schedule change.	4. ☐	4. ☐
5. Rewrite the TB medication prescriptions if patient does not have Medicaid and notify TB Services if this occurs.		5. ☐	5. ☐
6. Review TB prescriptions with MD.		6. ☐	6. ☐
B. RN:	B. Patient acknowledges understanding of medication regimen.	B. ☐	B. ☐
1. Review with patient TB medication regimen.		1. ☐	1. ☐
2. Enter patient. info and list of meds into the computer.		2. ☐	2. ☐

Beth Israel Medical Center
MULTIDISCIPLINARY ACTION PLAN
DAY 1   Date: _____
DIAGNOSIS: *TUBERCULOSIS*

Last Name: _____
First Name: _____
RUID: _____
MR: _____
DOB: _____

MULTIDISCIPLINARY INTERVENTIONS	PATIENT GOALS OR EXPECTED OUTCOMES	ACHIEVED	IF NOT EXPLAIN ON REVERSE SIDE
MEDICAL MANAGEMENT			
A. RPA: 1. Examine patient and review medical data and documentation of diagnosis. 2. Where indicated order tests. 3. Confer with primary care provider for additional info. 4. Confer with Clinic MD.	A. Patient describes signs or symptoms attributable to progression of TB disease or TB medications.	A. 1. ☐ 2. ☐ 3. ☐ 4. ☐	A. 1. ☐ 2. ☐ 3. ☐ 4. ☐
B. MD: Review patient MMTP chart for TB information.	B. Data correct in TB section MMTP chart.	B. ☐	B. ☐
C. RN: 1. Review documentation for diagnosis. 2. Confer with RPA on medical DOT treatment plan.	C. Meets with RPA, discuss documentation and DOT treatment plan.	C. ☐	C. ☐
CASE MANAGEMENT			
A. RPA, MD, RN, SW, CLINIC SUPERVISOR, COUNSELOR: 1. Reinforce adherence to TB Contract and consequences as established during ICC. 2. Assess patient needs and develop treatment plan.	A. Patient meets with clinic staff to develop a treatment goal, patient agrees to conditions of the contract.	A. ☐	A. ☐
B. COUNSELOR: 1. Review/update patient's psychosocial. 2. Contact Social Worker. 3. Notify HIV Health Coordinator of all newly diagnosed TB patients. 4. Ensure Medicaid is active.	B. Patient meets with staff and agrees to keep necessary outside appointments.	B. 1. ☐ 2. ☐ 3. ☐ 4. ☐	B. 1. ☐ 2. ☐ 3. ☐ 4. ☐
PATIENT EDUCATION			
A. RPA: Review with patient TB modes of transmission, determine contact risk in patient environment, and prevention.	A. Patient understands issues of TB transmission, treatment, and prevention.	A. ☐	A. ☐
B. RN: 1. Assess patient knowledge of TB, medications, treatment adherence & HIV infection. 2. Initiate TB education and encourage patient to express emotional and physical concerns.	B. Patient understands TB treatment plan.	B. 1. ☐ 2. ☐	B. 1. ☐ 2. ☐
C. COUNSELOR: Reinforce with patient need for adherence to treatment and TB Contract.	C. Patient meets with counselor to discuss importance of adherence to treatment and encourages patient to express feelings.	C. ☐	C. ☐
D. HIV HEALTH COORDINATOR: Counsel and recommend HIV testing, if indicated.	D. Patient meets with HIV Health Coordinator and is referred for HIV counseling and testing.	D. ☐	D. ☐
ADMINISTRATIVE (TB SERVICES)			
A. CASE MANAGER: TB Services notified of any new TB patient.	A. TB Coordinator notifies TB Services Case Manager of newly diagnosed TB patient.	A. ☐	A. ☐
B. SW: TB Services SW notified of newly diagnosed TB patient.	B. Case Manager conveys patient info to TB Services, SW & outreach workers.	B. ☐	B. ☐

A multidisciplinary
approach to quality
care

MPC

Multidisciplinary Patient Care

BETH ISRAEL MEDICAL CENTER

MULTIDISCIPLINARY ACTION PLAN

DIAGNOSIS: <u>WELL NEWBORN</u>

UNIT: <u>NEWBORN NURSERY</u>

DATE OF BIRTH: _____/_____/_____ **TIME:** _____:_____ am/pm

ADMISSION DATE: _____/_____/_____ **TIME:** _____:_____ am/pm

DATE MAP INITIATED: _____/_____/_____ **TIME:** _____:_____ am/pm

DRG #: <u>391/620/627/628/629/630</u>

EXPECTED LENGTH OF STAY: <u>24 TO 48 HOURS</u>

FOLLOWED BY PATIENT CARE MANAGER: YES ☐   NO ☐
(If Yes) Name: _____

FOLLOWED BY SOCIAL WORKER: YES ☐   NO ☐
(If Yes) Name: _____

GOALS MUTUALLY SET WITH PARENTS AND/OR SIGNIFICANT OTHER

_____ **YES**

_____ **NO**   **EXPLAIN** _____

PRENATAL HISTORY: _____

_____

_____

_____

APPENDIX G-2

Beth Israel Medical Center
MULTIDISCIPLINARY ACTION PLAN
DAY 1/0-8°

MD: _____

DIAGNOSIS: <u>WELL NEWBORN</u> _____

DATE: _____

TIME: FROM_____ TO_____

MAP DOES NOT REPLACE MD ORDERS

		NOTES
PHYSICAL ASSESSMENT:	Complete Newborn Admission Assessment (MD and RN) and Maternal Assessment Record. Initiate D/C summary.	
TESTS:	1. Check if following blood work done in labor and delivery; if not draw blood and send to lab: i.e. blood type, RH, Coombs, RPR, Bilirubin (T&D)PRN,Hep B$_8$A$_9$ 2. Glucose screening as per policy: Screen infants over 4000 or less than 2500 grams, infants born to diabetic mothers, postmature infants and infants with Intrauterine Growth Retardation.	
TREATMENTS:	Maintain infant under warmer or skin/skin on mother's chest until temperature stable. Rectal temp x1 on admission, then axillary temperature Q30 minutes until stable. Vital signs on admission. Clean cord with providine iodine x1, then with alcohol TID. Weight and measure on admission.	
MEDICATION:	Medication _____: See MAR Engerix/hepatitis B vaccination per MD order.	
CONSULTS:	As needed.	
NUTRITION EVALUATION:	Breastfeeding: 1. Frequency and duration of feedings. 2. Offering breast in response to hunger cues. 3. Alternating breasts and burping infant. 4. Importance of draining first breast before offering second. 5. Risks of limiting length of feedings and bottles use. 6. Use of pillows to aid positioning. 7. Football/clutch, transition and cradle positions. 8. Correct head, neck, and body alignment. 9. Repositioning for proper latch on and comfort. Evaluate for latching, suck, swallow, tolerance. Bottlefeeding: 10. Correct positioning of infant. 11. Frequency and amount of feedings. 12. Choice and preparation of formula. 13. Burping of infant. Evaluate for suck, swallow, tolerance.	
SOCIAL WORK:	At 9:00 a.m. rounds. Refer any newborns who meet Social Work high risk criteria for Social Work assessment.	
DISCHARGE PLANNING:		

SHIFT	INITIALS	PRINT NAME	SIGNATURE

MAP 070 (Rev 9/94)

APPENDIX G-3

Beth Israel Medical Center
MULTIDISCIPLINARY ACTION PLAN
DAY 1/0-8°

MD: _____

DIAGNOSIS: <u>WELL NEWBORN</u>_____

DATE: _____

TIME: FROM_____ TO_____

PATIENT PROBLEM AND NURSING INTERVENTIONS	EXPECTED PATIENT OUTCOME AND/OR DISCHARGE OUTCOME	ASSESSMENT/EVALUATION	
1. AT RISK FOR THERMO-REGULATION INSTABILITY → STABLE THERMOREGULATION			
A. Assess/observe for signs of cold stress: 1. Poor peripheral perfusion; 2. Cool extremities; 3. Peripheral cyanosis.	A. No signs of cold stress.	A. See Flowsheet	A. See Flowsheet
B. Place in warmer until stable temperature.	B. T° range: 97.6° - 98.6°F	B. See Flowsheet	B. See Flowsheet
2. AT RISK FOR MAL ADAPTATION TO EXTRAUTERINE LIFE → MAINTAIN NORMAL ADAPTATION TO EXTRAUTERINE LIFE			
A. Position on side after feeding.	A. No aspirations.	A.	A.
B. Assess/observe for signs of resp. distress: cyanosis, grunting, retracting, tachypnea, nasal flaring.	B. Regular/unlabored respirations.	B. See Flowsheet	B. See Flowsheet
C. If evidence of respiratory distress: 1. Administer oxygen. 2. Perform chest PT. 3. Suction mouth/nares.	C. Clear airway-normal breathing pattern resumes.	C.	C.
3. AT RISK FOR NUTRITION IMBALANCE LESS THAN BODY REQUIREMENT → MAINTAIN NUTRITIONAL BALANCE			
A. Assess/observe tolerance of feeding 1. Breastfeeding	A. Infant tolerates feedings: 1a. Latches on well to both breasts. b. Appropriate suck/swallow.	A. 1. See Flowsheet	A. 1. See Flowsheet
2. Bottlefeeding	2. Appropriate suck/swallow/nipple size.	2. See Flowsheet	2. See Flowsheet
B. Assess/observe hypoglycemia: Tremors, lethargy.	B. Blood glucose >40.	B. See Flowsheet	B. See Flowsheet
C. Assess daily weights and record.	C. Maintains desirable weight.	C. See Flowsheet	C. See Flowsheet
D. Record stools.	D. Stooling pattern 1-2x/24°.	D. See Flowsheet	D. See Flowsheet
E. Record voids.	E. Voiding pattern 5-6x/24°.	E. See Flowsheet	E. See Flowsheet
4. HIGH RISK FOR INFECTION R/T IMMATURE IMMUNE SYSTEM → INFECTION FREE			
A. Assess/observe for signs/symptoms of infection Hypothermia, lethargy, odor, redness, drainage, irritability feeding intolerance, fever.	A. No S/S of infection.	A.	A.
B. Apply iodine to cord on admission.	B. Cord remains dry and intact.	B.	B.
C. Apply alcohol to entire cord TID.	C. Cord remains dry and intact.	C.	C.
5. DISCHARGE PLANNING/PARENT'S TEACHING → MOTHER/S.O. INCREASED KNOWLEDGE OF INFANT CARE			
A. Assess mother/S.O. knowledge of infant care and instruct regarding the following as needed: 1. Cord care 2. Bathing 3. Breast/formula prep./feeding techniques 4. Burping 5. Diapering 6. Behavioral state of sleep-wake continuum.	A. Verbalize understanding/demonstrate successfully.	A	A
B. Instruct mother/S.O. regarding importance of parent infant attachment.	B. Mother/S.O. develop an attachment to infant.	B.	B.
C. Observe for objective signs of parental attachment: Eye contact, skin contact, cuddling, stroking, affectionate speech pattern.	C. Mother/S.O. exhibit bonding attachment.	C.	C.
D. Enc. mother/S.O. to participate in infant care.	D. Mother/S.O. participates in care.	D.	D.

MAP 070 (Rev 9/94)

APPENDIX G-4

Beth Israel Medical Center
MULTIDISCIPLINARY ACTION PLAN
DAY 1/9-16°

MD: _____
DIAGNOSIS: WELL NEWBORN _____
DATE: _____
TIME: FROM _____ TO _____

MAP DOES NOT REPLACE MD ORDERS

NOTES

PHYSICAL ASSESSMENT:	Continue newborn assessment. Continue D/C summary.	
TESTS:	Repeat blood work when indicated. Repeat Bilirubin (T&D) as indicated. Blood glucose screening as per policy. IMDS upon discharge. If D/C <24° old, F/U IMDS at 48° - 72°. Urine toxicology, as indicated.	
TREATMENTS:	Clean cord with alcohol TID; Vital signs every 12 hours; Consider circumcision; if circumcised apply petroleum gauze. Daily weight.	
MEDICATION:	Medication _____: See MAR Engerix/hepatitis B vaccination per MD order.	
CONSULTS:	As needed. Lactation specialist as indicated.	
NUTRITION EVALUATION:	Breastfeeding: 1. Frequency and duration of feedings. 2. Offering breast in response to hunger cues. 3. Awaken every 2° - 3° for feedings. 4. Alternating breasts and burping infant. 5. Importance of draining first breast before offering second. 6. Risks of limiting length of feedings and bottles use. 7. Use of pillows to aid positioning. 8. Clutch and transitional positions. 9. Correct head, neck, and body alignment. 10. Repositioning for proper latch on and comfort. Evaluate for latching, suck, swallow, tolerance. Bottlefeeding: 11. Correct positioning of infant. 12. Frequency and amount of feedings. 13. Choice and preparation of formula. 14. Burping of infant. Evaluate for suck, swallow, tolerance.	
SOCIAL WORK:	Refer any newborn who meets SW high risk criteria. Begin Social Work assessment for high risk patients. Consult with family, MD, RN, and HHIC as indicated.	
DISCHARGE PLANNING:	SW, RN or MD refer to HHIC for assessment of home care needs, if appropriate; If D/C scheduled for Day 1/24°, refer to HHIC for Early Maternity Discharge Program.	

SHIFT	INITIALS	PRINT NAME	SIGNATURE

MAP 070 (Rev 9/94)

APPENDIX G-5

<u>Beth Israel Medical Center</u>
MULTIDISCIPLINARY ACTION PLAN
DAY 1/9-16°

MD: _____

DIAGNOSIS: <u>WELL NEWBORN</u>

DATE: _____

TIME: FROM_____ TO_____

PATIENT PROBLEM AND NURSING INTERVENTIONS	EXPECTED PATIENT OUTCOME AND/OR DISCHARGE OUTCOME	ASSESSMENT/EVALUATION	
1. AT RISK FOR THERMO-REGULATION INSTABILITY → STABLE THERMOREGULATION			
A. Assess/observe for signs of cold stress: 1. Poor peripheral perfusion; 2. Cool extremities; 3. Peripheral cyanosis.	A. Vital signs WNL	A.See Flowsheet	A.See Flowsheet
B. Wrap baby well or put on mother's chest.	B. T° range: 97.6° - 98.6°F	B.See Flowsheet	B.See Flowsheet
2. AT RISK FOR MAL ADAPTATION TO EXTRAUTERINE LIFE → MAINTAIN NORMAL ADAPTATION TO EXTRAUTERINE LIFE			
A. Position on side after feeding.	A. No aspirations.	A.	A.
B. Assess/observe signs of resp. distress: cyanosis, grunting, retracting, tachypnea, nasal flaring.	B. Regular/unlabored respirations.	B. See Flowsheet	B. See Flowsheet
C. If evidence of respiratory distress: 1. Administer oxygen; 2. Perform chest PT.; 3. Suction mouth/nares.	C. Clear airway-normal breathing pattern resumes.	C.	C.
3. AT RISK FOR NUTRITION IMBALANCE LESS THAN BODY REQ. → MAINTAIN NUTRITIONAL BALANCE			
A. Assess/observe tolerance of feeding 1. Breastfeeding	A. Infant tolerates feedings: 1a. Latches on well to both breasts. b. Appropriate suck/swallow.	A. 1. See Flowsheet	A. 1. See Flowsheet
2. Bottlefeeding	2. Appro. suck/swallow/nipple size.	2. See Flowsheet	2. See Flowsheet
B. Assess/observe for hypoglycemia: Tremors, lethargy.	B. Blood glucose >40.	B. See Flowsheet	B. See Flowsheet
C. Assess daily weights and record.	C. Maintains desirable weight.	C. See Flowsheet	C. See Flowsheet
D. Record Stools.	D. Stooling pattern 1-2x/24°.	D. See Flowsheet	D. See Flowsheet
E. Records voids.	E. Stooling pattern 5-6x/24°.	E. See Flowsheet	E. See Flowsheet
4. HIGH RISK FOR INFECTION R/T IMMATURE IMMUNE SYSTEM → INFECTION FREE			
A. Assess/observe for signs/symptoms of infection Hypothermia, lethargy, odor, redness, drainage, edema, irritability, feeding intolerance, fever.	A. No S/S of infection.	A.	A.
B. Apply alcohol to entire cord TID.	B. Cord remains dry and intact.	B.	B.
C. If circumcised: 1. Assess/observe circumcision site for S/S of infection: Unusual discharge, foul odor, poor feeding, fever. 2. Bleeding present-apply gentle pressure with sterile gauze. 3. Apply petroleum gauze around penis upon diaper change. 4. Gently clean penis to remove urine & feces. 5. Notify MD if infant hasn't voided >12°.	C. Circumcision site remains dry and intact/no complications.	C.	C.
5. D/C PLANNING/PARENT'S TEACHING → MOTHER/S.O INCREASED INFANT CARE KNOWLEDGE			
A. Assess mother/S.O. knowledge of infant care and instruct as needed: 1. Infant safety; 2. Car safety; 3. Reinforce previous teaching.	A. Verbalize understanding 1. Mother/S.O familiar with infant safety. 2. Aware of NYS car seat law.	A	A
B. If circumcised instruct mother/S.O on Post circumcision care.	B. Verbalize understanding/return demonstration.	B.	B.
C. Give mother/S.O. written instructions and lifetime health record.	C. Verbalize understanding.	C.	C.
D. Assess familiarity with medical follow-up. 1. Follow-up appt.2. Date of first well baby check-up 3. Discuss S/S that must be reported to MD.	D. Mother/S.O verbalize understanding of follow-up appointment and S/S of infection.	D.	D.

MAP 070 (Rev 9/94)

APPENDIX G-6

Beth Israel Medical Center
MULTIDISCIPLINARY ACTION PLAN
DAY 1/17-24°

MD: _____

DIAGNOSIS: WELL NEWBORN _____

DATE: _____

TIME: FROM_____ TO_____

MAP DOES NOT REPLACE MD ORDERS

		NOTES
PHYSICAL ASSESSMENT:	Observe baby. Complete D/C summary.	
TESTS:	Repeat blood work when indicated. Repeat Bilirubin (T&D) as indicated. Blood glucose screening as per policy. IMDS upon discharge. If D/C < 24° old, F/U IMDS at 48° - 72°. Urine toxicology, as indicated.	
TREATMENTS:	Clean cord with alcohol TID. Vital signs Q12H. Circumcision care as indicated. Daily weight. <u>Hypothermia</u> - Return to warmer. - Blood glucose x1 and PRN.	
MEDICATION:	Medication _____ : See MAR	
CONSULTS:	As needed; Lactation specialist as indicated.	
NUTRITION EVALUATION:	<u>Breastfeeding:</u> 1. Frequency and duration of feedings. 2. Offering breast in response to hunger cues. 3. Awakes every 2°-3° for feedings. 4. Alternating breasts and burping infant. 5. Importance of draining first breast before offering second. 6. Risks of limiting length of feedings and bottles use. 7. Use of pillows to aid positioning. 8. Clutch and transitional positions. 9. Correct head, neck, and body alignment. 10. Repositioning for proper latch on and comfort. Evaluate for latching, suck, swallow, tolerance. <u>Bottlefeeding:</u> 11. Correct positioning of infant. 12. Frequency and amount of feedings. 13. Choice and preparation of formula. 14. Burping of infant. Evaluate for suck, swallow, tolerance.	
SOCIAL WORK:	- Cont. assessment, intervention & planning as indicated. If D/C is scheduled for Day 1/24° ensure necessary forms & referrals have been completed & that necessary services are available. - If PT has been or is being reported to Child Welfare Administration, document report. If CWA involved notify CWA when PT medically cleared for discharge. Should CWA place a protective hold on the PT notify medical staff. Document all pertinent material. PT can not be discharged until CWA notifies social work who will coordinate discharge.	
DISCHARGE PLANNING:	If discharge is scheduled for Day 1/24°; confirm all home care plans with HHIC, patient and family.	

SHIFT	INITIALS	PRINT NAME	SIGNATURE

MAP 070 (Rev 9/94)

APPENDIX G-7

Beth Israel Medical Center
MULTIDISCIPLINARY ACTION PLAN
DAY 1/17-24°

MD: _____

DIAGNOSIS: <u>WELL NEWBORN</u>_____

DATE: _____

TIME: FROM_____ TO_____

PATIENT PROBLEM AND NURSING INTERVENTIONS	EXPECTED PATIENT OUTCOME AND/OR DISCHARGE OUTCOME	ASSESSMENT/EVALUATION	
1. AT RISK FOR THERMO-REGULATION INSTABILITY → STABLE THERMOREGULATION			
A. Assess/observe for signs of cold stress: 1. Poor peripheral perfusion; 2. Cool extremities; 3. Peripheral cyanosis. B. Wrap baby well or put on mother's chest.	A. Vital signs WNL B. T° range: 97.6° - 98.6°F	A.See Flowsheet B.See Flowsheet	A.See Flowsheet B.See Flowsheet
2. AT RISK FOR MAL ADAPTATION TO EXTRAUTERINE LIFE → MAINTAIN NORMAL ADAPTATION TO EXTRAUTERINE LIFE			
A. Position on side after feeding. B. Assess/observe signs of resp. distress: cyanosis, grunting, retracting, tachypnea, nasal flaring. C. If evidence of respiratory distress: 1. Administer oxygen 2. Perform chest PT. 3. Suction mouth/nares.	A. No aspirations. B. Regular/unlabored respirations. C. Clear airway-normal breathing pattern resumes.	A. B.See Flowsheet C.	A. B.See Flowsheet C.
3. AT RISK FOR NUTRITION IMBALANCE BODY REQ. → MAINTAIN NUTRITIONAL BALANCE			
A. Assess/observe tolerance of feeding 1. Breastfeeding 2. Bottlefeeding B. Assess/observe for hypoglycemia: Tremors, lethargy. C. Assess daily weights and record. D. Record stools. E. Record voids.	A. Infant tolerates feedings: 1a. Latches on well to both breasts. b. Appropriate suck/swallow. 2. Appro. suck/swallow/nipple size. B. Blood glucose >40. C. Maintains desirable weight. D. Stooling pattern 1-2x/24°. E. Voiding pattern 5-6x/24°.	A. 1.See Flowsheet 2.See Flowsheet B.See Flowsheet C.See Flowsheet D.See Flowsheet E.See Flowsheet	A. 1.See Flowsheet 2.See Flowsheet B.See Flowsheet C.See Flowsheet D.See Flowsheet E.See Flowsheet
4. HIGH RISK FOR INFECTION R/T IMMATURE IMMUNE SYSTEM → INFECTION FREE			
A. Assess/observe for signs/symptoms of infection Hypothermia, lethargy, odor, redness, drainage, edema, irritability, feeding intolerance, fever. B. Apply alcohol to entire cord TID. C. If circumcised: 1. Assess/observe circumcision site for S/S of infection: Unusual discharge, foul odor, poor feeding, fever. 2. Bleeding present-apply gentle pressure with sterile gauze. 3. Apply petroleum gauze around penis upon diaper change. 4. Gently clean penis to remove urine and feces. 5. Notify physician if infant hasn't voided >12°.	A. No S/S of infection. B. Cord remains dry and intact. C. Circumcision site remains dry and intact/no complications.	A. B. C.	A. B. C.
5. D/C PLANNING/PARENT'S TEACHING → MOTHER/S.O.INCREASED KNOWLEDGE INFANT CARE			
A. Reinforce mother/S.O. knowledge of infant care and instruct as needed: 1. Infant safety; 2. Car safety; 3. Reinforce previous teaching. B. If circumcised instruct mother/S.O on Post circumcision care. C. Give mother/SO written instructions and lifetime health record. D. Assess familiarity with medical follow-up. 1. Follow-up appt.; 2. Date of first well baby check-up; 3. Discuss S/S that must be reported to MD. E. Reinforce mother/S.O. knowledge of infant care.	A. Verbalize understanding 1. Mother/S.O familiar on infant safety 2. Aware of NYS car seat law. B. Verbalize understanding/return demonstration. C. Verbalize understanding. D. Mother/S.O verbalize understanding of follow-up and S/S of infection. E. Verbalize understanding demonstrate successfully.	A B. C. D. E.	A B. C. D. E.

APPENDIX G-8

<u>Beth Israel Medical Center</u>
MULTIDISCIPLINARY ACTION PLAN
DAY 2/25-48°

MD: _____

DIAGNOSIS: <u>WELL NEWBORN</u>_____

DATE: _____

TIME: FROM_____ TO_____

MAP DOES NOT REPLACE MD ORDERS

		NOTES
PHYSICAL ASSESSMENT:	Complete D/C summary.	
TESTS:	IMDS.	
TREATMENTS:	Clean cord with alcohol TID. Vital signs Q12H. Circumcision care as indicated. Daily weight.	
MEDICATION:	Medication _____: See MAR	
CONSULTS:	As needed. Lactation specialist as indicated.	
NUTRITION EVALUATION:	Breastfeeding: 1. Frequency and duration of feedings. 2. Offering breast in response to hunger cues. 3. Awaken every 2° - 3° for feedings. 4. Alternating breasts and burping infant. 5. Importance of draining first breast before offering second. 6. Risks of limiting length of feedings and bottles use. 7. Use of pillows to aid positioning. 8. Clutch and transitional positions. 9. Correct head, neck, and body alignment. 10. Repositioning for proper latch on and comfort. Evaluate for latching, suck, swallow, tolerance. Bottlefeeding: 11. Correct positioning of infant. 12. Frequency and amount of feedings. 13. Choice and preparation of formula. 14. Burping of infant. Evaluate for suck, swallow, tolerance.	
SOCIAL WORK:	Continue involvement in discharge planning; on-going consultation with family, MD, RN and HHIC as indicated. Ensure that necessary forms and referrals have been completed and that necessary services are available. If patient has been or is being reported to Child Welfare Administration, document report. If CWA involved notify CWA when patient medically cleared for discharge. Should CWA place a protective hold on the patient notify medical staff. Document all pertinent material. Patient can not be discharged until CWA notifies social work who will coordinate discharge.	
DISCHARGE PLANNING:	Confirm all home care plans with HHIC, patient and family referral to.	

SHIFT	INITIALS	PRINT NAME	SIGNATURE

MAP 070 (Rev 9/94)

APPENDIX G-9

<u>Beth Israel Medical Center</u>
MULTIDISCIPLINARY ACTION PLAN
DAY 2/25-48°

MD: _____

DIAGNOSIS: <u>WELL NEWBORN</u>_____

DATE: _____

TIME: FROM_____ TO_____

PATIENT PROBLEM AND NURSING INTERVENTIONS	EXPECTED PATIENT OUTCOME AND/OR DISCHARGE OUTCOME	ASSESSMENT/EVALUATION	
1. *AT RISK FOR THERMO-REGULATION INSTABILITY → STABLE THERMOREGULATION*			
A. Assess/observe for signs of cold stress: 1. Poor peripheral perfusion; 2. Cool extremities; 3. Peripheral cyanosis.	A. Vital signs WNL	A. See Flowsheet	A. See Flowsheet
B. Wrap baby well or put on mother's chest.	B. T° range: 97.6° - 98.6°F	B. See Flowsheet	B. See Flowsheet
2. *AT RISK FOR MAL ADAPTATION TO EXTRAUTERINE LIFE → MAINTAIN NORMAL ADAPTATION TO EXTRAUTERINE LIFE*			
A. Position on side after feeding.	A. No aspirations.	A.	A.
B. Assess/observe signs of resp. distress: cyanosis, grunting, retracting, tachypnea, nasal flaring.	B. Regular/unlabored respirations.	B. See Flowsheet	B. See Flowsheet
C. If evidence of respiratory distress: 1. Administer oxygen; 2. Perform chest PT.; 3. Suction mouth/nares.	C. Clear airway-normal breathing pattern resumes.	C.	C.
3. *AT RISK FOR NUTRITION IMBALANCE BODY REQ. → MAINTAIN NUTRITIONAL BALANCE*			
A. Assess/observe tolerance of feeding 1. Breastfeeding	A. Infant tolerates feedings: 1a. Latches on well to both breasts. b. Appropriate suck/swallow.	A. 1. See Flowsheet	A. 1. See Flowsheet
2. Bottlefeeding	2. Appro. suck/swallow/nipple size	2. See Flowsheet	2. See Flowsheet
B. Assess/observe hypoglycemia: Tremors, lethargy.	B. Blood glucose >40.	B. See Flowsheet	B. See Flowsheet
C. Assess daily weights.	C. Maintains desirable weight.	C. See Flowsheet	C. See Flowsheet
D. Record stools.	D. Stooling pattern 1-2x/24°.	D. See Flowsheet	D. See Flowsheet
E. Record voids.	E. Voiding pattern 5-6x/24°.	E. See Flowsheet	E. See Flowsheet
4. *HIGH RISK FOR INFECTION R/T IMMATURE IMMUNE SYSTEM → INFECTION FREE*			
A. Assess/observe for signs/symptoms of infection Hypothermia, lethargy, odor, redness, drainage, edema, irritability, feeding intolerance, fever.	A. No S/S of infection.	A.	A.
B. Apply alcohol to entire cord TID.	B. Cord remains dry and intact.	B.	B.
C. If circumcised: 1. Assess/observe circumcision site for S/S of infection: Unusual discharge, foul odor, poor feeding, fever. 2. Bleeding present-apply gentle pressure with sterile gauze. 3. Apply petroleum gauze around penis upon diaper change. 4. Gently clean penis to remove urine and feces. 5. Notify physician if infant has not voided >12°.	C. Circumcision site remains dry and intact/no complications.	C.	C.
5. *D/C PLANNING/PARENT'S TEACHING → MOTHER/S.O. INCREASED KNOWLEDGE OF INFANT CARE*			
A. Assess mother/S.O. knowledge of infant care and instruct as needed: 1. Infant safety; 2. Car safety; 3. Reinforce previous teaching.	A. Verbalize understanding 1. Mother/SO infant safety familiar. 2. Aware of NYS car seat law.	A	A
B. If circumcised instruct mother/S.O on Post circumcision care.	B. Verbalize understanding/return demonstration.	B.	B.
C. Give mother/S.O. written instructions and lifetime health record.	C. Verbalize understanding.	C.	C.
D. Assess familiarity with medical follow-up. 1. Follow-up appt.; 2. Date of first well baby check-up; 3. Discuss S/S that must be reported to MD.	D. Mother/S.O verbalize understanding of follow-up appointment and S/S of infection.	D.	D.

Beth Israel Medical Center
MULTIDISCIPLINARY ACTION PLAN
DAY 3/49-72°

MD: _____

DIAGNOSIS: WELL NEWBORN _____

DATE: _____

TIME: FROM_____   TO_____

MAP DOES NOT REPLACE MD ORDERS

NOTES

PHYSICAL ASSESSMENT:	Complete D/C summary.
TESTS:	IMDS.
TREATMENTS:	Clean cord with alcohol TID. Vital signs Q12H. Circumcision care as indicated. Daily weight.
MEDICATION:	Medication _____ : See MAR
CONSULTS:	As needed. Lactation specialist as indicated.
NUTRITION EVALUATION:	Breastfeeding: 1. Frequency and duration of feedings. 2. Offering breast in response to hunger cues. 3. Awaken every 2° - 3° for feedings. 4. Alternating breasts and burping infant. 5. Importance of draining first breast before offering second. 6. Risks of limiting length of feedings and bottles use. 7. Use of pillows to aid positioning. 8. Clutch and transitional positions. 9. Correct head, neck, and body alignment. 10. Repositioning for proper latch on and comfort. Evaluate for latching, suck, swallow, tolerance. Bottlefeeding: 11. Correct positioning of infant. 12. Frequency and amount of feedings. 13. Choice and preparation of formula. 14. Burping of infant. Evaluate for suck, swallow, tolerance.
SOCIAL WORK:	Continue involvement in discharge planning; on-going consultation with family, MD, RN and HHIC as indicated. Ensure that necessary forms and referrals have been completed and that necessary services are available. If patient has been or is being reported to Child Welfare Administration, document report. If CWA involved notify CWA when patient medically cleared for discharge. Should CWA place a protective hold on the patient notify medical staff. Document all pertinent material. Patient can not be discharged until CWA notifies social work who will coordinate discharge.
DISCHARGE PLANNING:	Confirm all home care plans with HHIC, patient and family referral to.

SHIFT	INITIALS	PRINT NAME	SIGNATURE

MAP 070 (Rev 9/94)

APPENDIX G-11

Beth Israel Medical Center
MULTIDISCIPLINARY ACTION PLAN
DAY 3/49-72°

MD: _____

DIAGNOSIS: <u>WELL NEWBORN</u> _____

DATE: _____

TIME: FROM_____ TO_____

PATIENT PROBLEM AND NURSING INTERVENTIONS	EXPECTED PATIENT OUTCOME AND/OR DISCHARGE OUTCOME	ASSESSMENT/EVALUATION	
1. AT RISK FOR THERMO-REGULATION INSTABILITY → STABLE THERMOREGULATION			
A. Assess/observe for signs of cold stress: 1. Poor peripheral perfusion; 2. Cool extremities; 3. Peripheral cyanosis.	A. Vital signs WNL	A. See Flowsheet	A. See Flowsheet
B. Wrap baby well or put on mother's chest.	B. T° range: 97.6° - 98.6°F	B. See Flowsheet	B. See Flowsheet
2. AT RISK FOR MAL ADAPTATION TO EXTRAUTERINE LIFE → MAINTAIN NORMAL ADAPTATION TO EXTRAUTERINE LIFE			
A. Position on side after feeding.	A. No aspirations.	A.	A.
B. Assess/observe signs of resp. distress: cyanosis, grunting, retracting, tachypnea, nasal flaring.	B. Regular/unlabored respirations.	B. See Flowsheet	B. See Flowsheet
C. If evidence of respiratory distress: 1. Administer oxygen; 2. Perform chest PT.; 3. Suction mouth/nares.	C. Clear airway-normal breathing pattern resumes.	C.	C.
3. AT RISK FOR NUTRITION IMBALANCE BODY REQ. → MAINTAIN NUTRITIONAL BALANCE			
A. Assess/observe tolerance of feeding 1. Breastfeeding 2. Bottlefeeding	A. Infant tolerates feedings: 1a. Latches on well to both breasts. b. Appropriate suck/swallow. 2. Appro. suck/swallow/nipple size	A. 1. See Flowsheet 2. See Flowsheet	A. 1. See Flowsheet 2. See Flowsheet
B. Assess/observe hypoglycemia: Tremors, lethargy.	B. Blood glucose >40.	B. See Flowsheet	B. See Flowsheet
C. Assess daily weights.	C. Maintains desirable weight.	C. See Flowsheet	C. See Flowsheet
D. Record stools.	D. Stooling pattern 1-2x/24°.	D. See Flowsheet	D. See Flowsheet
E. Record voids.	E. Voiding pattern 5-6x/24°.	E. See Flowsheet	E. See Flowsheet
4. HIGH RISK FOR INFECTION R/T IMMATURE IMMUNE SYSTEM → INFECTION FREE			
A. Assess/observe for signs/symptoms of infection Hypothermia, lethargy, odor, redness, drainage, edema, irritability, feeding intolerance, fever.	A. No S/S of infection.	A.	A.
B. Apply alcohol to entire cord TID.	B. Cord remains dry and intact.	B.	B.
C. If circumcised: 1. Assess/observe circumcision site for S/S of infection: Unusual discharge, foul odor, poor feeding, fever. 2. Bleeding present-apply gentle pressure with sterile gauze. 3. Apply petroleum gauze around penis upon diaper change. 4. Gently clean penis to remove urine and feces. 5. Notify physician if infant has not voided >12°.	C. Circumcision site remains dry and intact/no complications.	C.	C.
5. D/C PLANNING/PARENT'S TEACHING → MOTHER/S.O. INCREASED KNOWLEDGE OF INFANT CARE			
A. Assess mother/S.O. knowledge of infant care and instruct as needed: 1. Infant safety; 2. Car safety; 3. Reinforce previous teaching.	A. Verbalize understanding 1. Mother/SO infant safety familiar. 2. Aware of NYS car seat law.	A	A
B. If circumcised instruct mother/S.O on Post circumcision care.	B. Verbalize understanding/return demonstration.	B.	B.
C. Give mother/S.O. written instructions and lifetime health record.	C. Verbalize understanding.	C.	C.
D. Assess familiarity with medical follow-up. 1. Follow-up appt.; 2. Date of first well baby check-up; 3. Discuss S/S that must be reported to MD.	D. Mother/S.O verbalize understanding of follow-up appointment and S/S of infection.	D.	D.

MAP 070 (Rev 9/94)

APPENDIX H-1

The Long Island College Hospital
Division of Nursing

<u>Position Description/Criteria-based Performance Appraisal</u>

Title: Clinical Nurse Specialist - Case Manager

Division: Nursing

Responsible to: Director of Case Management/
                                Assistant Director of Nursing - Case Management

Date: June, 1995
                                Revised September, 1995/February, 1996

<u>General information:</u>
On the following pages is an outline of the essential duties and supplemental responsibilities of this job. Even though the job description is broad, every effort has been made to make this outline as complete as possible.

<u>Performance evaluation:</u>
This form includes space for one appraisal period. Evaluations must be completed by the department supervisor at the end of the probationary period and annually thereafter.

<u>Scope:</u>
The practice of the profession of nursing as a registered professional nurse is defined as "diagnosing and treating human responses to actual or potential health problems through such services as case finding, health teaching, health counseling, and provision of care supportive to or restorative of life and well-being, and executing medical regimens prescribed by a licensed or otherwise legally authorized physician or dentist." A nursing regimen shall be consistent with and shall not vary any existing medical regimen.

<u>General summary:</u>
The Clinical Nurse Specialist (CNS) is a Master's prepared, advanced practice professional who, as a result of comprehensive education and extensive clinical experience, possesses the knowledge and skills necessary to promote expert nursing. It is the CNS's responsibility to demonstrate this clinical expertise to patients, families and staff. His/her scope of practice includes prevention, health promotion, maintenance, restoration and education. The CNS has an advanced understanding of the physiological and psychosocial dimensions of illness-wellness for the client, his/her significant others and the community. He/she exhibits an in-depth knowledge of the concepts and theories of nursing science and applies this knowledge to the subspecialty. The CNS is responsible for maintenance/improvement of quality, clinical nursing practice. He/she is also responsible for the coordination, development, implementation, monitoring and evaluation of interdisciplinary plans of care for selected patient populations. He/she, utilizing managed care principles, works collaboratively with all members of the health team to insure efficient, cost-effective care for these identified individuals. The CNS is self-directed and accountable for the development of this role.

<u>Identified competencies:</u>
*Clinical practice
*Education
*Consultation
*Research

APPENDIX **H-2**

Clinical Nurse Specialist-Case Manager
Position Description/Criteria-Based Performance Appraisal (continued)

Name: _____ Appraisal date: _____

Department: _____ Performance period: _____

Director's/ADN's name: _____

Section One: Competency Assessment Summary:
This section is required for all patient care areas

		Yes	No
1)	Demonstrates competence during initial employment and orientation process and meets department/unit standards.	[ ]	[ ]
2)	Maintains competence during the year in accordance with department/unit policy and standards, and includes in-service and continuing education.	[ ]	[ ]
3)	Demonstrates competence during the year in accordance with department/unit policy and standards.	[ ]	[ ]
4)	Maintains competence in regulatory agencies and hospital mandated programs	[ ]	[ ]
5)	Other: _____ _____ _____	[ ]	[ ]

Section Two: Age(s) of Patients Served:
This section is required for all patient care areas

[ ] Neonate - birth to 1 mo.   [ ] Infant - 1 mo. to 1 yr.

[ ] Early childhood - 1 yr. to 5 yrs.   [ ] Late childhood - 6 yrs. to 12 yrs.

[ ] Adolescence - 13 yrs. to 17 yrs.   [ ] Adult - 18 yrs. to 54 yrs.

[ ] Senior Adult - 55 yrs. to 64 yrs.   [ ] Geriatric - 64 yrs. and above

[ ] All age groups

APPENDIX H-3

<u>Clinical Nurse Specialist-Case Manager</u>
<u>Position Description/Criteria-Based Performance Appraisal (continued)</u>

Performance Criteria
Instructions to Director, Assistant Director, and/or Designee: Use the key below to rate each performance criteria. Give your rating utmost care and thought. Use the comments section to delineate specific instances that are typical of the individual's work and performance capability. Comments must be made for ratings of 1 and 3. *Performance Level Achieved (PLA):* 1 = Does not meet expectations   2 = Meets expectations 3 = Exceeds expectations   4 = Not applicable

Clinical Practice Component		
Criteria	1,2,3, or 4	Comments
1. Demonstrates clinical expertise through participation in direct patient care activities for a selected population of clients.		
Maintains clinical expertise. Maintains knowledge of scientific progress in nursing and the subspecialty, and incorporates this into practice.		
Assumes ongoing responsibility for the nursing care of patients in a caseload which has been selected according to specific criteria developed by the CNS. Caseload patients will have complex needs and problems requiring sustained intervention by the CNS.		
Assesses biopsychosocial needs of the client based on history and physical examination.		
Analyzes and interprets data, makes nursing diagnoses, and explains the same to client and significant others.		
With the client and significant others, formulates a plan of care to promote, maintain and restore health.		
Selects nursing interventions which reflect an understanding of patient and family care requirements throughout the stages of the patient's illness.		
Assists the patient and family in identifying and implementing strategies to cope with the events and stresses of hospitalization or to adapt to illness and promote wellness as the patient and family learn to live with a chronic illness.		

APPENDIX **H-4**

Clinical Nurse Specialist-Case Manager
Position Description/Criteria-Based Performance Appraisal (continued)

Clinical Practice Component (continued)		
Criteria	1,2,3, or 4	Comments
1. Demonstrates clinical expertise through participation in direct...(continued).		
Utilizing knowledge of the health care system, assists the patient in gaining access to the services essential to continuity of care.		
Facilitates continuity of care after patients are discharged. Manages acute and chronic health problems by providing appropriate follow-up in the Ambulatory Care Department; educates patients and families, and initiates referrals for the treatment and management of complex medical, surgical and psychiatric conditions.		
Identifies and documents patient outcomes, nursing interventions and evaluation criteria.		
In collaboration with the NM and the nursing staff, initiates planned change and evaluates outcomes to improve the quality of patient care.		
Serves as a role model by demonstrating the integration of nursing theory into practice.		
2. Demonstrates clinical expertise by coordinating managed care to target populations.		
Participates in the development/ refinement/revision/modification/ implementation of standards, protocols, guidelines and interdisciplinary MAP's for selected patient populations as necessary.		
In conjunction with the NM and staff nurses, participates in the selection of appropriate patient populations for placement on MAP's.		
Assists the staff in the integration of nursing theory into practice by observing, guiding, and directing the staff's practice.		
Assists nursing staff in planning for complex or unusual patient/family needs.		

APPENDIX **H-5**

Clinical Nurse Specialist-Case Manager
Position Description/Criteria-Based Performance Appraisal (continued)

Clinical Practice Component (continued)		
Criteria	1,2,3, or 4	Comments
2. Demonstrates clinical expertise by coordinating managed care...(continued).		
Identifies/tracks/trends/analyzes selected variations (variances—patient/family, practitioner, system or community) which effect patient care or length of stay.		
Presents significant findings related to managed care/MAP's to interdisciplinary team members and members of Hospital Administration.		
Implements corrective actions when possible.		
3. Communicates effectually with members of the interdisciplinary team to effectively utilize MAP's.		
Coordinates interdisciplinary communication to facilitate usage of MAP'S.		
Identifies interdisciplinary issues and uses a collaborative approach to resolve conflicts.		
Participates in rounds/meetings with other disciplines as necessary.		
Processes feedback from all disciplines to make needed changes in MAP's.		
Education Component		
Criteria	1,2,3, or 4	Comments
1. Participates in the assessment, development, implementation, and evaluation of educational programs designed to enhance the delivery of nursing care services by staff.		
Identifies learning needs through medical record reviews and communication with staff.		
Utilizes adult teaching/learning principles in providing formal and informal educational opportunities.		

APPENDIX **H-6**

Clinical Nurse Specialist-Case Manager
Position Description/Criteria-Based Performance Appraisal (continued)

Education Component (continued)		
Criteria	1,2,3, or 4	Comments
1. Participates in the assessment, development, implementation,...(continued)		
Fosters an educational environment in which sharing of expertise is encouraged.		
Collaborates with the NM in implementation of stuff development/ educational programs related to case management and the subspecialty.		
Assures the implementation of the nursing process and resolution of patient problems by guiding and directing the clinical activities of the nursing staff (e.g., participating in intershift reports, clinical care conferences, patient care rounds, and service conferences). Demonstrates an understanding of group dynamics.		
Incorporates principles of health maintenance, health promotion, disease prevention, symptom management, patient education and counseling as well as family, crisis, and nursing theories.		
Assists nursing staff in the assembly and development of appropriate resources and staff/patient/family teaching materials. Incorporates growth/development theory and cultural/psychosocial considerations.		
Identifies and utilizes community resources as necessary.		
Acts as a facilitator for new appointees to advanced practice roles.		
Facilitates practicums for graduate students, collaborates with faculty members, and/or participates as faculty in graduate nursing programs.		
Participates in interdisciplinary educational programs for health professionals and the community.		

APPENDIX **H-7**

Clinical Nurse Specialist-Case Manager
Position Description/Criteria-Based Performance Appraisal (continued)

Consultation Component		
Criteria	1,2,3, or 4	Comments
1. Acts as a consultant to all disciplines regarding issues related to quality patient care.		
Serves as liaison between colleagues in nursing, medicine, ancillary disciplines and the patient/family unit.		
Serves as advocate for patient/family unit's concerns in the health care system.		
Participates in the formulation/ implementation of policies, procedures, standards, protocols, guidelines and interdisciplinary MAP's necessary to provide quality patient care.		
Participates in departmental, divisional and institutional committees and councils dealing with clinical practice issues.		
Advises nursing personnel on strategies to facilitate collaboration with other disciplines.		
Makes necessary referrals to peers and/or other members of the health team as necessary. Seeks consultation from nursing colleagues and others in problematic situations.		
Provides consultation to other colleagues when needed.		
Shares specialized knowledge and experience in clinical practice through discussion with other nurses in the institution, colleagues, students, and other health professionals.		
Participates in selection process for appointment of candidates to the clinical ladder and assists the NM with the evaluation of clinical performance.		
Acts as a resource to Nursing Administration for clinical issues and/or problem resolution.		

APPENDIX **H-8**

Clinical Nurse Specialist-Case Manager
Position Description/Criteria-Based Performance Appraisal (continued)

Consultation Component (continued)		
Criteria	1,2,3, or 4	Comments
2. Acts as a consultant to all disciplines regarding issues specific to managed care/case management.		
Serves as advisor for development of/ongoing progress toward a managed care approach.		
Consults with staff nurses regarding foci, goal setting, progression of MAP's and variances.		
Facilitates use of MAP's in daily unit operations by providing guidance to all departments as necessary.		
Research Component		
Criteria	1,2,3, or 4	Comments
1. Participates in or conducts nursing research related to quality patient care issues.		
Initiates, conducts and participates in clinical nursing research. Identifies researchable problems in clinical nursing practice. Formulates research questions, contributes to the development of a research design and implementation.		
Assists with other clinical research projects when appropriate and feasible.		
Conducts patient and family interviews/assessments/surveys and medical record reviews on an on-going basis.		
Utilizes research findings to assist nursing staff to modify theory and improve quality of care by incorporating such findings into nursing practice.		
Participates in the Quality Improvement Program for the Division of Nursing.		

Clinical Nurse Specialist-Case Manager
Position Description/Criteria-Based Performance Appraisal (continued)

Professional Responsibilities		
Criteria	1,2,3, or 4	Comments
Continuously assesses and evaluates knowledge and practice. Maintains and develops professional competence through self-directed participation in professional organizations and advanced, continuing education programs. Maintains professional knowledge of physiological, psychological, social and developmental theories and issues affecting patients and families.		
Contributes to professional growth of members of the nursing staff.		
In collaboration with the NM and immediate supervisor, formulates goals for the enhancement of practice.		
Formulates goals and objectives, evaluates self and shares progress with immediate supervisor.		
Maintains open lines of communication with Vice President Patient Care Services/Director of Nursing-Nursing Services/Administrator-Special Projects/Director of Case Management/Assistant Director of Case Management/Case Management Coordinator/Divisional Assistant Directors of Nursing/Assistant Directors of Nursing.		
Assures that available resources are utilized effectively. Works with interdisciplinary team members to identify cost-savings measures in service-line operations and patient care.		
Participates in intramural and extramural activities (e.g., lectures, presentations and community projects).		
Maintains awareness of current legislation affecting nursing practice; current issues/trends within the nursing profession.		
Develops and implements strategies that maximize the role of the Clinical Nurse Specialist and have positive effects on the health care system.		
Performs professional and related duties as required.		

Clinical Nurse Specialist-Case Manager
Position Description/Criteria-Based Performance Appraisal (continued)

Adherence to Institution/Department Policies and Regulations			
	Meets expectations	Needs improvement	Comments
1. Punctuality			
2. Attendance			
3. Dress code/professional appearance			
4. Safety			
5. Infection control practices			
6. Compliance with employee health protocol			
7. Efficient use of supplies/ resources			

Clinical Nurse Specialist-Case Manager
Position Description/Criteria-Based Performance Appraisal (continued)

Knowledge, Skills and Abilities				
Consider the extent to which the employees' demonstrated knowledge, skills and abilities appear to meet or fall short of the expectations of his/her current job. These ratings should be consistent with the results indicated in performance appraisal.				
	Exceeds expectations	Meets expectations	Needs improvement	Not applicable
Job knowledge/skills The understanding of the principles, techniques, skills, practices, and procedures required by the job. The ability to use the materials and equipment required by the job.				
Planning and organizing The ability to logically and effectively structure tasks, plan the work, establish priorities, and accomplish work activities.				
Communication The ability to organize and present information clearly and concisely. The ability to keep supervisors, peers and visitors (if appropriate) informed about progress, problems and developments.				
Teamwork The ability to work effectively with supervisors and co-workers and to appropriately respond to requests for assistance as a productive team member.				
Initiative The ability to act independently and offer suggestions and new ideas for improving performance and operations.				
Problem solving The ability to analyze situations, identify problems, identify and evaluate alternative courses of actions, and to take appropriate actions. The willingness to be flexible and resourceful.				
Customer service The demonstration of a courteous and helpful manner during interactions with others, such as patients, families, visitiors, and other employees.				
Behavior The ability to conduct oneself in a positive, respectful, professional manner.				
Critical thinking The ability to retain acquired knowledge and exercise appropriate judgement.				

Clinical Nurse Specialist-Case Manager
Position Description/Criteria-Based Performance Appraisal (continued)

Overall Performance

Comments:

[ ] Exceeds expectations

_____
_____
_____

[ ] Meets expectations

_____
_____
_____

[ ] Does not meet expectations

_____
_____
_____

Employee Development

Identify areas for development and specific actions to be taken during the next appraisal period. These may include on the job training, specific developmental assignments, off-site training, etc.:

Comments and Signatures

Employee comments and signature (The employee's signature indicates only that the appraisal has been discussed with the employee and may not indicate agreement with the appraisal):

Signature: _____   Date: _____

Evaluator comments (optional) and signature:

Signature: _____   Date: _____

Second-level reviewer comments and signature (optional):

Signature: _____   Date: _____

APPENDIX **H-13**

<u>Clinical Nurse Specialist-Case Manager</u>
<u>Position Description/Criteria-Based Performance Appraisal (continued)</u>

Position Requirements

<u>Physical demands:</u>
Definitions:
- Constant - Activity or condition exists 2/3 of the time or more
- Frequent - Activity or condition exists form 1/3 to 2/3 of the time
- Occasional - Activity or condition exists up to 1/3 of the time

Work requires:
- Frequent sitting, walking
- Occasionally lifts patients/objects from 10 lbs to 150 lbs.
- Occasionally pushes objects up to 200 lbs.
- Occasional stooping, bending, pulling, pushing, turning, stretching
- Occasionally lifts with assistance objects greater than 150 lbs.
- Occasionally carries objects weighing up to 50 lbs.

Mental demands:
- Ability to memorize details
- Visual acuity for reading and preparing reports
- Speech and hearing utilized in contacts with other health care professionals, patients and visitors.

<u>Education and experience:</u>
- Graduate of a NLN accredited School of Nursing.
- Masters Degree in Nursing.
- Current enrollment in post-graduate, advanced practice certificate program desirable.
- Current New York State Licensure.
- Current BCLS Certification.
- Effective teaching, leadership and interpersonal/communication skills.
- Clinical competence in subspecialty.
- Experience as outcome coordinator/case manager and/or in an advanced practice role desirable.
- Current ANA Certification preferred.

<u>Working conditions:</u>
Works indoors in well-lighted and ventilated rooms with direct patient contact. Possibility of cuts or minor burns from instruments and equipment. Some direct exposure to contagion. Possibility of strains due to moving patients or injury from irrational patients. Risk is minimal when proper precautions are used.

<u>Reporting relationship:</u>
The Clinical Nurse Specialist is directly accountable to the Assistant Director of Nursing-Case Management/Director of Case Management.

<u>Additional work requirements:</u>
Work requires availability to work such hours as required to assure proper functioning of the institution. Must report for duty when called in for emergent situations.

A P P E N D I X **I-1**

The Long Island College Hospital
Department of Case Management
Case Manager — Monthly Report

Name: _____

Month/year: _____

Critical pathways initiated: _____

Unit(s): _____

Days worked this month: _____

Patients case managed: _____

Progress: _____
_____
_____
_____
_____
_____
_____
_____
_____
_____
_____
_____
_____

Problems: _____
_____
_____
_____
_____
_____
_____
_____
_____
_____
_____
_____
_____

Goals for next month: _____
_____
_____
_____
_____
_____
_____
_____

Due the 5th of the month

The Long Island College Hospital
Case Management Data Flow Record

Completed by: _____

Month/year: _____

Patient name & Medical record number	Reason for admission	Admission date	Discharge date	ICU or other transfer (# days)	Clinical service	MAP used (name)	Case managed? (yes or no)	Service or private	Physician name

Due the 5th of the month

GLOSSARY OF TERMS

access to care The ability and ease of patients to obtain health care when they need it.

actuarial study Statistical analysis of a population based on the utilization and demographic trends of the population. Results used to estimate health care plan premiums or costs.

algorithm The chronological delineation of the steps in, or activities of, patient care to be applied in the care of patients as they relate to specific conditions/situations.

alternate delivery system (ADS) Any of the health care benefit plans other than the traditional fee-for-service reimbursement systems. Examples include PPOs and HMOs.

ancillary services Other diagnostic and therapeutic hospital services that may be involved in the care of patients other than nursing or medicine. Includes respiratory, laboratory, radiology, nutrition, physical and occupational therapy, and pastoral services.

appeal The formal process or request to reconsider a decision made not to approve an admission or health care services; or a patient's request for postponing the discharge date and extending the length of stay.

approved charge The amount Medicare pays a physician based on the Medicare fee schedule. Physicians may bill the beneficiaries for an additional amount, subject to the limiting charge allowed.

assumption of risk The voluntary exposure to a known risk. It involves the comprehension that a peril is to be encountered, as well as the willingness to encounter it.

beneficiary An individual eligible for benefits under a particular plan. In managed care organizations beneficiaries may also be known as members (HMO) or enrollees (PPO).

benefits The amount payable by an insurance company to a claimant or beneficiary under their specific coverage.

capitation The amount of money per-member-per-month (PMPM) paid to a provider for covered services. The typical reimbursement method used by HMOs.

caregiver The person responsible for caring for a patient in the home setting. Can be a family member, friend, volunteer, or an assigned health care professional.

carrier An insurance company or administrator of benefits under an insurance contract.

carve out Services excluded from a provider contract that may be covered through arrangements with other providers. Providers are not financially responsible for services carved out of their contract.

case-based review The process of evaluating the quality and appropriateness of care based on the review of individual medical records to determine whether the care delivered is acceptable. It is performed by health care professionals assigned by the hospital or an outside agency (e.g., Island Peer Review Organization [IPRO]).

case management Patient care delivery system that focuses on meeting outcomes within identified time frames using appropriate resources. Case management follows an entire episode of illness, from admission to discharge, crossing all health care settings in which the patient receives care.

case management plan A time line of patient care activities and expected outcomes of care that address the plan of care of each discipline involved in the care of a particular patient. It is usually developed prospectively by an interdisciplinary health care team in relation to a patient's diagnosis or surgical procedure.

case manager Responsible for coordinating the care delivered to an assigned group of patients based on diagnosis or need. Other responsibilities include patient/family education and outcomes monitoring and management.

case mix complexity An indication of the severity of illness, prognosis, treatment difficulty, need for intervention, or resource intensity of a group of patients.

case mix index (CMI) The sum of all DRG-relative weights, divided by the number of cases.

certification The approval of patient care services, admission, or length of stay by a health benefit plan (e.g., HMO, PPO) based on information provided by the health care provider.

coding A mechanism of identifying and defining patient care services/activities as primary and secondary

247

diagnoses and procedures. The process is guided by the ICD-9-CM coding manual, which lists the various codes and their respective descriptions.

comorbidity A preexisting condition (usually chronic) that, because of its presence with a specific condition, causes an increase in the length of stay.

complication An unexpected condition that arises during a hospital stay or health care encounter that prolongs the length of stay and intensifies the use of health care resources.

concurrent review A form of utilization review that tracks the consumption of resources and the progress of patients while being treated.

consensus Agreement in opinion of experts. Building consensus is a method used when developing case management plans.

co-payment A cost-sharing arrangement between the member and the insurer, in which the member pays a specific charge for a specified service. Co-payments may be flat or variable amounts and may be for such things as physician office visits, prescriptions, or hospital services.

credentialing A review process to approve a provider who applies to participate in a health plan. Specific criteria are applied to evaluate participation in the plan.

database An organized, comprehensive collection of patient care data. Sometimes it is used for research or for quality improvement efforts.

diagnosis-related group (DRG) A patient classification scheme that provides a means of relating the type of patient a hospital treats to the costs incurred by the hospital. DRGs demonstrate groups of patients using similar resource consumption and length of stay.

discharge outcomes Clinical criteria to be met before or at the time of the patient's discharge. They are the expected/projected outcomes of care that indicate a safe discharge.

discharge planning The process of assessing the patient's needs of care after discharge from a health care facility and ensuring that the necessary services are in place before discharge. This process ensures a patient's timely, appropriate, and safe discharge.

discharge status Disposition of the patient at discharge (e.g., left against medical advice, expired, discharged home, transferred to a nursing home).

effectiveness of care The extent to which care is provided correctly (i.e., to meet the patient's needs, improve quality of care, and resolve the patient's problems).

efficiency of care The extent to which care is provided to meet the desired effects/outcomes to improve quality of care and prevent the use of unnecessary resources.

enrollee An individual who subscribes for a health benefit plan provided by a public or private health care insurance organization.

exclusive provider organization (EPO) A managed care plan that provides benefits only if care is rendered by providers within a specific network.

fee-for-service (FFS) Providers are payed for each service performed, as opposed to capitation. Fee schedules are an example of fee-for-service.

fee schedule A listing of fee allowances for specific procedures or services that a health plan will reimburse.

gatekeeper A primary care physician (usually a family practitioner, internist, pediatrician, or nurse practitioner) to whom a plan member is assigned. Responsible for managing all referrals for specialty care and other covered services used by the member.

global fee A predetermined all-inclusive fee for a specific set of related services, treated as a single unit for billing or reimbursement purposes.

health benefit plan Any written health insurance plan that pays for specific health care services on behalf of covered people/enrollees.

health maintenance organization (HMO) An organization that provides or arranges for coverage of designated health services needed by plan members for a fixed prepaid premium. There are four basic models of HMOs: group model, individual practice association, network model, and staff model. Under the Federal HMO Act an organization must possess the following to call itself an HMO: (1) an organized system for providing health care in a geographical area; (2) an agreed-on set of basic and supplemental health maintenance and treatment services; and (3) a voluntarily enrolled group of people.

hospital days/1000 The number of inpatient hospital days per 1000 health plan members.

ICD-9-CM International Classification of Diseases, Ninth Revision, Clinical Modification, formulated to standardize diagnoses. It is used for coding medical records in preparation for reimbursement.

individual practice association (IPA) model HMO An HMO model that contracts with a private practice physician or health care association to provide health care services in return for a negotiated fee. The individual practice association then contracts with physicians who continue in their existing individual or group practice.

integrated delivery network (IDN) A single organization or group of affiliated organizations that provides a wide spectrum of ambulatory and tertiary care.

intensity of service An acuity of illness criteria based on the evaluation/treatment plan, the interventions, and anticipated outcomes.

intermediate outcome A desired outcome that is met during a patient's hospital stay. It is a milestone in the care of a patient or a trigger point for advancement in the plan of care.

length of stay The number of days that a health plan member stays in an inpatient facility.

liability Legal responsibility for failure to act appropriately or for actions that do not meet the standards of care, inflicting harm on another person.

litigation A contest in a court for the purpose of enforcing a right, particularly when inflicting harm on another person.

malpractice Improper care or treatment by a health care professional. A wrongful conduct.

managed care A system that provides the generalized structure and focus when managing the use, cost, quality, and effectiveness of health care services. Links the patient to provider services.

Medicaid A federal program administered and operated individually by state governments that provides medical benefits to eligible low-income persons needing health care. The costs of the program are shared by the federal and state governments.

medical loss ratio (MLR) The ratio of health care costs compared to revenue received. Calculated as total medical expense/total revenue.

Medicare A nation-wide, federally administered health insurance program that covers the cost of hospitalization, medical care, and some related services for eligible persons. Medicare has two parts. Part A covers inpatient hospital costs (currently reimbursed prospectively using the DRG system). Medicare pays for pharmaceuticals provided in hospitals but not for those provided in outpatient settings. Also called Supplementary Medical Insurance Program. Part B covers outpatient costs for Medicare patients (currently reimbursed retrospectively).

negligence Failure to act as a reasonable person. Behavior is contrary to that of any ordinary person facing similar circumstances.

nursing case management A process model using the components of case management in the delivery aspects of nursing care.

other weird arrangements (OWA) Acronym sometimes used to describe new or hybrid types of managed care arrangements.

outcome The result of a health care process. A good outcome is a result that achieves the expected goal.

outcomes management The use of information and knowledge gained from outcomes monitoring to achieve optimal patient outcomes through improved clinical decision making and service delivery.

outcomes measurement The systematic, quantitative observation, at a point in time, of outcome indicators.

outcomes monitoring The repeated measurement over time of outcome indicators in a manner that permits causal inferences about what patient characteristics, care processes, and resources produced the observed patient outcomes.

outlier threshold The upper range (threshold) in length of stay before a patients stay becomes an outlier. It is the maximum number of days a patient may stay in the hospital for the same fixed reimbursement rate. The outlier threshold is determined by the Health Care Finance Administration (HCFA).

per diem A daily reimbursement rate for all inpatient hospital services provided in one day to one patient, regardless of the actual costs to the health care provider.

plaintiff A person who seeks a lawsuit in court because of a belief that his or her rights have been violated or a legal injury has occurred.

point-of-service (POS) plan A type of health plan allowing the covered person to choose to receive a service from a participating or a nonparticipating provider, with different benefit levels associated with the use of participating providers.

precertification (prior approval) The process of obtaining and documenting advanced approval from the health plan provider before obtaining the medical services needed. This is required when services are of a nonemergent nature.

preferred provider organization (PPO) A program in which contracts are established with providers of medical care. Providers under a PPO contract are referred to as preferred providers. Usually the benefit contract provides significantly better benefits for services received from preferred providers, thus encouraging members to use these providers.

prepaid health plan   Health benefit plan in which a provider network delivers a specific complement of health services to an enrolled population for a predetermined payment amount (*see* capitation).

principal diagnosis   The condition that chiefly required the patient's admission to the hospital for care.

principal procedure   A procedure performed for definitive treatment rather than diagnostic, or one that is necessary for treating a certain condition. It is usually related to the principal diagnosis.

prior authorization (precertification)   The process of obtaining and documenting advance approval of health services to an enrolled population for a predetermined payment amount (capitated rate).

relative weight   An assigned weight that is intended to reflect the relative resource consumption associated with each DRG. The higher the relative weight, the greater the payment to the hospital.

retrospective review   A form of medical records review that is conducted after the patient's discharge to track appropriateness of care and consumption of resources.

severity of illness   An acuity of illness criteria that identifies the presence of significant/debilitating symptoms, deviations from patient's normal values, or unstable/abnormal vital signs or lab findings.

target utilization rates   Specific goals regarding use of medical services, usually included in risk-sharing arrangements between managed care organizations and health care providers.

third-party payor   An insurance company or other organization responsible for the cost of care so that individual patients do not directly pay for services.

utilization   The frequency with which a benefit is used during a 1-year period, usually expressed in occurrences per 1000 covered lives.

utilization management   Review of services to ensure that they are medically necessary, provided in the most appropriate setting, and at or above quality standards.

variance   Any expected outcome that has not been achieved within designated time frames. Categories include system, patient, and practitioner.

withhold   A portion of payments to a provider held by the managed care organization until year end, which will not be returned to the provider unless specific target utilization rates are achieved. Typically used by HMOs to control utilization of referral services by gatekeeper physicians.